DO YOU KNOW...

- why fat may often be the real culprit in diabetes?
- the risks of diuretics and other commonly used drugs that when used unnecessarily may actually make the patient worse?
- why carbohydrates should sometimes be increased, not reduced?
- why consuming too much protein may be damaging to your kidneys?
- when fish oil supplements may be substituted for aspirin to reduce the risk of dangerous blood clots?
- that diet and exercise alone sometimes eliminate the need for insulin shots, pumps, and pills?

Reversing Diabetes

is based on sound nutritional principles and a conservative method of treatment shown to be effective in research studies available to doctors for decades. An important book, it will help diabetic patients better understand their condition and may significantly improve the overall health and well-being of millions.

Also by Julian M. Whitaker, M.D.

REVERSING HEART DISEASE
REVERSING HEALTH RISKS

Reversing Diabetes

Julian M. Whitaker, M.D.

WARNER BOOKS

A Time Warner Company

DISCLAIMER

If you are a diabetic patient or have a diabetic member of the family the advice in this book can be a valuable addition to your doctor's advice, and is designed for your use under his care or direction.

Copyright © 1987 by Julian M. Whitaker, M.D.
All rights reserved.
Warner Books, Inc., 1271 Avenue of the Americas, New York, NY 10020
Visit our Web site at http://warnerbooks.com

W A Time Warner Company

Cover design: Anne Twomey
Book design: H. Roberts

Printed in the United States of America
First trade paperback printing: November 1990
20   19   18   17   16

Library of Congress Cataloging-in-Publication Data

Whitaker, Julian M.
  Reversing diabetes.

  Bibliography: p.
  Includes index.
  1. Diabetes—Diet therapy.   2. Exercise therapy.
3. Diabetes—Diet therapy—Recipes.   I. Title.
[DNLM: 1. Diabetes Mellitus—therapy—popular
works. WK 850 W577r]
RC662.W46   1987   616.4′620654   86-40416
ISBN 0-446-38563-8

I would like to dedicate this book to any diabetic patient who reads it, puts it to use, and benefits from it.

ACKNOWLEDGMENTS

This book, as with any book that tries to touch a lot of bases, is the result of the efforts of many.

To start with I would like to acknowledge all of the physicians, both research scientists and clinicians, who went through the effort to publish their work which forms the basis of the material contained in this book.

Second, I would like to acknowledge the editorial staff at Warner Books, particularly Lillian Rodberg, copy editor, who worked very hard in rewording sections of the manuscript, making the concepts more understandable.

I would like to acknowledge James W. Anderson, M.D., Chief Metabolic Endocrinology Section, VA Medical Center and Professor of Medicine and Clinical Nutrition, University of Kentucky Medical Center; Thaddeus E. Prout, M.D., Chairman, Department of Medicine, Greater Baltimore Medical Center at Johns Hopkins School of Medicine; and John K. Davidson, M.D., Ph.D., Professor of Medicine (Endocrinology) Emory University School of Medicine and Director of the Diabetes Unit, Greater Memorial Hospital, Atlanta, Georgia, for reviewing all or sections of the manuscript and offering critical suggestions.

I would also like to acknowledge Patricia Mercado and Valerie Close for their assistance in typing, retyping, and yet retyping again, this book. Even though they are proficient on an advanced word processor, the effort and time was still substantial.

And also, Mrs. Barbara Tancredi, who put together the all-important diet regimen of this book. Her efforts are most obvious.

CONTENTS

Much has been written about the consumption of too much sugar, but it seems to us that there is an equal or more serious tendency at present toward the overconsumption of fat.

—Dr. W. D. Samsum,
—*Journal of the American Medical Association,* 1926

PREFACE

In 1979, I opened the Whitaker Wellness Institute.* The Institute was designed to provide patients who have diabetes, heart disease, and high blood pressure with a training ground where they could get the education and motivation needed to put what may be the strongest available therapeutic tool to work for them. The program combines a low fat diet with vigorous exercise. By the time I founded the Institute, I had concluded that most physicians were ignoring the appropriate use of diet and exercise in treating diabetes and other degenerative conditions. This was happening despite the fact that for the last 50 years, researchers and medical publications had been screaming, "Diet and exercise are the most powerful tools available for helping patients with these diseases. Why not use them?"

Somewhere along the line, we in the medical profession seem to have dropped the ball. We keep looking for "*the* answer," that single technological breakthrough that will make everything all right for our patients. And with the current explosion of technology, we stand convinced that the answer is just around the corner.

While we are waiting, however, our patients continue to suffer not because the breakthrough is yet to come, but because we ignore what would be the only "answer" necessary for many of

*4400 MacArthur Blvd., Suite 630, Newport Beach, CA 92660 (714) 851-1550

them: a disciplined program of diet and exercise that the *patient* views as the most important part of his or her treatment. The high-tech climate of modern medicine continues to foster high hopes of a technological miracle that will spare the patient from making a lifestyle change.

Hopes for a Single Answer Fade

For example, in the mid-1960s, research began on transplanting donor pancreas cells into diabetic patients, an approach that was inconceivable 40 years ago. The researchers hoped, and some even assumed, that these transplanted cells would function just like the body's own normal cells, manufacturing and secreting the insulin that is lacking in one type of diabetes (see Chapter 1). With the donor cells successfully implanted, the diabetic condition, with all its problems, was expected simply to go away: *The* answer would be found!

However, anytime a foreign material is placed inside a human body, complications both foreseen and unforeseen surface. Complications are especially likely when the foreign substance is living cells that are expected to function just like the body's own cells.

When cell transplantation research was started, I did not think the approach would live up to anyone's expectation of benefit. I felt sorry for the diabetic patients who read newspaper reports of this "breakthrough" and were waiting for it to cure them. I was right. Like so many other searches for single answers to a degenerative disease, pancreas transplant research has hit some rough water.

At the 1986 meeting of the American Diabetes Association (ADA) in Anaheim, California, the major researchers with pancreatic cell implants appeared quite discouraged. Under the headline "Hopes for Whole Pancreas, Islet Cell Transplant Falter" the *Internal Medicine News* reported that "a large problem with whole or partial pancreatic transplantation is that long term immunosuppression is required, and side effects of the drugs can be more serious than the complications of the disease." (September 1–14, 1986, p. 3.)

Even though the need for immunosuppression had long been recognized as a serious obstacle to use of transplanted tissue, this did not stop the initial enthusiasm for pancreatic transplants. Dr. David Sutherland, Director of the Pancreas Transplantation Program at the University of Minnesota Hospital in Minneapolis, stated that initially "everyone thought islet transplantation was just around the corner."

It's not, and as Kevin J. Lafferty, Ph.D., Research Director of the Barbara Davis Center for Childhood Disease at the University of Colorado in Denver, stated "we must understand more about what is going on before we go too far ahead. Let the basic scientists work a little longer to sort these things out in animals before we rush in to the clinical [use of this procedure]."

Before I am accused of being antitechnology, let me say that I am not opposed to this research. However, when we are *not* doing nearly enough to help diabetic patients today with the simpler, less dramatic tools of diet and exercise, then the false hopes and dreams pinned to some future research just get in the way!

Why wait for some yet to be discovered "answer"? A "miracle cure" is already available for helping hundreds of thousands, perhaps even millions, of diabetics in this country to become drug free and healthier in every measurable respect. They simply need education and motivation to follow a diet very high in complex carbohydrate calories and fiber combined with an exercise program. The following case of a patient who spent two weeks with us illustrates this point.

CASE STUDY: MR. R.K.

Mr. R.K., a very successful 66-year-old businessman, came to our institute in May of 1984 to receive and learn about diet and exercise treatment for his diabetes and high blood pressure. He had known about our approach for several years but was not interested, because he was convinced he was getting the best possible medical care. True, he was seeing two very competent and respected physicians in his community, but his treatment had been focused only on the use of multiple drugs.

His condition had been deteriorating for a year, and his wife wanted the two of them to come to the institute to get more detailed instructions in diet. R.K. was skeptical. He couldn't see that a treatment program that emphasized diet could do much. He had been "dieting" all his life!

When he finally did check in for treatment, R.K. was taking the following medications. First of all, he was injecting 90 units of NPH insulin in the morning and 40 units in the evening, totaling 130 units a day. He was taking hydrochlorothiazide, a diuretic often used for high blood pressure, twice a day. Because he had developed a cardiac arrythmia, or irregular heartbeat, he was also taking 40 milligrams of Verapamil four times a day. Since he had been losing too much potassium in his urine while taking hydrochlorothiazide, a "potassium sparing" diuretic, Midamor, was added to his regimen. Lanoxin, a heart drug, was being used to control intermittent irregularities of his heart rhythm. Lastly, he was taking potassium chloride to replace the potassium being lost in his urine.

His problems had begun six years earlier when he was found to have mild high blood pressure (hypertension). For this he was given the diuretic hydrochlorothiazide. His blood pressure fell to some extent, but his blood sugar level elevated; that is, he developed a diabetic condition. His potassium level fell. Elevation of the blood sugar and depletion of potassium have both been associated with the use of thiazide diuretics in some patients. Adequate potassium in the blood and tissues of the heart is essential for maintenance of normal heart rhythms. Mr. K.'s low potassium levels led to heart-rhythm irregularities.

Digoxin was prescribed to correct the irregular heart rhythms, and the oral drug Orinase (later switched to Diabinese) was prescribed for his diabetes. In addition, the drug Inderal was added in an attempt to control his blood pressure, since the diuretic had not reduced the pressure adequately. Inderal was later dropped because Mr. K. experienced significant side effects, primarily depression.

Even though he was taking Diabinese, his blood sugar gradually went up. Insulin therapy was started, even though Mr. K. had the form of diabetes that is not insulin dependent (see Chapter 2). Gradually, the insulin dosage was increased, until he was taking 130 units a day in two injections.

Mr. K.'s doctor monitored his condition carefully. Three times a week, Mr. K. went to the hospital to have his blood sugar measured. He was having three or four episodes a week in which he would become confused, sweaty, and dizzy and would have to quickly drink some juice or eat something sweet. These reactions, known as "insulin shock" or hypoglycemic reactions, are almost *always* a part of insulin treatment (see Chapter 6).

To treat his potassium wastage problem, another diuretic, Midamor, was prescribed, along with potassium supplements. His heart irregularities worsened and he was given Verapamil. He had been on the combined regimen described for close to 18 months. He felt lousy.

Help for Mr. R.K.

When Mr. K. and his wife arrived at the institute, we immediately put him on a high carbohydrate, low fat, high fiber diet combined with mild exercise. He responded rapidly. Because we knew that this regimen would lower his insulin requirement (it almost always does) we cut his insulin dose in half on the first day to avoid hypoglycemic reactions. On the second day, his blood sugar in the normal range, we discontinued the insulin altogether. Such a rapid reduction in insulin is unusual, however. Any reduction in insulin dosage must be combined with frequent measurements of the blood sugar level under close control by a health professional. Total elimination of insulin can be achieved only in the non-insulin dependent form diabetes that Mr. K. had (see Chapters 1 and 2).

Remarkably, this patient's blood sugar never went back up. His blood pressure also normalized, and within twelve days he was able to stop taking both diuretics. Eventually he could stop taking the potassium supplement. Since his arrythmia had not occurred during his two weeks at the institute, the Lanoxin and Verapamil were also stopped on a trial basis with close monitoring.

Table 1 compares laboratory findings when Mr. K. arrived at the institute and after two weeks of our diet and exercise program, when he left. The initial laboratory readings were obtained while he was taking all the medications listed. After only two weeks on the diet regimen with mild exercise, he was taking *no medication at all,* yet he showed improvement in most findings.

TABLE 1
Summary of Mr. R.K.'s Progress

Measurement	Initial	2 Weeks
Height	5 feet 9 inches	
Weight	187	180
Blood pressure	126/88	128/89
Fasting glucose (blood sugar)	93	102
Total cholesterol	190	159
HDL cholesterol	31	36
Cholesterol:HDL ratio	6.1	4.4
Uric acid level	4.8	8.0
Serum triglycerides (fats)	347	142
Blood urea nitrogen (BUN)	19	15

Six months later Mr. R.K. was still taking no medications for diabetes or high blood pressure. His heart arrhythmia had recurred, so he resumed taking the Digoxin. Possibly this irregularity was related to the extended potassium depletion that occurred while he was on diuretic therapy. One year later, his fasting blood sugar was a normal 91, his blood pressure a youthful 117/80, and his total cholesterol level a respectable 159.

His diabetes and high blood pressure had disappeared—a miracle cure! But this was done without transplanted pancreas cells, new drugs, the insulin pump, or any of the other "technology breakthroughs" that are so much a part of modern medicine.

Ironically, if you could credit Mr. K.'s results to a pill or a machine, it would be heralded as the biggest medical breakthrough since computerized billing. But since it comes from something as simple as a doctor and patient sitting down and finally getting serious about what the patient puts into his mouth, the cure has no pizzazz. After all, most physicians have been telling their patients "to diet" for years.

Mr. K.'s case not only demonstrates the power of low fat nutrition in the treatment of diabetes and high blood pressure, but more importantly, it illustrates how dangerous it can be to chase symptoms with drugs. In his case, each time a drug was prescribed, a new condition developed and had to be treated with a new drug.

What was lacking in this patient's initial treatment was any serious attempt to use life-style changes to control the problems. Relying solely on drug therapy, he developed more and more problems.

Here at the Institute, diet and exercise are given the highest priority. Drugs and invasive techniques are used only to supplement the diet program, *not the other way around.*

With this shift in emphasis, the amount of medications that can be eliminated is startling.

INTRODUCTION

Diabetes mellitus is a major cause of mortality and morbidity in the United States, and thus a considerable amount of resources have been directed to its control and cure. It has been estimated by the U.S. Department of Health and Human Services that approximately $15 billion are spent annually on this disease. Additionally, in the U.S., diabetes is the third cause of death by disease and the leading cause of blindness in adults, nontraumatic amputations, renal failure, and thus kidney transplantation and the second leading cause of peripheral nerve disease.

Because of these important health care statistics and the psychosocial implications, the United States government and the agencies involved with diabetes have developed several natural resources in an attempt to arrest this disease. Thus, through a variety of federal agencies there are diabetes research centers, a variety of scholarships and fellowships to help train investigators in diabetes. At the Center for Disease Control in Atlanta, Georgia, financial and scientific resources are directed to most states in the Union to control diabetes.

These activities have not yet had a significant impact upon the general population of diabetic patients in the U.S. In fact, only in 1987 did the Department of Health and Human Services officially recognize in a policy statement the usefulness of home blood glucose monitoring.

It has been impossible to inform health care providers of new findings related to diabetes care for a variety of reasons, one of which is the information explosion. Certainly, our understanding of the disease has advanced, and it is hoped that in the near future these advancements may result in direct application to the general population of diabetic patients through health care–provided education. One method of education is through books such as Dr. Whitaker's *Reversing Diabetes*.

One of the major approaches to the control of diabetes has been to improve blood sugar control in the patient with diabetes. There are a variety of data in animals, and suggestive data in humans, that blood sugar control is directly related to the chronic complications of diabetes which result in significant morbidity and mortality. Although the prevention and early intervention strategies against chronic diabetic complications have not been proven beyond a shadow of doubt, virtually all diabetes clinics in the United States and Europe have developed intensive strategies to control blood sugar levels.

One study, being performed in the United States using federal sponsorship, the Diabetes Control and Complications Trial (DCCT), is probably going to be the only study of its kind to evaluate the prevention and treatment of chronic diabetic complications. The results of this study will require five to ten years. Because of animal data and current data in humans, the diabetes medical community in general has elected not to wait for all the results of the DCCT study. Thus, most patients in diabetes centers have a specific goal that is also endorsed by the American Diabetes Association: near normalization of blood sugar levels.

Although these goals are very difficult to achieve currently, there is a sizeable percentage of patients, probably 20–40 percent, who can achieve normal blood sugar control. In an attempt to encourage all physicians to improve the control of their diabetic patient's blood sugar, the American Diabetes Association has issued policy statements related to the treatment of diabetes, and strongly encourages improvement of blood sugar control with the goal of having a positive impact upon chronic diabetic complications. The American Diabetes Association has also issued specific nutritional guidelines for the treatment of diabetes, since this organization recognizes the profound significance of nutrition in this fundamentally nutritional disorder.

Diabetes results from the absence and/or ineffectiveness of

insulin. Insulin is primarily a nutritional storage hormone or a food storage hormone. After one ingests a mixed meal containing fat, carbohydrate and protein, insulin is secreted in response to a variety of internal stimuli. The food is then broken down or digested in the intestine, absorbed through the intestinal wall and then delivered to a variety of body tissues, either for direct utilization or for fuel storage for future energy requirements. Insulin is the primary hormone mediating these storage events. There are no other recognized hormones involved in this process, and thus the absence of insulin results in a rather significant disease.

If diabetes is primarily nutritional, it seems appropriate that the first mode of treatment with many cases of diabetes would also be nutritional. Dr. Whitaker has recognized this fact, but more importantly, he has recognized that the health care-providing community has virtually forgotten the nutritional aspects of the treatment of diabetes. The lack of nutritional attention has resulted in overuse of drug therapies such as oral hypoglycemic agents or insulin. Dr. Whitaker is correct in his analysis of the nutritional impact of all diabetic patients and thus his book is most germane to current-day diabetes management.

For the 6 million Americans who have diabetes and their health care providers, *Reversing Diabetes* would be excellent reading material as it correctly points out the relative role of nutrition in the treatment of the disease. The points made in *Reversing Diabetes* do not eliminate the need for other forms of treatment of diabetes, but explicitly emphasizes nutrition which in many patients is the only suitable treatment, whereas in other patients certain drug treatment may also be required.

Dr. Whitaker's background in diabetes and the nutritional treatment of a variety of other significant diseases such as heart disease is broad-based. His Wellness Institute is dedicated to what is needed for the diabetic patients in this country—nutritional therapy with more clinics stressing and emphasizing dietary treatment. Since *Reversing Diabetes* accomplishes a similar goal, it is strongly recommended as routine reading material for all diabetic patients and their families.

In *Reversing Diabetes* Dr. Whitaker points out the dangers of prescribing machines and other highly technical treatment in diabetes without a similar degree of attention to the nutritional aspects of the disease. For the treatment of the blood sugar disorder, he is exactly correct. It should be stressed that for certain chronic complications such as retinopathy, high technology is the only form of diagnosis and treatment that has been documented. Thus, a balance of nutrition and other aspects of diabetes treatment is essential in the overall treatment of the disease.

Dr. Whitaker correctly points out that insulin's effectiveness is strongly modified by diet and there are a variety of studies that support that conclusion. With that fact in mind, the strength of nutritional therapy in diabetes is extremely important. He also alertly points out that certain diets that we thought important in diabetes just a few years ago currently are now under re-evaluation, especially with regards to excessive protein in the diet. What was originally felt to be reasonable amounts of protein, such as 80-100 grams per day, appears now to be excessive for the typical diabetic patient. Thus changes are occurring in this arena which he describes.

Reversing Diabetes is not simply a nutritional "how-to" book. In fact, he describes diabetes, its impact in this country, and discusses major forms of therapies. He uses a very critical style which ensures that readers of *Reversing Diabetes* will be careful before jumping to the routine drug therapies of diabetes.

Dr. Whitaker's *Reversing Diabetes* also describes exercise and its significance in diabetes. Exercise has been linked with nutrition as perhaps the two most important aspects of diabetes treatment. Without these two treatments properly aligned, most patients will have difficulties in the management of sugar control diabetes.

In addition to exercise, certain nutritional supplements such as fish oil, vitamins, and garlic have been described in *Reversing Diabetes*. The significance of these dietary ingredients in diabetes is interestingly presented and hopefully will be more thoroughly evaluated scientifically because it appears that these forms of therapy may offer some major advantages to diabetic patients.

No textbook of diabetes would be complete without a discussion of insulin and Dr. Whitaker thoroughly reviews the use of insulin in the diabetic patient. Again he emphasizes the precautions associated with insulin. Understanding the toxicity of insulin is important for all insulin using diabetic patients and health care providers and there are very few similar descriptions available. Most textbooks describe the "how-to" use of insulin rather than the potential complications associated with insulin. Thus, *Reversing Diabetes* is fresh and full of a variety of useful pieces of information.

Reversing Diabetes is somewhat dated, however, it is difficult to prepare textbooks during an information explosion. Recent information since the preparation of the text has indicated that for pregnancy, improvement of metabolic or sugar control into the normal range is strongly associated with a striking decrease of congenital anomalies. In fact, the decrease drops the rate of anomalies into the normal range in offspring born of diabetic mothers. This is the first major evidence that good metabolic control associated with nutrition, exercise and drug therapy can really prevent and reverse a chronic diabetic complication. These data make this book even more important since nutritional treatment in the state of pregnancy is again vitally important.

Although I do not agree to all aspects of Dr. Whitaker's approach to the treatment of diabetes, this book is, on the whole, an excellent piece of educational material for all diabetic patients and health care providers.

M. Arthur Charles, M.D., Ph.D.
Professor of Medicine and Physiology
University of California, Irvine
Clinical Director, Focused Research Program in Diabetes
Director, UCI/AMI Diabetes Research Center

PART I
Knowing What to Expect

1

What to Expect
If You Have Diabetes

The disease known as diabetes mellitus affects close to 5 percent of the U.S. population, and about 10 percent of those over 60. It is estimated that there are about 12 million diabetics in the country both diagnosed and undiagnosed.

What Is Diabetes?

Medical dictionaries actually list many forms of diabetes, but when we talk about diabetes in common terms we use the term to mean the disease *diabetes mellitus*, sometimes called "sugar diabetes." "Diabetes" is a combined term that comes from the Greek words for "to go through"—and indeed, frequent urination is a major symptom of this disease. "Mellitus" comes from the Greek word for honey.

Basically, diabetes mellitus is a disorder of the body's means of utilizing sugar, or glucose—the body's basic fuel. Before the food we eat can be used as fuel by our muscles and other body tissues, it must first be converted into glucose. Then, the glucose must enter the individual cells where it is metabolized, or "burned" to provide energy for the cell's functions. The hormone insulin, which is manufactured by the islet cells of the pancreas, is necessary for glucose utilization to occur.

There are two basic kinds of diabetes mellitus, type 1 and type 2. Type 1 diabetes used to be called "juvenile diabetes" because its symptoms often become apparent in childhood or infancy. Type 2 diabetes most often becomes apparent in middle age or later and was once called "maturity onset diabetes." Type 1 diabetes arises because of a lack of insulin in the body and is therefore known as *insulin dependent diabetes mellitus* (IDDM). Type 2 diabetes does not reflect a lack of insulin but rather the inability of the body to use it effectively. Therefore, type 2 diabetes is called *noninsulin dependent diabetes mellitus* (NIDDM). We'll discuss these two varieties later in this chapter. These two types differ in several respects. In order to understand these differences, you must first understand how insulin functions in your body.

What Is Insulin?

Insulin is a hormone produced in patches of specialized cells scattered throughout the pancreas. These insulin-producing "islands" were named the Isles of Langerhans in honor of the German pathologist Paul Langerhans, who first described them in 1869. He had no idea that they produced insulin or had anything to do with the diabetic condition; insulin was to be discovered half a century later.

As described above, insulin is necessary for glucose circulating in the bloodstream to enter the cells, where it supplies the energy to run the functions of your body. If glucose does not enter the cells, it is virtually useless, and the cells of the body starve. In short, the body's cells require insulin to maintain a constant energy supply. There are two exceptions to this general rule: (1) Insulin is not necessary for glucose to enter the cells of the brain, and (2) when you are exercising, the muscle cells can extract glucose from the blood without insulin.

For the most part, however, if insulin is not present, or *if its action is blocked* (a concept that is very important for the purpose of this book), glucose is not removed from the bloodstream, the glucose level rises, the cells begin to starve, and the diabetic condition results.

If the blood sugar level elevates markedly, the metabolism is thrown off completely, and the blood becomes more acidic. This is called diabetic hetoacidosis. There is danger that the patient could go into a diabetic coma and die.

Insulin works like a key, opening the cell door for glucose to enter. The diabetic condition is present if there is an inadequate supply of insulin keys (type 1), or if the insulin keys are present but the keyholes have been plugged (type 2).

Type 1 (Insulin Dependent) Diabetes

Type 1 diabetes occurs when the pancreas loses its ability to produce insulin, leading to an acute "key shortage." Usually, this occurs at an early age and manifests itself with the four classic symptoms of the condition:

- The individual urinates frequently and excessively (polyuria).
- The individual becomes excessively thirsty and drinks large amounts of fluids (polydipsia) to replace the water lost through the excessive urination.
- The individual becomes ravenously hungry and eats excessively (polyphagia) in an attempt to feed the starving cells.
- The individual loses weight despite excessive food ingestion because the cells cannot utilize the food.

These four symptoms are all related to the elevated levels of glucose in the blood and the body's inability to clear the blood of this glucose and use it for energy. People with diabetes must urinate frequently because the very high blood glucose level stimulates the kidneys to excrete a large volume of urine that contains glucose. At normal levels of blood glucose, the kidney "conserves" glucose, and there is none in the urine. With diabetes, the high levels of glucose in the blood overwhelm the kidney's conservation ability.

Thirst and excessive water drinking develop not only because the type 1 diabetic loses copious amounts of water, but also because the high level of glucose in the blood makes the blood thicker—that is, more concentrated. This sets off all the "thirst" sensors, making it impossible for the diabetic to pass the water fountain.

The combination of weight loss with excessive food intake is characteristic of type 1 diabetes. Because the glucose in the blood cannot enter the cells and be used, the cells are starving—in an ocean of plenty—and weight loss rapidly occurs. To combat this unhealthy state, the diabetic person eats more, but to no avail, as the energy contained in the food simply passes through the body and is lost in the urine.

Often, type 1 diabetics are first diagnosed in a hospital emergency room where they appear with very high blood sugar levels, usually in the range of 350 to 750 milligrams per milliliter of blood. The normal blood sugar ranges between 80 and 110 milligrams per milliliter. Sometimes the patient is in a diabetic coma. (This *hyperglycemic* coma, which results from excessively *high* blood sugar levels of uncontrolled diabetes, must be distinguished from the *hypoglycemic* shock resulting from low blood sugar brought on by too much insulin.) Diabetic coma is a life-threatening condition that must be treated with insulin to correct the basic problem and fluids to replace those that are lost. Persons with type 1 diabetes will almost always require insulin injections, but the amount of insulin can usually be reduced by following the principles in this book. Type 1 diabetes is the more serious form but also the less common, accounting for only 10 percent of those with the diabetic condition.

Type 1—What Causes It?

In type 1 diabetes, the cells that produce insulin have been damaged or destroyed and can no longer produce enough insulin to regulate the blood sugar. Though we do not know exactly what causes type 1 diabetes, it seems usually to result from the *interaction* of three factors: (1) an inherited vulnerability, plus (2) acute damage to the islet-cells, which (3) stimulates the body's immune system to attack these cells, severely damaging them or destroying them all together. However, it remains possible for any of these factors to operate alone, also.

The Inherited Tendency It has now been well established that *susceptibility* to type 1 diabetes is inherited. Studies of twins are often used to determine whether a condition is inherited, because the genetic makeup of identical twins is the same. In various studies of twins in which one of the pair had type 1 diabetes, the disease also developed in the second twin 30 to 50 percent of the time—but not 100 percent. That means that it is not diabetes itself that is inherited but some condition that increases a person's risk of developing it. Severe type 1 diabetes can develop in people with *no* family history of the condition.

Next, Acute Damage to the Islet Cells Acute damage to the islet cells can result from a variety of environmental factors. First on the list would be virus infections. In the *New England Journal of Medicine* (300:1173–79, 1979) Dr. J.W. Yoon reported a case of a boy of 10 who developed severe type 1 diabetes after having the flu. The virus that had caused the boy's illness was isolated and injected into an experimental animal, where it destroyed the pancreatic cells. The animal developed diabetes.

Mumps, measles, chickenpox and other viral diseases are often reported as antecedents to the development of type 1 diabetes. There are also reports of the disease following exposure to various pesticides and other chemical compounds found in our environment.

Some of my patients who have type 1 diabetes report that a very stressful life event occurred six months to a year before they developed the diabetes. Some had lost a close family member, others had moved abruptly, still others had a particularly stressful time at work or school. Recent studies indicate that stress can alter the immune system. If that is so, stress could reasonably be considered as the initiating event that brought on diabetes, particularly in someone with an inherited tendency.

The Body's Immune System: The Final Straw One of the major functions of the body's immune system is to produce *antibodies*. These specialized cells are powerful agents in helping ward off bacteria, viruses, or other foreign or threatening substances. When type 1 diabetes develops, however, these antibodies attack the body's own damaged islet cells. For some reason, the body's defense system looks upon these damaged cells as "foreign." It begins producing antibodies against them, which "finishes them off." Current medical literature is loaded with reports of antibodies to the insulin-producing cells being found in patients with type 1 diabetes. Ake Lernmark of the University of Chicago Diabetes Research and Training Center reported in the *New England Journal of Medicine* that he found antibodies to the insulin-producing cells in 32 percent of type 1 diabetics (299:375–380, 1978).

Dr. S. Srikanta of the Joslin Diabetes Center in Boston studied a set of twins and a set of triplets; one child in each set had developed diabetes, indicating a high probability that it would develop in the others. Diabetes did develop in one of the triplets and in the second twin. But years before the condition surfaced in these children, Dr. Srikanta's team found antibodies to the islet cells in their bloodstreams. These antibodies were *not* found in the triplet who did not develop diabetes (*New England Journal of Medicine, 308*:322–325, 1983).

Type 2—Non-Insulin Dependent Diabetes

By far the larger percentage (90%) of diabetics have the type 2 variety, which in many respects is a different condition entirely. Often the type 2 has none of the classic diabetes symptoms, and the disease is usually *discovered* during a routine laboratory exam. Typically, the patient is middle-aged and overweight. Usually he or she is inactive. A routine laboratory reveals an elevated blood sugar of 150 to 300 milligrams per milliliter of blood. The patient is informed that he or she has diabetes and is often put on a diet and/or the oral antidiabetes pills (to be discussed in chapter 7).

Usually, the type 2 diabetic has *no defect in insulin production*. Instead, *there is some kind of block in the cells' sensitivity to the insulin that is produced*. The insulin just doesn't work. There are plenty of keys that could open the cells to let in glucose, but the *keyholes have been plugged!* This form of diabetes is more subtle than type 1 and usually responds very well to treatment methods designed to increase the cells' sensitivity to insulin.

Causes of Insulin Insensitivity

Unfortunately, the concept of insulin sensitivity is usually not discussed with diabetic patients today. Yet this concept is almost as important as insulin replacement for the type 1 diabetic. It is *all*-important for the type 2 patient. Insulin insensitivity *causes* diabetes in 90% of those with the condition. The process by which the insulin "key" unlocks the cell so that it can enter is too complex to discuss here. It involves incredibly small structures of the cell membrane called insulin receptors. Several conditions can render these receptors a "poor fit" for the key.

• In the United States, *inappropriate diet* is probably the major factor associated with insulin insensitivity and thus the major cause of diabetes. Dietary factors leading to insulin sensitivity are important in both type 1 and type 2 varieties. Diet is discussed in detail in Chapter 3.

• *Obesity*, or too high a proportion of fat in body tissues, is associated with marked insulin insensitivity. In obese people, type 2 diabetes is as common as a 42-inch waist. It is important to realize the effect that obesity has on the cells' sensitivity to insulin, because it means that even if insulin injections are given—as they sometimes are, even to type 2 diabetics—they will not work.

• *Inactivity* or a very low level of activity in itself may destroy insulin sensitivity for some people and may bring on type 2 diabetes. Also, inactivity usually leads to obesity. An exercise program dramatically increases insulin sensitivity and lowers the blood sugar.

• *Deficiencies of certain vitamins and minerals* may lead to insulin insensitivity. This issue is discussed in Chapter 5.

The association between decreased insulin sensitivity and the diabetic condition was demonstrated over 60 years ago, and treatment methods to improve insulin sensitivity were demonstrated at that time. For the most part, however, physicians concentrate almost exclusively on insulin replacement instead of working out ways to improve insulin sensitivity. This is a mistake. In fact, it is the reason for this book.

The Diabetic Condition

Whether you have type 1 or type 2 diabetes it is best to think of your problem as a *condition*, not a *disease*. Thinking in terms of disease tends to lead to arbitrary parameters by which we classify anyone with a fasting blood sugar (FBS) over 115 to 120 as "sick," leading those whose blood sugar is 114 or less to think of themselves as "well." But unlike pregnancy, diabetes is anything but an "all or nothing" phenomenon. The condition moves along a spectrum that begins with only slight elevations of blood sugar (120 to 140 mg/dl) all the way to the severe elevations (700 to 800 mg/dl) associated with diabetic coma.

Often, patients with only slight elevations of blood sugar in the 130 to 150 range may worry as much about this "disease" as do patients whose blood sugars shoot to 350 even while taking insulin. Yet there are so many things you can do to improve the diabetic condition, regardless of which type you have! That is the focus of this book. To think of diabetes as a "disease" is psychologically crippling. As you will see in Chapter 2, this book gives you a program to enhance your sensitivity to insulin, whether it is your own or you inject it.

2

What to Expect of This Book

This book is a "how-to" book with a program diabetic patients can follow with their physician's approval. *You must be under the care of your physician because your medication requirements are likely to change rapidly.* The diet recommendations differ from those that, before 1979, were routinely given to diabetic patients and that some physicians and patients still follow. The difference is that the proportions of carbohydrate and fiber in the diet are increased, while fat is decreased. The reasons for change are explained throughout this book.

This Program Protects Against Today's Mistakes

Regardless of what you, I, or your doctor thinks, we really do not know the long-term effects of most of the drugs or invasive techniques we use today. Many may turn out to be more harmful than beneficial. We in the medical profession often forget that medical history consists as much of failures abandoned as it does of successes built upon. Sometimes we look back in disbelief. For instance:

A Mistake of Yesteryear

In 1799, Benjamin Rush, a prominent physician of his day, was called to the bedside of George Washington. George had developed the flu and was running a fever. Dr. Rush had popularized bleeding therapy for febrile illnesses and it had become widely accepted. Dr. Rush was the leading expert whose advice was sought by many. George, still pretty bright, wanted nothing to do with this therapy and protested loudly. His concerned friends and family, however, wanted him to have the best treatment possible and overruled him. He was bled into shock and died.

Despite this highly visible and tragic result, the practice of bleeding continued for the next fifty years before it was finally abandoned. There were physicians who openly questioned whether bleeding was the best approach for febrile illness, but they were either ignored or castigated for their nonconformity.

The moral of this story is that every era has its mistakes that only history reveals. The purpose of this book is to bring about the maximum benefit from a low-fat diet and exercise to reduce the chances that you will be harmed by today's mistakes—we really do not know what they are.

This Material Is Not New and Is Used in Some Medical Centers Today

Nothing contained in this book is new. In fact, much of the diet material was already worked out 60 years ago. In addition, Chapter 3 describes recent studies by James Anderson, M.D., Professor of Medicine at the University of Kentucky. Dr. Anderson demonstrated that a high carbohydrate, high fiber diet similar to the diet regimen recommended in this book reduced blood sugar levels without insulin or the oral drugs in close to 70 percent of type 2 diabetics. These were patients who had been following today's more commonly used diet regimen. Dr. Anderson has written and lectured widely on the power of a high carbohydrate, high fiber diet as a treatment tool that is often ignored.

John Davidson, M.D., Ph.D., Professor of Medicine (Endocrinology) at Emory University and Director of the Diabetes Unit at Grady Memorial Hospital, Atlanta, Georgia, has been advocating a low fat, high carbohydrate diet for years. He also stopped the use of all oral medications for diabetes at Emory University in 1971 and has been a vocal critic of their use ever since (see Chapter 8). Dr. Davidson recently published a medical textbook, *Clinical Diabetes Mellitus, A Problem Oriented Approach* (New York: Thieme, Inc., 1986). This text emphasizes the appropriate use of low fat nutrition and even short-term fasting as powerful tools for eliminating the need for medications in diabetics. Hopefully this textbook will find its way into the office of every physician who treats diabetic patients.

I wrote this book to bring this information directly to those interested in diabetes and to encourage you to put it to use. Often diabetics are motivated and will follow diet instructions, but the diets used most often are too high in fat and too low in fiber, and the benefits that can be derived from diet are not accomplished.

In addition, the benefits of exercise are often ignored completely, particularly with the middle-aged, moderately obese, type 2 diabetic who could benefit the most from a prescribed exercise regimen. Rarely does a diabetic patient enter this Institute with a previously prescribed exercise program. Few of our incoming patients are aware that exercise is necessary for optimum diabetic control.

If the Material Is Not New, Why Has It Been Ignored?

This question is asked by almost every patient who uses the principles in this book to reduce medication and improve. Why aren't all physicians enthusiastically educating and motivating their patients to make the diet changes necessary to eliminate, as much as possible, the need for medications?

That is a difficult question to answer, but there seem to be three aspects of modern medicine that work together to discourage the use of diet and exercise as *primary* tools of treatment for diabetes. First, physicians are trained to prescribe. Second, we are in the midst of a technology rush. Third, there is widespread conformity of physician thought and practices.

The Drug Orientation of Physicans

Modern physicians are trained to prescribe. We learned in medical school that prescription drugs are the most powerful tools we have for treating disease. Since diet changes were almost never presented as therapeutic tools, drugs are usually viewed as the only *significant* therapeutic options available.

If diet and exercise used vigorously fail to solve the problem and medications are needed, then the medications are indeed helpful. However, the accepted way of doing things today is to prescribe first and recommend a diet as an afterthought.

The pressures on physicians to use medications are almost insurmountable. Not only have they been taught that drugs are necessary, but the drug companies exert enormous influence on physicians' treatment patterns.

The next time you are in a doctor's office, thumb through one of the professional journals such as the *Journal of the American Medical Association* (JAMA) or the *New England Journal of Medicine*. Look only at the advertisements. Virtually every one of them is for a prescription drug, and the most elaborate and expensive ads are for the newest drugs. The effort here is to induce the physician to switch from an older, usually less expensive medication, to a newer one, implying that the newer one is better simply because it is new.

Many physicians claim that they are not influenced by the ads appearing in medical journals but rely only on the scientific literature contained within. That doesn't make sense. If advertising by the pharmaceutical companies were not effective, *it would not be done*.

Even for those physicians who do rely only on the scientific articles, the bulk of that literature deals with the use of drugs and drug comparisons. In short, because the pharmaceutical companies exert enormous influence on medical education, medical research, and the medical literature, today's physicians look to prescription drugs to solve their patients' problems, almost to the exclusion of anything else.

For the overwhelming majority of type 2, non-insulin dependent diabetics, the condition can be handled with a strict life-style change only. However, today's reliance on medications has reduced the flexibility physicians need to change from *prescriber* to *educator* when it is appropriate. There is just too much confidence in drugs.

The Rush of Technology

Modern medicine is in a state of enormous change. There is an explosion of technology from which a myriad of diagnostic and treatment alternatives for heart disease and diabetes have sprung. In the diabetic treatment field today, the excitement is over the insulin pump, the permanently placed insulin pump, pancreatic tissue transplants and extremely close monitoring of the blood sugar level with machines that the patient can use at home to measure the blood glucose in a matter of seconds. In the heart disease treatment field, which is important to all patients with diabetes because of the increased frequency of heart disease associated with the diabetic condition, physicians can now call upon diagnostic tools such as the angiogram, the echocardiogram, the thallium scan, and the CAT scan. These techniques were not even imagined 40 years ago. This kind of diagnostic power funnels patients into increasingly more aggressive therapies including bypass surgery, angioplasty, and down the road some form of laser treatment of the cholesterol plaques deposited in the arteries.

What is not recognized by most patients and doctors is that the use of this high technology has not been shown, in most cases, to be superior to more conservative, less dangerous, methods. However, because the procedures are new and "high tech," they have enormous appeal to both physician and patient.

As an example, take Mr. R.K., whose case was described in the introduction. He was hesitant to come to our facility for it seemed like a "step backward" from the sophisticated drug approach used for him. How could the simple tools of diet and exercise possibly have the potential for his benefit equal to those dished out in today's modern hospitals?

In spite of the seductive nature of rapidly expanding

technology, there are physicians, including myself, who feel that the extensive use of technology for treating degenerative disease is often inappropriate, with the potential for doing more harm than good. However, the availability of technology almost demands that it be used.

Obviously, the appropriate use of technology that *has* been scientifically documented as beneficial is helpful. So often, though, the controlled studies necessary to prove the benefit of the myriad of procedures used today are pending or not even on the drawing board! Yet the technology is used as if it had already been proven!

You should be aware that new surgical techniques and diagnostic procedures are not subjected to the rigorous research protocols required for new drugs. Before a new drug reaches the general population, it must first be subjected to a battery of animal and controlled human experiments designed to demonstrate its effectiveness and dangers. These controls serve to protect patients from drugs that are more harmful than beneficial. Even though, as we shall see, these safeguards do not prevent the use of some drugs that ultimately do more harm than good, at least the safety net is in place.

Surgical procedures or invasive diagnostic procedures, which can be as dangerous as a new drug, are not required to be tested for their safety or efficacy before being used with patients. If the procedure seems "to make sense," it will quickly find its way into the hospitals and doctors' offices before it has been subjected to the controlled trials necessary to demonstrate that it is better than the older methods of handling the problem. We confuse technology with science. In order for any technical procedure to qualify as a scientific improvement, it must be subjected to scientific studies designed to demonstrate that improvement. All too often, the technology is accepted before any studies are done.

One thing we do know about the explosion of technology, however: it dramatically increases the danger of modern medicine. Benjamin Rush may have been a menace running around and bleeding people with colds, but the *potential* danger of doctors today is far greater, because of the vast diversity of techniques available to today's physicians and the tremendous power of those techniques.

How history will treat all the drugs, catheters, machines, and other tools currently used—tools that can alter every function of the human body—is frightening to contemplate.

A medical dictum dating back to Hippocrates states: *Prima non nocere* (first, do no harm). Technology has made it almost impossible to practice medicine today and abide by this dictum.

Conformity of Thought Among Doctors

More than any other profession, medicine breeds—even demands—conformity among its practitioners. The concept of "accepted practices" carries considerable weight in the medical profession. There may seem to be "controversies" within the profession, but most doctors are predictably uniform in the approaches taken with any given problem.

For the young physician, the pressures of conformity start in medical school and are intensified in the training programs that follow. The amount of material that a medical student or a training physician is expected to master, in addition to the time that he or she must spend caring for patients, is so large that little time can be spent asking whether what is being taught is the best approach to a particular problem. Since there is general conformity of medical practices and education across the country (with a few notable exceptions), there is little reason for the physician in training to have any doubts that he or she is learning the superior, if not the only, method of treating our common diseases.

After completion of medical training, conformity is necessary to receive hospital privileges and to garner patients by referral from other doctors. The fear of disapproval from other physicians may sometimes be greater than the desire to do what seems best for the patient. This fear is justified, for nonconforming physicians can be stripped of their ability to practice medicine regardless of the benefit their patients may be receiving from their particular approach.

Therefore, conforming to today's norms guarantees a degree of safety for the physician. Regardless of the outcome of a therapy, good or bad, physicians are above censure if they have complied with the currently accepted approaches. They can take comfort knowing that they did "what was considered best." This of course could be true, but what was thought best at any time in history is only just that—what was *thought* best at that time.

It bears repeating: The history of medicine, even to the present day, is as much a sequence of failures abandoned as successes built upon. Yet each "abandoned failure" was strongly believed in and practiced in its day.

Even modern medicine is constantly cleaning house. It is estimated that 50 percent of all medical practices are abandoned or replaced by safer or more effective ones every 20 years! Until then, whatever is the "accepted practice" of the day will be dispensed with enthusiasm and confidence by most physicians.

For better or for worse, however, conformity of thought within any group guarantees a form of unconsciousness. The late journalist Walter Lippmann once said, "When all think alike, no one thinks very much." Albert Einstein noted that "Few people are capable of expressing with equanimity opinions which differ from the prejudices of their social environment. Most people are even incapable of forming such opinions."

It is not hard to see, therefore, how something as simple as looking to diet and exercise as the first-line, even superior, therapy for the diabetic could be ignored, even reviled, given the present enthusiasm for drugs and technology that is engendered by medical training and perpetuated by the forces of professional conformity.

About the Author

For me, the treatment of diabetes is a matter of priorities. When faced with a diabetic patient, I look to diet and exercise before drugs or technology.

How did I come to appreciate the power of life-style change as a treatment tool for diabetes? It was a moderately tortuous path, and should be explained.

All of my medical training had been geared toward a surgical speciality. I graduated from Emory University Medical School in

1970, took a medical/surgical internship at the Emory University Hospitals in Atlanta, and then entered a surgical residency program in San Francisco at the University of California. Two-and-a-half years into this residency program, I took some time off to reevaluate my long-term goals. I wanted a year or two to think about that direction. I fully intended at that time to continue my training in surgery.

Until then, I had absolutely no interest in nutrition. Having had only about two credit hours of "nutrition," consisting of a few lectures on the properties of proteins, fats, and carbohydrates, I was convinced that the afflictions of man were either *acts of God*, *bad luck*, or *both*, and could only be handled with appropriate drugs or surgery.

I signed on as an emergency room physician in Southern California. One day a woman, about 34 or 35, who had sprained her ankle came in for an evaluation. Except for a minor injury to her ankle, she glowed with good health. Suddenly, it dawned on me: Healthy people don't see doctors.

Like that of most physicians, the major portion of my training dealt with patients in crisis. I was curious about this healthy patient and asked her about her habits. She explained her program of diet, exercise, and vitamin and mineral supplements. This woman believed that the way she lived determined her physical well being. I had been studying medicine for six-and-one-half years, but this patient was the first practitioner of *preventive* medicine I had encountered.

I read materials that she gave me and subsequently went to work with Dr. Wilbur Currier in Pasadena, California. Dr. Currier was a former ear, nose, and throat surgeon who had abandoned surgery to specialize in preventive medicine. Low-fat nutrition was his primary tool. While working with Dr. Currier, I read some monographs of a then little-known inventor, Nathan Pritikin. Mr. Pritikin, as many of you know, was a passionate crusader for the benefits of a low fat diet and exercise.

I'll never forget my surprise upon reading sections of a monograph he had written dealing with diabetes. It contained research published in the 1920s and 1930s that clearly demonstrated how excessive fat in the diet could bring on diabetes. This astounded me, for in medical school it was never taught that the *type* of food someone ate had anything to do with the onset of diabetes.

To learn more about low fat nutrition in treating diabetes and other degenerative diseases, I worked on the medical staff of the Longevity Center directed by Mr. Pritikin from 1975 to 1976. I was amazed at the power of life-style changes.

I left the Longevity Center to return to my own practice, and in 1979 I opened the Whitaker Wellness Institute, offering patients with diabetes, heart disease, and high blood pressure a two-week live-in program that taught them how to change their life-style. Since then, over 4,000 patients have come through the Institute, and my experiences with diabetes are the subject of this book.

What to Expect From This Program

This is a program designed to make your body more *sensitive* to insulin, whether it is injected or produced in the pancreas. Most diabetic patients can reasonably expect to lower their insulin dose or eliminate the oral diabetic medications. Some patients may be able to stop injecting insulin altogether. In addition, those who need to lose weight will do so on this regimen.

This program should substantially lower your blood cholesterol levels, as well as your blood pressure. Lowering blood pressure and cholesterol reduces the risk of heart or blood vessel problems.

These improvements are accomplished by incorporating three aspects of the program into your life-style: (1) changes in diet, (2) aerobic exercise, and (3) vitamin and mineral supplementation.

Diet Changes. The diet recommendations at the end of the book provide a substantial increase in the amount of carbohydrate calories and a substantial reduction in the amount of fat calories. In simplest terms, calories generally consumed in the form of fat are replaced with carbohydrate calories. The caloric percentage of the diet is 70 to 80 percent carbohydrate, 10 to 15 percent protein, and 10 to 15 percent fat.

The program is purposely high in dietary fiber. By increasing the fiber content of a diabetic's diet, the insulin requirement is reduced. Often diabetics are not given any recommendation to increase the dietary fiber. Although the ADA has recommended less fat and more fiber in its exchange diets since 1979, many physicians do not stress the importance of these changes.

This diet program represents a major change in the diet of most Americans and many diabetics as well. The average American diet is composed of 40 percent carbohydrate calories, 20 percent protein calories, and 40 percent fat calories. As discussed in Chapters 3 and 4, this kind of diet appears to be a major cause of diabetes.

As we all know, we Americans have a strong bias toward animal protein: meat, eggs, and cheese. Almost every meal features some form of animal protein food. This bias automatically increases the amount of fat we consume, since animal protein foods are composed of only fat and protein calories (with the exception of some dairy products that contain lactose, a milk sugar). In addition, animal protein foods contain no fiber. Dietary fiber is present only in foods derived from vegetable sources.

Aerobic Exercise. As discussed in Chapter 5, aerobic exercise enhances the body's sensitivity to insulin and is recommended because it significantly lowers the insulin requirement. Exercise is work, but people with diabetes should understand that the rewards are great. An exercise program should be prescribed for the diabetic patient in the same way that medication or diet is prescribed.

Vitamins and Mineral Supplements. This book recommends vitamin and mineral supplements. This recommendation will surely be controversial. That controversy and the rationale behind the prescription are addressed in Chapter 6.

An additional part of this program is to understand that long-term dangers are associated with the aggressive use of insulin (Chapter 7), and the oral diabetes drugs (Chapter 8). Harmful side effects have also been associated with the additional drugs often used to treat elevated blood pressure and heart disease that so often are part of the diabetic picture (Chapter 9). Obviously, the more that can be accomplished with diet and exercise to minimize the need for medication, the better.

This program requires a shift of some of the responsibility

from the doctor to the patient. This shift is certainly compatible with our changing attitudes about health. Today, we realize more and more that the diseases and disability we suffer are related more to what we do each day, the food we eat, the amount of exercise we get, and the way we handle our lives, than to almost any other factor.

This Book Is Meant to Stimulate Questions

This book was meant to stimulate questions. For instance, is it truly best to shoot for very close control of the blood sugar level? Most authorities certainly believe in close control, but the evidence supporting such a belief is not nearly so strong as the belief itself.

For instance, a very large controlled study is currently in progress to determine if very close control of the blood sugar level with insulin reduces the frequency of eye problems, kidney problems, heart disease, and deterioration of the nerves associated with diabetes. Yet the overwhelming majority of physicians *already* believe that close control is best.

If close control is best, why is there a study going at this late date asking that very question? The reason: We may believe that close control is best, but we really don't know.

What we do know is that the medications used to obtain close control have enormous dangers, and studies already published have shown that in some patients, close control of blood sugar levels with insulin actually *accelerated* destruction of the eyes (Chapter 7).

Another question. Why are the oral drugs still on the market when the *only major long-term controlled study* of their usefulness found them to be so toxic that the researchers stopped the study before the scheduled completion (Chapter 8)?

To be quite frank, this book does not and cannot definitively answer these or other questions that it raises. Instead, it is intended to stimulate thought about some of the beliefs that are more or less universally accepted.

It also offers the guidelines to a diet regimen that seems to be best for the diabetic patient, based upon both early and recent medical literature.

It is intended to be used for your improvement *while under your doctor's care*. Please use it that way.

PART II
The Basis of the Diet Solution

3

How Diet Can Improve Insulin Sensitivity

Before insulin was discovered in 1921, there was simply no effective treatment for the type 1 diabetic, whose body does not produce insulin. The patient was usually put on a starvation diet with no carbohydrates (starches and sugars) at all. But without insulin, the result was invariably rapid weight loss and early death. Then insulin was discovered and rightly heralded as one of this century's greatest breakthroughs. However, the idea that diabetics must *restrict carbohydrates* has been carried over from the preinsulin era into today's treatment approaches.

The reasoning behind carbohydrate restriction goes like this: The basic problem in diabetes is elevated blood glucose. Since carbohydrates are broken down into glucose and enter the blood as such, carbohydrates obviously should be restricted—even eliminated from the diet. Another part of this reasoning is the *assumption* that carbohydrates bring on the diabetic condition by flooding the blood with glucose, making the pancreas work so hard to produce more insulin that it ultimately "wears out."

Unfortunately for millions of diabetics, these "obvious assumptions" were absolutely wrong! Carbohydrates should not be restricted in treating diabetes; they should be increased. Also, carbohydrates not only do not bring on diabetes, but restricting carbohydrates can bring it on. The culprit is not carbohydrates. *It is fat!*

After the discovery of insulin, however, patients with severe

27

type 1 diabetes no longer followed the traditional path to emaciation and death. Astute scientists began to challenge the dogma of carbohydrate restriction. One of the first to publish better results with diabetic patients using a high-carbohydrate, low-fat diet was Dr. W.D. Samsum, of Santa Barbara, California. In the *Journal of the American Medical Association* of January 16, 1926, he reported how he simply stumbled onto the reality in the process of treating a patient:

Ever since the discovery of insulin by Banting and Best, we have hoped to be able to use better diets. . . . Our first experiment was instigated, however, to satisfy a discontented patient:

A man, aged 51, who, in the past, had been able to do big things in the business world, was admitted to the clinic from Denver, March 9, 1924, with the usual symptoms of a mild diabetes. His weight was normal at 140 pounds (63.5 kg.) net. There were no complications except for a very mild chronic interstitial nephritis, as evidenced by an occasional hyaline cast in the urine. The highly intelligent cooperation of both him and his wife enabled them to learn the diabetic routine rapidly. At the end of three weeks, he was discharged from the hospital on a diet containing 120 gm. of carbohydrate, 80 gm. of protein and 195 gm. of fat, totaling 2,555 calories. [The caloric composition of this diet regimen was carbohydrate 19%, protein, 13%, and fat, 68%. See Part IV for the explanation of how to calculate caloric percentage.] He was sugar free, had a normal blood sugar and did not take insulin, nor did we advise its use.

He returned to the clinic October 20, to be carefully checked up, stating frankly that he had gained nothing by the six months of treatment, and that there must be something wrong either with him or with our diet. He had adhered faithfully to the weighed diet prescribed. He had remained constantly sugar-free, and his blood sugar had been normal whenever it had been taken. His weight had remained constant. We felt that he had managed his case as well as it could have been done. For theoretical reasons, we advised the use of a diet with a slightly higher proportion of carbohydrate to fat and small doses of insulin, although his diet then did not contain as much fat as was usually given. He refused, however, to be annoyed with insulin injections and returned home after a stay of seven days.

The patient returned to the clinic, November 16, with the intention of staying many months in a warmer climate at a lower altitude, in the hope that a long rest would bring about the desired improvement. In the meantime, although sugar-free, his blood sugar had risen slightly above normal, and on our advice he had reduced the carbohydrate and raised the fat so that his diet contained 80 gm. of carbohydrate, 88 gm. of protein and 207 gm. of fat, totaling 2,535 calories. [Carbohydrate calories 13%, protein 14%, fat 73%] This diet brought about no improvement in his blood sugar, and he felt even worse than he did before. On this admission, we again advised the slightly higher carbohydrate diet with small doses of insulin. This he willingly agreed to. We gave him a diet consisting of 119 gm. of carbohydrate, 78 gm. of protein and 200 gm. of fat, totaling 2,588 calories, with 30 units of insulin daily. [Carbohydrate 18%, protein 12%, fat 70%] He reported that on this diet he felt better, and with his approval we planned a radical experiment with a high carbohydrate diet. December 26, we gave him a diet containing 278 gm. of car- bohydrate, 85 gm. of protein and 117 gm. of fat, totaling 2,505 calories. [Carbohydrate 44%, protein 14%, fat 42%] Within twenty-four hours, he noticed a change, and eight days later he felt so much better that he left the hospital and re- turned to work. We found that on this diet, 112 units of insulin was required to keep him sugar-free and with a normal blood sugar. He has written us a letter each month, and again and again has asserted that the diet with insulin has fully restored him to his former pre-diabetic state of mental and physical activity. He has been able to reduce his insulin dosage gradually, and Aug. 16, 1925, still using the same diet, he was taking only 34 units a day.

Dr. Samsum went on to use carbohydrate-rich diets in 150 diabetic patients and found significant improvement in almost all his cases:

In many instances, both with insulin and non-insulin patients, we have frequently substituted carbohydrate for fat without the appearance of sugar in the urine in the non-insulin cases or without raising the insulin dosage in the insulin cases. . . . From the patients' standpoint, the most striking advantage gained by the use of these high carbohydrate diets has been the improvement in physical and mental activity.

The typical diabetic diet used by many physicians when Dr. Samsum was active was the Woodyatt formula, which had a caloric composition of 14% carbohydrate calories, 7% protein calories, and 79% fat calories.

The almost immediate improvement of his diabetic patients when put on a much higher carbohydrate, lower fat diet stimulated Samsum to experiment with two of his lab assistants. These unfortunate volunteers

ate the typical diabetic diet, balanced according to the Woodyatt formula . . . and within a few days they began to complain of a diminution in their mental and physical powers. This was associated with acetone in the urine and considerable indigestion, doubtless due to the large amounts of fat. Following this experiment, it required some time to restore them to normal.

Much has been written about the consumption of too much sugar, but it seems to us that there is an equal or more serious tendency at present toward the overcompensation of fat, or rich (fat) foods.

Considering the time when Samsum was making these changes and observations, his departure from the dogma of the day was remarkable. According to almost all the "experts" at that time, the "best" diet for diabetics consisted of large quantities of animal lard, fatty meats, and high cholesterol foods including copious amounts of mayonnaise and egg yolks, while such foods as breads, fruits, and vegetables were forbidden.

The Diabetic Diet Shown to Cause Diabetes

In 1927, shortly after Dr. Samsum published his findings, Dr. J. Shirley Sweeney demonstrated that the high fat, low carbohydrate diet used in treatment of diabetic patients, would *cause* diabetes in normal people as demonstrated by the glucose tolerance test (Dietary Factors That Influence the Dextrose Tolerance Test, *Archives of Internal Medicine 40*: 818–830, 1927). The glucose or dextrose (the tests are the same) tolerance test does just what the name implies: measures someone's "tolerance" to glucose. On an empty stomach, usually in the morning, the patient is given about 100 grams of glucose dissolved in water to drink. The patient's blood sugar level is measured at intervals of 30 to 60 minutes, and the fluctuations are indicative of the presence or absence of diabetes. Sweeney, like Samsum, like all true contributors to scientific knowledge, was curious:

> It occurred to me that perhaps the character of the food and
> the amount of water that a person had been consuming for a
> few days prior to the time of the tolerance test was made
> might be factors that would influence the dextrose tolerance
> curve.

So he rounded up 23 "young, healthy, male medical students" and divided them into four groups giving each group a different diet for two days before doing the glucose tolerance test:

• Group 1, High fat diet, consumed only "olive oil, butter, mayonnaise made with egg yolk, and 20% cream." This diet would be generally accepted by diabetic experts as a *good diet* for patients with diabetes.
• Group 2, High protein diet, received only "lean meat and egg whites."
• Group 3, High carbohydrate diet, received only "sugar, candy, pastry, white bread, baked potatoes, syrup, bananas, rice, and oatmeal."
• Group 4, Starvation, "did without food for two days."

Sweeney found that volunteers on any diet that *restricted carbohydrate*—the high fat, high protein, and the starvation diets—

all had diabetes demonstrated by glucose tolerance curves as shown in Table 2.

TABLE 2
Average Dextrose Tolerance Curves of the Students in the Four Different Dietary Groups

Diet Groups	Fasting	Blood Sugar (milligrams per 100 milliliter) After Dextrose		
		30 min	60 min	120 min
High Fat	83	170	206	173
High Protein	69	143	167	145
High Carbohydrate	84	118	113	96
Starvation	67	145	188	184

He then switched the volunteers around and found that when those who had blood sugar levels indicative of diabetes while on the high fat or high protein diet were put on the high carbohydrate diet, the diabetes *disappeared*! Likewise, when those who had normal blood sugar levels while on the high carbohydrate diet were put on any of the other three diets, they immediately developed diabetes as demonstrated by the glucose tolerance test.

Sweeney concluded that it was "plain from the foregoing experiments that the dextrose tolerance test may be significantly affected by the character of food taken prior to the test." If you want a quick case of diabetes as demonstrated by the glucose tolerance test, just eliminate the carbohydrates from your diet for a couple of days and then take the test. It will demonstrate diabetes.

In the early 1930s, H.P. Himsworth published several articles that should be required reading for all physicians, particularly those who treat patients with diabetes. Like Sweeney, he demonstrated that in a normal individual, a fat-rich diet could bring on diabetes which could be eliminated by a carbohydrate-rich diet. He showed clearly that when a normal individual was given a high-fat diet prior to taking the glucose tolerance test, the test

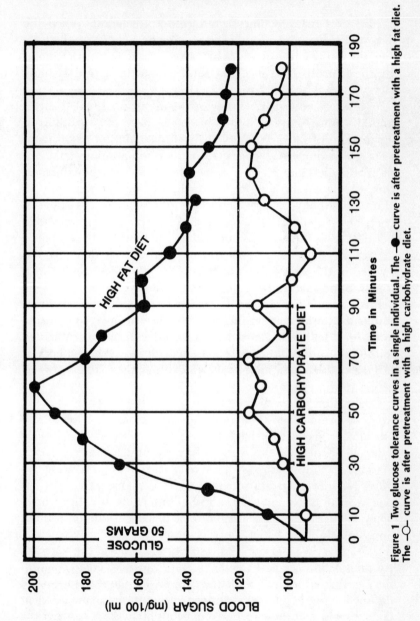

Figure 1 Two glucose tolerance curves in a single individual. The —●— curve is after pretreatment with a high fat diet. The —○— curve is after pretreatment with a high carbohydrate diet.

would show marked glucose intolerance (diabetes). When the same individual was then shifted to a low-fat, high-carbohydrate diet, the test results were normal ("The Dietetic Factor Determining the Glucose Tolerance and Sensitivity to Insulin of Healthy Men," *Clinical Science* 2:67–94, 1935).

In the same article, Himsworth demonstrated that diabetes could be induced in individuals in various degrees depending on the amount of fat in the diet. His volunteers in this experiment were given one of seven different diet compositions. Table 3 shows the diets and Figure 1 shows the blood-sugar fluctuations. Diet #1 was a very high fat, low carbohydrate diet with only 50 grams of carbohydrates (which equals 200 calories), 240 grams of fat (which equals 2160 calories), and 80 grams of protein (320 calories). This diet composition is almost identical to the diet used in treating diabetic patients during Himsworth's time. (It was revived in the 1970s as a treatment for "hypoglycemia.") Himsworth found that individuals who consumed this diet for a week before taking the glucose tolerance test would have positive results on the test, indicating the presence of impaired glucose tolerance. He then began replacing the fat with carbohydrate and found that with each increase in carbohydrate, at the expense of fat, the diabetic condition as shown by the glucose tolerance test began to disappear.

Himsworth demonstrated clearly what the patient eats in the week before a glucose tolerance test will determine the result. Obviously this meant that using the test without first strictly controlling the diet the week before the test leads to extreme inaccuracy. Himsworth's work (as well as that of others during this time) has not been appreciated. In fact, many physicians are unaware of the significant contributions made by Himsworth. They still use the GTT to diagnose the diabetic condition without imposing significant diet controls before the test.

Dr. Marvin Siperstein, Professor of Medicine at the Veterans Administration Medical Center in San Francisco, pointed out in the *Family Practice News* of October 15, 1979, that physicians were *still* relying on the glucose tolerance test to make the diagnosis of diabetes and that they were wrong about 80 to 90 percent of the time (9[20]:1). Speaking at a conference on diabetes sponsored

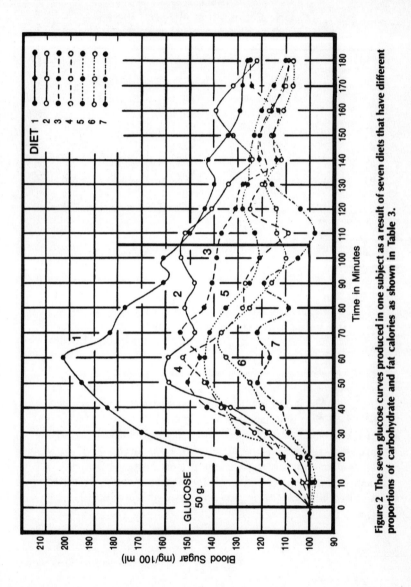

Figure 2 The seven glucose curves produced in one subject as a result of seven diets that have different proportions of carbohydrate and fat calories as shown in Table 3.

TABLE 3
Caloric Composition of Seven Diets
Used in Himsworth's Experiment

Diet No.	Carbohydrate Calories	Protein Calories	Fat Calories	TOTAL
1	200	320	2160	2680
2	500	320	1800	2680
3	800	320	1560	2680
4	1100	320	1260	2680
5	1400	320	960	2680
6	1700	320	660	2680
7	2000	320	360	2680

by the University of California School of Medicine in San Francisco, Dr. Siperstein pointed out that only 17 percent of a group of 9- to 25-year-olds with abnormal tests had gone on to develop true diabetes by the time they were 50 to 60 years old. In another study, an abnormal glucose tolerance test in subjects over 26 was 100 percent inaccurate as a predictor of diabetes in later years. At the meeting, Dr. Siperstein stated quite bluntly:

> Thus, whether glucose tolerance is high or low (on the GTT), it has no value. The test is wrong 80–90% of the time resulting in a grossly absurd number of patients who are misdiagnosed and wrongly tagged with the label "diabetic" for the rest of their lives. Many of these nondiabetic patients are inappropriately treated with oral agents and even insulin.
>
> Other disadvantages of inaccurately being labeled as diabetic include a doubling of life insurance rates, job discrimination, and problems in retaining a driver's license.

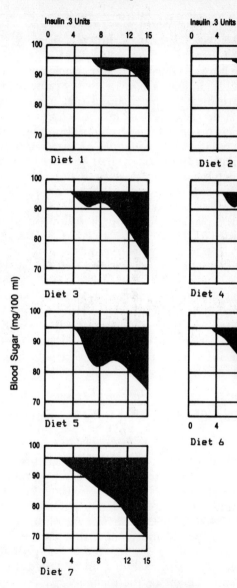

Figure 3 Seven insulin depression curves after injection of 3 units of insulin intravenously in a single subject after pretreatment with the seven different diets that varied in carbohydrate and fat calories.

Insulin Tolerance Test:
The Reverse Glucose Tolerance Test

Insulin Insensitivity Proven Himsworth also clearly answered the question of *why* a high-fat, low-carbohydrate diet caused chemical diabetes long before most people realized that it did. He performed what is best described as an "insulin tolerance test." He put several volunteers on one of the seven different diet compositions in Table 3. These diets ranged from very high fat/low carbohydrate to low fat/high carbohydrate. Then, with the volunteer in a fasting state in the morning he gave each an injection of 3 units of insulin. He then measured the effect of insulin on the blood sugar over a three-hour period.

As you would expect, an injection of insulin in a normal individual caused the blood sugar to drop. However, the rapidity and the degree of drop in the sugar level was dependent on the type of diet the individual had been eating before the test was done.

In my opinion, neither the insulin tolerance test nor the glucose tolerance test is very useful. There are too many factors that can alter the test, including the patient's diet, weight, and exercise pattern. However, if it is done, the patient should definitely be on an increased carbohydrate diet before the test.

Low Fat, High Carbohydrate Diet Put to Use in the 1930s

I.M. Rabinowitch put the high carbohydrate diet to work in patients and published numerous articles on its benefits. In 1930, he outlined his departure from the generally accepted methods of the day ("Experiences with a High Carbohydrate–Low Calorie Diet for the Treatment of Diabetes Mellitus," *Canadian Medical Association Journal 23*:489–98, 1930). He was one of the first to use increasing amounts of bread and to note that the insulin level often went down instead of up. He stated that "fat-protein diets from which carbohydrates are excluded find no logical place in the present day management of the diabetic."

Like many of the pioneers during that time, Rabinowitch was baffled that his observations and results were so different from the accepted beliefs. In 1932, he wrote:

The interesting question which arises is—Why is this diet successful? Experiences with it are incompatible with our present conception of the metabolism of diabetes. . . . In as yet some unknown manner, exposure to this diet appears to lead to an increase in the available supply of insulin. The view held generally at present is that in diabetes, there is defective production of insulin. Much of our experimental data to date fail to support this view. Diabetes does not appear to be due to defective production of insulin but to interference with the action of normal supply.

From our experiences with the above mentioned routine procedure in determining whether patients do or do not require insulin, our conclusion is that the great majority do not; diet in the majority of cases still remains the most important factor in the treatment of diabetes, and it is my opinion, that providing individuals follow prescribed treatment, the high carbohydrate low calorie diet can do much in not only keeping the patient alive, but in keeping him relatively more comfortable. ("The Present Status of the High Carbohydrate–Low Calorie Diet for the Treatment of Diabetes," *Canadian Medical Association Journal* 26:46–148, 1932.)

In 1935, Rabinowitch summarized his results in 50 diabetic patients who had been followed closely on the high carbohydrate/ low calorie diet for five years ("Effects of the High Carbohydrate– Low Calorie Diet Upon Carbohydrate Tolerance in Diabetes Mellitus," *Canadian Medical Association Journal* 26:136–144, 1935). Twenty-four percent of these patients were successfully withdrawn from insulin. Insulin requirements were reduced in almost all who still required it. The patients felt better, had more energy, and lived more comfortably. He concluded: "I believe that in the data presented here there is incontestable evidence that the high carbohydrate–low calorie diet is more effective in controlling diabetes than all other methods of treatment reported hitherto." (When was the last time you saw the word "hitherto" used in a sentence? The benefits of high carbohydrate nutrition in treating diabetes were documented a *long* time ago.)

The American Diabetes Association and Lag Time

Most diabetics, at one time or another, have followed the diet recommendations offered by the American Diabetes Association (ADA). Just the mention of "exchanges" or an "exchange list" conjures up a familiar picture for the diabetic patient: six exchanges—milk, fruits, vegetables, breads, meat, and fat. Instructions were to eat from each exchange in a balanced way to provide a specified amount of calories each day.

Up until 1979, the balance of calories recommended in the ADA diet did not differ significantly from the balance of calories contained in the average American diet. The diet served only to control the number of calories consumed; it did not alter their composition. In short, it simply ignored all the research, some of it published in the 1920s and 1930s, showing that the balance, or composition, of calories is one of the most important aspects of the diet to the diabetic, far more important than the mere number of calories.

For instance, if the exchange list of the pre-1979 2000 calorie ADA diet were followed correctly, it provided 200 grams of carbohydrate, 95 grams of protein, and 90 grams of fat. To understand the consequences (good or bad) of these recommendations, you must first know how to calculate what percentage of the calories in a food or a diet come from carbohydrates, proteins, and fats—probably the most important bit of mathematical knowledge the diabetic person can have.

At first glance, the ADA diet appears high in carbohydrates, certainly in comparison to fat, but this is not the case. One gram of carbohydrate or protein contains only 4 calories, while one gram of fat contains 9 calories, *two and a quarter times as many calories per gram!* To calculate the caloric composition, you must first convert the grams of each to calories. Let's start with carbohydrates:

- Each gram (g) of carbohydrate contains *4 calories* (kcal).
- Therefore, 200 g × 4 kcal per g = 800 kcal.
- This means that out of the 2000 calories recommended in this diabetic diet, only 800, or 40 percent, are carbohydrate calories.

Now let's calculate the percentage of fat calories in the recommended diet. Each gram of fat contains 9 calories. (A gram of fat contains 225 percent of the calories that a gram of carbohydrate does.) Therefore 90 grams of fat contains (91g × 9 kcal): 810 calories or about 41 percent of the 2000 calories.

Protein, like carbohydrate, contains 4 calories per gram. 95 grams of protein contains (95 g × 4 kcal): 380 calories or about 18 percent. Therefore the above ADA diet recommendations are:

- 40 percent carbohydrate calories
- 18 percent protein calories
- 41 percent fat calories

(Note that the total percentage adds up to 99 instead of 100 because some values have been "rounded off.")

This calculation method is very important to remember, because every nutrition label displayed on packaged food lists the calories per serving, followed by the grams of carbohydrate, protein, and fat in the serving. With a little practice, you can very easily make a quick calculation of the caloric percentage of the three nutrients right there in the supermarket aisle. Some will surprise you. For instance, some of the "low fat" dairy products that list their product as containing only 2 percent fat by weight actually derive around 30 percent of their calories from fat. The 2 percent refers to the *weight* percentage, not the *caloric* percentage.

The caloric percentage calculated above is identical to the caloric percentage of the usual American diet. In general, the only way the ADA recommendations alter the diabetic's diet from what he or she would normally be eating is to control calories and perhaps to reduce the amount of simple sugar. There was little if any scientific rationale for the diet recommendations.

This diet did not incorporate any of the research demonstrating that improved insulin sensitivity can be derived from carbohydrates. Neither did it incorporate research demonstrating the benefits derived from increased dietary fiber.

In short, it was no more scientific than simply taking the average American diet that may well be the *cause* of diabetes, putting the foods in an exchange list, and giving the diet back to those who had developed the diabetes condition. Yet this diet was in use for decades.

Beginning in 1979, the ADA began changing its recommendations for both the caloric composition and amount of dietary fiber. The current recommendation is for 60 percent carbohydrates, about 30 percent fat, and 20 percent protein. In addition they emphasize the importance of more fiber, to be discussed next. These improvements are definitely in the right direction, but, in my opinion, these recommendations fall short of the optimum carbohydrate percentage, which seems to be about 65 to 80 percent of the calories.

Fiber

Dietary fiber has finally come into its own. It is hard to believe that the importance of fiber was all but ignored until the early 1970s. Since then, many people are aware of the host of benefits to be derived by increasing the fiber in one's diet. Fiber plays a role in colon cancer prevention, cholesterol control, weight loss, and smooth functioning of the intestinal tract. It is hard to believe that only a few years ago, physicians would actually advise *reduction* of fiber in a patient's diet for a variety of reasons!!

Fiber is essential for the best glucose control for the diabetic. It seems to hold nutrients in the intestinal tract longer, allowing a slower absorption rate and reducing the ups and downs of blood sugar levels characteristic of poor control.

Perla M. Miranda, R.D., M.S., and David L. Horwitz, M.D., Ph.D., F.A.C.P., studied the effect of increased fiber on eight insulin-dependent diabetics ("High-Fiber Diets in the Treatment of Diabetes Mellitus," *Annals of Internal Medical 88*:482–486, 1978). Each diabetic subject consumed either 20 grams of dietary fiber per day in the form of a very high fiber bread or 3 grams of fiber. All other factors of the diet were kept constant, as was the insulin dosage. On the low fiber intake, the mean (average) blood glucose level of the patients was 169.4 milligrams per 100 milliliters of blood, plus or minus 11.7. During the period of higher fiber intake, the mean blood sugar level was 120.8 plus or minus 10.1. In seven of the eight patients, the blood sugar level was substantially lower. These patients had hypoglycemic reactions (episodes of excessively low blood sugar) much more often while

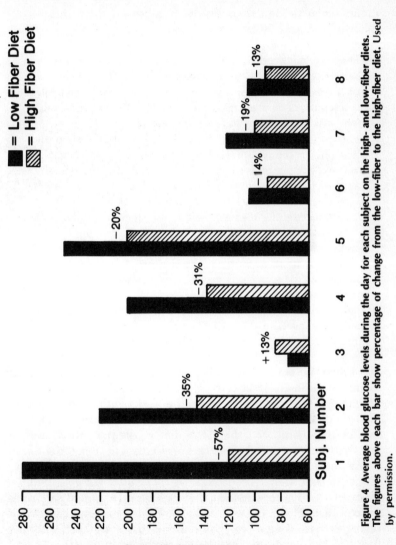

Figure 4 Average blood glucose levels during the day for each subject on the high- and low-fiber diets. The figures above each bar show percentage of change from the low-fiber to the high-fiber diet. Used by permission.

consuming the increased fiber than they did on the low fiber intake—even though their insulin dosage was the same.

Miranda and Horwitz concluded:

> These results also point out that a marked change in dietary fiber content may lead to a substantial change in diabetic control. In particular, there was a significant increase in hypoglycemic episodes on the high-fiber diet. This finding is actually more striking than the data would suggest, for two of the eight patients had such severe and frequent insulin reactions when put on the high-fiber diet and given their usual insulin dose that their protocol had to be restarted after they had stabilized on a lower insulin dose. Thus the physician must be aware that if the dietary fiber is increased for any reason in an insulin-requiring diabetic patient, a change in insulin requirement may be needed.
>
> Because of the above considerations, it may no longer be adequate to think in terms of the traditional diabetic "exchange" lists, where foods may be freely substituted if equal in calories, carbohydrate, fat, and protein. We must also now think of the fiber content of the individual foods. For instance, apple juice contains 0.1 g of fiber per serving; an apple contains close to 10 g of fiber.

James W. Anderson, M.D., and his group at the Veterans Administration Hospital at the University of Kentucky College of Medicine in Lexington have been the leaders in bringing to light the best diet composition for the diabetic patient. In one of their studies they compared the ADA diet recommendations with a high-carbohydrate, high-fiber diet on 13 diabetic men ("Beneficial Effects of a High Carbohydrate, High Fiber Diet on Hyperglycemic Diabetic Men," *American Journal of Clinical Nutrition 29*:895–899, 1976). These patients were all receiving medication to control their blood glucose: eight were on insulin, and five were taking the oral drugs. They were not newcomers to diabetes; they had had the condition for an average of eight years.

At the hospital, these patients were first stabilized for one week on the ADA diet recommendations, which contained only 43 percent carbohydrate calories and about 4.7 grams of crude fiber. They were then shifted to a diet containing 75 percent carbohydrate calories, only 9 percent fat calories, and 14.2 grams of crude fiber.

The results were almost unbelievable. Of the eight who had required insulin injections, four (50%) were rendered insulin free and one reduced his insulin requirement from 28 units to 15. Three patients who had been taking 40 to 55 units experienced no reduction in insulin requirement. Of the five who required the oral diabetic medications, all were rendered drug free! All this occurred in just two weeks!

It is hard to underestimate the significance of this study. In this group of stable, long-term diabetic patients, all of whom needed medication for control while on the diet recommendations of the ADA, a simple diet shift rendered nearly 70 percent drug free, with 50 percent of those taking insulin coming off it completely! This suggests that of the 6 million or so diabetics in the country who are taking some kind of diabetic medication, about 4.3 million could become drug free if they were given a high-carbohydrate, high-fiber diet!

Therefore, the optimal diet composition for the diabetic individual would contain between 70 and 80 percent complex carbohydrates, 10 to 15 percent fat calories, and 10 to 15 percent protein calories. It should also contain about 30 to 40 grams of dietary fiber derived from grains, succulent fruits, and bran, particularly oat bran. Once this composition has been achieved, calories should be controlled to stimulate weight loss if necessary.

This rationale is the basis of the diet used here at the Institute and described in detail in the latter portion of this book.

4

Too Much Protein Can Be Dangerous

Most of the degenerative diseases in this country can be traced to our meat-based diet, and diabetes is no different. We Americans eat meat as if we were a nation of dogs and cats, and this food preference floods our system with protein and fat calories that make us sick. Meat, eggs, chicken, and almost all other animal protein foods are void of carbohydrates, providing protein and fat calories *only.* There are some carbohydrates in dairy products, but even here the majority of calories are fat and protein. Second, there is no fiber in any animal protein food; fiber is found only in vegetable foods. An animal protein diet is just plain wrong for the human system, which is designed for the clean burning carbohydrates and fiber found only in vegetable foods. "Vegetable" does not mean only salads. The term "vegetable foods" also applies to grain products, such as breads and pastas, and potatoes, sweet potatoes, and all varieties of beans and bean dishes.

If the foregoing statements contradict everything you "know," then you grew up as I did, being taught that milk and meat are absolutely essential to growth, strong healthy bones and teeth, and glowing health. Right? **Wrong!** In fact, the opposite is the case. Substantial amounts of milk, meat, and other animal protein foods set the stage for degenerative diseases, with diabetes being only one of them.

How can this be true? Where did we go wrong?

Let's dismantle our dangerous nutritional beliefs.

What Are Americans Eating and Why?

The food choices of Americans, like the food choices of any other culture, are arbitrary and are not even remotely related to what would be the most healthy choices. In no culture has anyone first stopped to figure out what food would be *best* for human health and then designed a diet to conform to those findings. We eat first and ask questions later. Dogs, cats, gorillas, lions, or tigers follow strict dietary patterns regardless of where they live. These animals have "instinctual barriers" that ordinarily prevent their eating foods that are not healthy for them. Humans, on the other hand, have no instinctual controls of their food intake. We learn "what is good" from cultural forces. Often we develop preferences for foods that are alien to our physiological makeup and are decidedly unhealthy.

Take the habit and tradition of drinking milk. Of the thousands of mammals that live on earth, only the human species continues to drink milk after weaning. This is strange! Not only do we continue to drink milk, but we drink the milk of different species. This is not to say that some dairy products cannot be a useful addition to our diet, but the manner in which they are incorporated into our food patterns has no precedent in nature.

Since the diet of humans is so diverse and not instinctively controlled, we can only estimate which food groups best suit the human system by comparing humans with the other mammals whose food patterns are instinctively controlled.

In terms of diet there are three types of mammals. The *carnivores*, such as lions, dogs, and cats, eat meat exclusively. The leaf, grain, and grass eaters include the herding animals like cows, horses, and antelopes. The fruit eaters include monkeys, gorillas, baboons, and chimpanzees, among others. Table 4 compares some basic physiological differences between these three groups of mammals and humans.

TABLE 4
Comparison of Humans With Three Types of Mammals in Terms of Diet

Meat Eater	Grass-and-Leaf Eater	Fruit Eater	Human Beings
Has claws	No claws	No claws	No claws
No pores on skin; perspires through tongue to cool body	Perspires through millions of pores on skin	Perspires through millions of pores on skin	Perspires through millions of pores on skin
Sharp, pointed front teeth to tear flesh	No sharp, pointed front teeth	No sharp, pointed front teeth	No sharp, pointed front teeth
Small salivary glands in the mouth (not needed to predigest grains and fruits)	Well-developed salivary glands, needed to predigest grains and fruits	Well-developed salivary glands, needed to predigest grains and fruits	Well-developed salivary glands, needed to predigest grains and fruits
Acid saliva; no enzyme ptyalin to predigest grains	Alkaline saliva; much ptyalin to predigest grains	Alkaline saliva; much ptyalin to predigest grains	Alkaline saliva; much ptyalin to predigest grains
No flat, back molar teeth to grind food	Flat, back molar teeth to grind food	Flat, back molar teeth to grind food	Flat, back molar teeth to grind food
Much strong hydrochloric acid in stomach to digest tough animal muscle, bone, etc.	Stomach acid 20 times less strong than meat eaters	Stomach acid 20 times less strong than meat eaters	Stomach acid 20 times less strong than meat eaters
Intestinal tract only 3 times body length so rapidly decaying meat can pass out of body quickly	Intestinal tract 10 times body length, leaf and grains do not decay as quickly so can pass more slowly through the body	Intestinal tract 12 times body length, fruits do not decay as rapidly so can pass more slowly through the body	Intestinal tract 12 times body length

*"What's Wrong With Eating Meat?" by Barbara Parham. Reprinted with permission of Ananda Marga Publications, 854 Pearl Street, Denver, CO 80203-3314.

It is obvious that the human physiology is similar, if not identical, to the fruit eaters, and that we are not designed to handle a lot of meat. Remember that the first humans, without tools or weapons, would have had trouble acquiring much meat.

The carnivore, on the other hand, is ideally suited for acquiring meat. It has an exceptionally strong jaw with sharp, pointed fangs that are used to kill other animals and tear their flesh into chunks to swallow. The carnivore does not chew its food, but swallows it whole. The carnivore's mouth and teeth structure are ideally suited for hunting and for defense.

A man in the wild without tools is more likely to be an animal's dinner, than to eat one himself. He is ideally suited for food gathering, and the structure of his mouth and teeth is designed for vegetable foods that must be chewed well and mixed with the digestive enzymes in his saliva.

There are other significant differences in the digestive system as well. The meat eater has 20 times the amount of hydrochloric acid in his stomach that fruit eaters do. Large amounts of protein require copious amounts of concentrated acid for digestion, while vegetable matter doesn't.

In addition, the intestinal tract of the meat eater is only about four times the length of his body trunk as measured from the hips to the shoulders. Therefore for a meat eater the size of man (the distance from hips to shoulders measures about four feet), the intestinal tract would be about 12 feet long. This relatively short intestinal tract is best suited for meat, which putrefies rapidly. The intestinal tract of the fruit eaters is proportionately longer, measuring about 12 times the body trunk length, which for man is about 48 feet. Vegetable matter, because of its fiber content, is slow to digest, requiring the significant increase in intestines for adequate assimilation.

Since lions are not partial to salad, why do we flood our system with meat? It is like putting diesel oil in the gasoline tank of your car. No one would do that. It is against the design specifications of the machine. However, that is exactly what we do when we regularly load each meal with animal protein foods.

Of course there will be detractors to this argument, but anyone who examines our food selection with its quantity of meat and fat and concludes that it is "best" for our system only kids himself.

How It Started

If we are so wrong in our food selection, how did it start? A large part of the blame can be laid at the feet of some prominent German scientists in the mid-1800s. Carl Voit studied German workers at that time. These men were already on a meat-based diet and most were taking in about 120 grams of protein, very much like today. Because he considered them to be in good health, Voit assumed that the optimum protein intake was 120 grams per day.

Justus von Leibig, another prominent German physiologist, made what seems even today to be a reasonable assumption: muscle strength depends on the amount of protein ingested. Voit and von Leibig were highly respected in their times, but we now know that their assumptions about the protein needs for humans were wrong. However, their ideas have echoed around the world ever since.

The mistakes of the great are far more damaging than the mutterings of the multitudes.

How Much Do We Need?

If we are eating too much protein, how much do we really need?

We can easily assess the protein requirements for adult men and women now. Most of the work is done with nitrogen balance studies. Protein contains nitrogen, and the amount of nitrogen that is eaten and the amount that is lost can be measured to give an accurate assessment of protein balance. As we become more sophisticated in our measurements of the amount of protein needed for optimum health, we find it to be exceedingly small, between 20 and 40 grams per day. Dr. W.C. Rose of the University of Illinois in 1950 found that 20 grams of high quality protein would sustain an adult in good protein balance if all other aspects of his diet were adequate. ("Amino Acid Requirements of Man," *Journal of Biological Chemistry*, 217:997–1004, 1955.)

A more conservative but still very low assessment of the protein needs for adults came from the World Health Organization (WHO) and the Food and Agriculture Organization (FAO) in

1967. These groups concluded that the adult needed only half a gram of protein per kilogram of body weight per day. The average man weighs about 150 pounds which is 70 kg. Therefore, his requirement for protein would be only 35 grams.

The actual requirements for protein are indeed very low in comparison to the 100 or more grams of protein that the average American eats each day. The reason so little is needed is that the body is very efficient in conserving proteins and synthesizing new proteins when needed.

One of the most widely held and truly dangerous beliefs is that protein is an "energy food." Protein is used exclusively for enzyme production and *maintenance* of other body proteins. Under ordinary circumstances, only carbohydrates and fats are used for energy; for protein to be burned, it must first be converted to sugar. This energy-inefficient process occurs only in times of starvation; that is, when no carbohydrates or fats are available to the body.

It is particularly self-defeating to have "a protein drink" in the morning thinking that this will increase your energy. In fact, the more protein you eat in excess of your requirements, the more energy you must use to get rid of the waste products.

Excessive Protein Causes Rapid Deterioration

When we eat too much carbohydrate or fat, the body can store this extra energy as fat. This is unsightly and unhealthy, but in many ways excessive protein causes more damage. The body cannot store the extra protein. It must be broken down, and its waste products must be excreted by the kidney. When we consistently eat 300 to 400 percent more protein than we need, we stress the body and cause accelerated ageing and disease. As John M. Hindhede, a Danish physiologist of the late 19th century, pointed out, there is a fundamental mismatch between the design of the human kidney and the amount of protein it is called upon to process with the usually excessive protein diets of most Western countries.

Protein and Kidney Failure
in the Diabetic Condition

In the case of diabetes, this mismatch is even more serious because the diabetic condition damages the kidney. With the added stress of a high protein intake, the diabetic individual is even more vulnerable to kidney destruction.*

Since the discovery of insulin, diabetics do not die from elevated blood sugar levels. Instead, they have to contend with long-term complications of their condition. One of the more serious is kidney failure. *Diabetes is the number one cause of kidney failure.* It accounts for the majority of patients receiving machine dialysis as well as most recipients of kidney transplants. The reason for the kidney damage brought on by diabetes is not clearly understood. It is thought that diabetes damages the small blood vessels in the kidney and the filtering process shuts down, ultimately failing completely.

Kidney failure does not come on all of a sudden. In the diabetic, you can see it coming from 40 miles down the road and in plenty of time to slow it down or stop it by restricting the protein intake. However, this is not usually done. Most diabetics are informed that their kidneys are deteriorating, but only rarely is the diabetic given any advice to lower the protein intake to slow down the process.

Kidney function can be accurately measured by the amount of protein breakdown products that are found in the blood and urine. In the blood, levels of urea nitrogen (BUN) and creatinine rise when the kidneys are failing. Perhaps the most sensitive test for kidney damage is the creatinine clearance test, in which the amount of creatinine excreted in the urine over 24 hours is measured. Because of the ease of measurement, however, the BUN and the blood creatinine levels are the most frequently monitored laboratory values.

The BUN test is not as accurate as the creatinine as a measure of kidney function. If you have been eating a lot of protein, the BUN level in the blood can rise as the kidney becomes a little backlogged in its filtering responsibilities. Also, dehydration elevates the BUN while excessive water intake lowers it.

---

*The ADA recommendation for protein intake is 0.8 g/kg based on the RDA and considers the risk of renal complications.

The creatinine, on the other hand, is not affected by these changes and is therefore a more accurate measure of kidney function. Therefore, when the level of creatinine in the urine goes up, the kidney has been damaged. The higher the level goes, the more damage has been done. Actually, one of the first signs of kidney damage is the presence of albumin (a protein) in the urine. This would be the time to reduce dietary protein.

Diabetic patients with slightly elevated creatinine levels are usually told that sometime down the line they will need the dialysis machine. A few years later, they do. At that time, they are put on a very low protein diet. When the dialysis machine is used instead of the kidney, the more protein you eat, the more frequently you require the machine to filter out the breakdown products. A thick steak dinner can land a patient with kidney failure in the hospital almost immediately.

The irony of this is that rarely, if ever, is the diabetic patient with *impending* kidney failure told to reduce his protein intake *before* kidney failure is a reality. For instance, a diabetic patient who has a creatinine level of 2 to 3 milligrams per 100 deciliters obviously has sustained some kidney damage, and once started, there is progressive kidney destruction until the kidney fails and the creatinine has risen to 10 to 15 milligrams per deciliter. At this stage the patient is put on a kidney dialysis machine and a diet very low in protein.

By not using a low-protein diet at the first sign of kidney damage, the patient has lost the opportunity to slow the rate of kidney damage, or, in some cases, to stop it all together.

William E. Mitch, M.D., of Harvard Medical Center, and Mackenzie Walser, M.D., of Johns Hopkins University, and others studied the effect of a very low protein diet on the progression of kidney failure in 17 patients ("The Effect of a Keto Acid–Amino Acid Supplement to a Restricted Diet on the Progression of Chronic Renal Failure," *New England Journal of Medicine 311*:623–629, 1984). These patients had kidney problems arising from a variety of causes—four from diabetes—and all were progressing toward complete kidney failure. They were given a very low protein, mostly vegetable diet with supplements of some amino acids and their analogues. (Proteins actually consist of chains of amino acid molecules.)

This regimen slowed the rate of kidney destruction in 10 patients and stopped it altogether in seven. The authors noted that the low protein diet was able to stop the progression of kidney failure in those in whom it had not already gone too far. That means that the earlier a low-protein diet is started in a diabetic patient with impending kidney failure the better are the chances of stopping the progression. The researchers concluded:

> If the findings of this study can be generalized and if progression in a large fraction of patients can be arrested for many years, the need for dialysis will be substantially reduced. Most patients with chronic renal failure are diagnosed before the creatinine level reaches 8 mg per deciliter, so that a majority may have at least a temporary arrest in progression.

In the fall of 1984, at the Ninth International Congress of Nephrology (nephrology is the study of kidney diseases), Dr. Carmelo Giordano of the University of Naples, Italy, noted:

> Up until a few years ago, dietary management of chronic renal failure was confined to those patients having little renal function—perhaps 10%—left. The new concept is to recommend dietary management not only for patients waiting to enter dialysis but for the estimated two million Americans who have a serum creatinine of 2 mg/dl (or higher).

His recommendations were for about 20 to 30 grams of protein per day, substantially lower than the protein consumption of most diabetics with progressive kidney failure.

Dr. Sergio Acchiardo, professor of medicine at the University of Tennessee Center for Health Sciences in Memphis, recommends a daily protein intake of .55 gram—about half a gram—per kilogram of body weight as a *low protein diet* for patients with impending kidney failure. This is precisely the recommendation of WHO for adequate protein intake for the adult!

The recipes and meals in this book are broken down into their nutrient components for easy calculation. From these analyses, you and your doctor can work out a nutrition regimen with very low protein intake that would be well suited for you if you have any evidence of kidney dysfunction. In fact, the condition of diabetes is reason enough for reducing your protein intake to spare your kidneys.

Excessive Protein:
A Main Cause of Osteoporosis

Part of the "milk and meat" myth is that these foods are necessary for building and maintaining strong bones and teeth. In reality, the opposite is true. It is milk and meat that *cause* the weakening of the bones called osteoporosis. The reason for this paradox is that calcium balance is determined not by the amount of calcium you eat but by the amount of protein. Here's why.

All protein foods contain nitrogen, and many contain sulphur and phosphorus as well. The body has no way of storing the extra protein we take in every day and must break it down to urea, creatinine, and uric acid and eliminate it through the kidneys. These breakdown products create an acid condition in the blood, which leaches calcium from the bones. This calcium is then lost in the urine along with the protein breakdown products.

Osteoporosis is epidemic in this country, and there are constant warnings that we should consume the recommended daily allowance of calcium that today is 800 mg. However, what is important is not how much calcium we consume daily but how much we are able to deposit into our bones. When we are on a high-protein diet, even "extra" calcium is lost in the kidneys.

There are other cultures who eat even more protein than we do, and they have more severe problems with weakening of the bones. Richard B. Mazess, Ph.D., using sophisticated methods of measuring bone density, found that the Eskimos, by age 40, had a 10 to 15 percent reduction in bone density compared to whites in the same area ("Bone Mineral Content of North Alaskan Eskimos," *American Journal of Clinical Nutrition,* 27:916–925, 1974). He concluded "that the most obvious factor in the 2 to 3% higher rate of bone loss [per year] in middle-aged Eskimos would be their meat diet." The Eskimos consume about 200 to 300 grams of protein per day, which is far greater than even the high protein intake of most Americans.

High Protein Equals Calcium Loss

Nancy E. Johnson, of the Department of Nutritional Sciences at the University of Wisconsin in Madison, found that a high protein diet would put healthy young men in negative calcium balance even if they were taking in more calcium than the Recommended Dietary Allowance (RDA) ("Effect of Level of Protein Intake of Urinary and Fecal Calcium and Calcium Retention of Young Adult Males," *Journal of Nutrition 100*:1425–1430, 1970).

Six young, healthy men, ages 18 to 20, were given 1400 mg of calcium daily plus either a low-protein diet of 48 g or a high-protein diet of 141 g. Calcium balance was determined, which means the amount of calcium taken in was compared with the amount of calcium lost either by lack of absorption or by urinary excretion.

Calcium balance

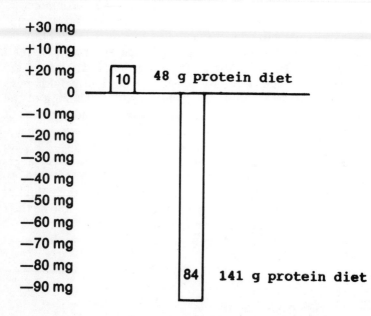

Figure 5 Bars represent calcium balance in 6 healthy men all taking 1400 mg of calcium and on a 48-gram protein diet, then a 141-gram protein diet.

On the lower protein diet, the young men were in positive calcium balance. They retained 10 mg per day to be deposited into their bones, increasing the bones' strength. On the high-protein diet, all the subjects were in negative calcium balance, losing on the average 85 milligrams per day (Figure 5). This means not only that all of the calcium they ingested was lost—1400 milligrams—but that an additional 85 milligrams was taken from their bones and lost as well!

Dr. Johnson pointed out that "the calcium loss of 84 mg daily, which occurred when the high protein diet was fed, was substantial and if continued over a period of time would result in considerable loss of body calcium."

Dr. Ruth Walker, from the same Department of Nutritional Sciences at the University of Wisconsin, carried the studies a step further ("Calcium Retention in the Adult Human Male as

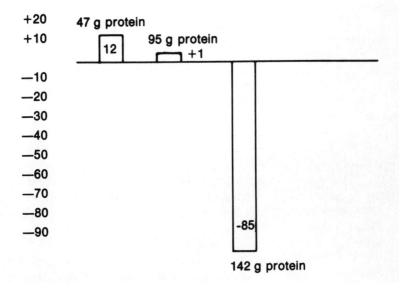

Figure 6 Bars represent calcium balance of nine healthy men given 800 milligrams of calcium and three different protein diets.

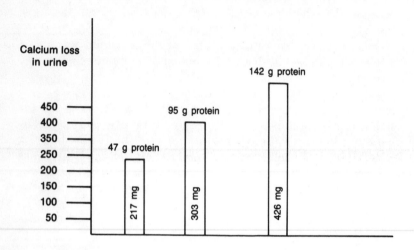

Figure 7 Calcium loss in urine of nine men all eating 800 milligrams of calcium a day and three different amounts of protein.

Affected by Protein Intake," *Journal of Nutrition 102*:1297–1302, 1972). She gave nine healthy young men 800 milligrams of calcium per day (RDA) and three separate diets containing 47, 95, or 142 grams of protein. On the average, the subjects were in positive calcium balance on the low protein intake (+12 mg) and on the medium protein intake (+1 mg). However, they were in severe negative calcium balance on the high-protein diet (−85 mg).

The major reason for the difference was the effect of protein on the average daily amount of calcium excreted by the kidneys. On the low-protein diet the average amount of calcium excreted by the kidneys was 217 mg. On the medium-protein diet it was 303 mg, and on the high-protein diet, it was 426 mg.

Dr. Walker demonstrated that the amount of protein in the diet had an immediate effect on the excretion of calcium by the kidney. As shown in Figure 8, the minute you go on a lower protein diet, your body begins to hang on to more calcium.

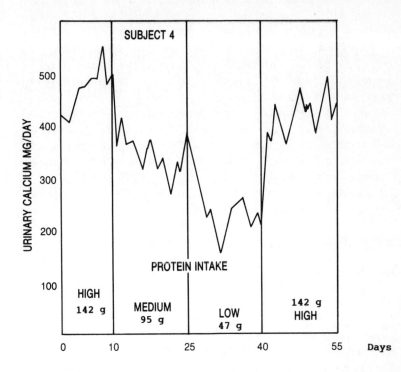

Figure 8 Effect of the protein level on the daily urinary calcium of a single subject. (Reprinted by permission from "Calcium Retention in the Adult Human Male as Affected by Protein Intake" by Dr. Ruth Walker, *Journal of Nutrition 102*, 1300, 1972.)

What is also interesting about these two studies is that increasing the calcium intake did not diminish the negative effect of protein on the calcium balance. In Nancy Johnson's study the intake of calcium was 1400 mg, and the low protein intake, 48 g, resulted in a positive calcium balance of 10 mg per day. On the high-protein (141 g) diet, a negative calcium balance (−84 mg per day) occurred, despite a calcium intake in excess of the RDA.

In Ruth Walker's study, substantially less calcium was used: 800 mg, which, until recently, was the recommended dietary allowance. Even so, the balances were almost identical: The low intake of 47 grams of protein resulted in a +12 mg positive calcium balance, while the high protein intake of 142 grams caused a negative calcium balance of −85 mg daily.

Every newspaper you pick up these days is admonishing us to get more calcium in our diet to avoid osteoporosis. But the amount of calcium we eat per day seems to have little if anything to do with osteoporosis.

At a recent meeting of the American Society for Bone and Mineral Research, two researchers presented strong evidence countering today's conventional wisdom that increasing the calcium intake wards off osteoporosis ("How Important Is Dietary Calcium in Preventing Osteoporosis," *Science 233*:519–520, 1986). Dr. Lawrence Riggs of the Mayo Clinic in Rochester, Minnesota, studied 107 women for 4.3 years and made regular measurements of their bone density. These women consumed a wide range of calcium—anywhere from 269 to 2000 mg a day. He found no difference in the degree of bone density loss related to the amount of calcium taken in.

To see whether those women who were taking in the most calcium had stronger bones than those women taking in the least, Dr. Riggs compared the bone density of the women whose daily consumption of calcium exceeded 1400 mg per day with that of those who were consuming less than 500 mg a day. He found that the rate of bone loss was essentially the same! In short, he "found no correlation at all between calcium intake and bone loss, not even a trend."

Dr. C. Christiansen of Golstrup Hospital in Denmark reported the results of a different sort of study. Forty-three women who were immediately postmenopausal were put on either 2000 mg of calcium, daily estrogen replacement, or placebo for two years. A placebo is a substance containing no active ingredient but appearing identical to the tested substance. He found that the calcium did no more than the placebo to retard bone loss, while the estrogen was effective. Again, the intake of calcium had no effect on the rate of bone loss.

Dr. Richard Mazess of the University of Wisconsin was not surprised at the results of these two studies. He cited numerous studies that demonstrate that people in countries where calcium intake is high have no stronger bones than populations with the least intake: "There is an abundance of data showing that calcium intake in a population is unrelated to bone density."

In spite of strong evidence that the amount of calcium in our diet has no relationship to the strength of our bones, we hear from the dairy industry almost daily about the need to get more calcium from dairy products to avoid osteoporosis. However, Dr. John McDougall points out in his excellent book, *McDougall's Medicine, A Challenging Second Opinion* (New Century Press, 1985), that the countries with the highest dairy consumption (the United States, Sweden, Israel, Finland, and the United Kingdom) have the most osteoporosis and the world's highest incidence of fractures of the hip. Countries with the least intake of dairy products (Hong Kong, Singapore, South Africa—Black Townships only) have the least osteoporosis and the lowest number of hip fractures.

The Irony of the Protein Myth

We believe that large amounts of protein are good for us, strengthening our bodies, when, in reality, excessive protein does just the opposite. As I have pointed out, our bodies were not designed for such protein excess, and our beliefs on the matter will not change that.

It is a fact that total vegetarians, at any age, have much stronger bones than those who eat meat, because of the lower and healthier protein intakes. In addition, they live longer: Numerous studies on the Seventh Day Adventists have shown that their vegetarian diet leads to far lower rates of heart disease and cancer and increases the average life span by several years.

It is particularly important for individuals with diabetes to keep protein consumption down, for the diabetic condition only accelerates the damage done by protein excess.

5

Exercise: A Must for the Diabetic

Exercise may get more lip service but less action than any other currently ignored therapy for the diabetic condition. Almost all of the articles written about treating diabetes mention exercise as a powerful therapeutic tool. However, among the vast numbers of diabetic patients who come to our Institute from all over the country, it is *exceedingly rare* to find one who already has an exercise prescription in hand.

Every diabetic individual regardless of age or type of diabetes should have an exercise program. This chapter will help you understand why exercise is both necessary and beneficial.

Exercise Clears the Blood of Glucose Without Insulin

In a sense exercise acts like an insulin shot to reduce blood levels of glucose. The cells of exercising muscle can extract glucose from the blood much more efficiently than resting muscles can. Diabetic individuals who exercise may be able to reduce their dosage of insulin or oral drugs that stimulate insulin production. In fact, exercise may entirely eliminate the need for insulin therapy or oral drugs. The glucose-reducing action of exercise was demonstrated a hundred years ago, though we still do not know exactly how it works.

One theory is that by dilating (opening) the blood vessels, exercise allows even small amounts of circulating insulin to be utilized, thus causing a fall in blood glucose. Another theory is that the exercising muscle may release some substance that acts like insulin in allowing the circulating glucose to enter the cells, but this substance has never been isolated. We do know exercising muscles produce lactic acid and carbon dioxide. Perhaps these substances somehow unlock the receptors in the muscle cells, letting glucose come in. Finally, it is known that the level of calcium within the muscle cell increases during exercise. It is thought that, in some way, this allows glucose to enter.

The glucose-lowering effect of exercise is probably a combination of all these factors plus some we do not yet recognize. It will be a source of interest for another 100 years. The bottom line for today's diabetic individual is that *exercise is a powerful tool to lower the blood sugar level* and reduce the amount of insulin necessary.

D. M. Klachko and others from the University of Missouri explored the effects of exercise by taking continuous measurements of blood sugar levels in normal and insulin-dependent diabetic subjects during measured activity ("Blood Glucose Levels During Walking in Normal and Diabetic Subjects," *Diabetes 21*:89–100, 1972). The subjects took half-mile "walks" on a treadmill at the relatively brisk but not too strenuous pace of 4 miles per hour. The treadmill was elevated at either 2.5 or 5 degrees.

For the nondiabetic subjects, the less strenuous walk at the 2.5 degree elevation dropped the blood sugar level an average of 5.3 mg/dl. The more strenuous produced an average drop of 11.7 mg/dl. The diabetic subjects, however, recorded an average drop of 24.5 mg/dl with the less strenuous walk and 30.0 mg/dl for the more strenuous walk.

After the exercise, the blood sugar in the diabetic subjects went back up, but not to the level recorded before the walk. In the normal subjects, the blood sugar level went back to the preexercise level. In some, it went above this level.

These little bursts of exercise took only 7½ minutes, but the drop in blood sugar was substantial. The researchers concluded:

Our study shows that moderate exercise has a more profound effect on blood glucose levels in insulin-dependent diabetics than in normal individuals. The amount of fall appears to depend mainly on the level of blood glucose at the onset of exercise as well as on the amount of exercise taken. In addition, following the exercise, there is absence of the rise in blood glucose concentration which is frequently seen in normal individuals. These factors support the clinical observations of the marked effect of exercise in bringing down blood glucose levels in insulin-treated diabetics, and thus its important role in diabetes control.

A Word of Warning

In the true insulin-dependent diabetic (thin, active, yet still requiring insulin), exercise can make matters worse if the patient is too tightly *or* too loosely controlled.

First, with too much insulin (very tight control) exercise may cause a severe drop in blood sugar (hypoglycemia). Insulin-dependent diabetic patients should know that *they must substantially reduce their insulin dose* on the days they plan vigorous activity. It is important not to start exercise with blood sugars in the low-normal range. The patient should always carry some source of carbohydrate to be eaten if signs of hypoglycemia occur. The reduction in insulin dosage when embarking on an exercise program should be worked out under a physician's care.

For a controlled type 1 diabetic the reduction could be as much as 80 percent on the mornings when a long bike ride or some other form of protracted activity is planned.

For the type 2 diabetic treated with diet and exercise only, exercise is not likely to cause hypoglycemia. If the individual is taking oral hypoglycemic drugs or if he or she has been put on insulin therapy, hypoglycemia can occur. Again, professional supervision is needed.

If the type 1 diabetic starts exercise with very high blood sugars, the blood sugar may not fall. In fact, the exercise could cause the blood sugar to rise even more. This sequence could bring on the dangerous condition known as *ketoacidosis,* which could lead to hospitalization.

The danger of ketoacidosis with exercise applies only to the thin insulin-dependent diabetic. For the obese type 2 diabetic, there is no danger that exercise will cause an elevation in the blood sugar leading to ketoacidosis. For the type 2 diabetics who constitute 90 percent of the diabetic population, exercise, if started and carried out properly, is an unmitigated plus.

Exercise Increases the Cells' Sensitivity to Insulin

Besides having the immediate effect of clearing the blood of glucose, exercise has long-range benefits for diabetic individuals. A program of aerobic conditioning definitely increases the body's sensitivity to insulin whether it is produced by the person's own pancreas or injected. This increased insulin sensitivity has both short-term and long-term effects that work together to lower the insulin requirement.

Short-Term Sensitivity

It has been shown that exercise after eating tends to lower the blood glucose level. Here at the Institute, we see to it that all diabetic clients get some exercise—8 to 12 minutes' worth—directly after each meal. We instruct them to continue this practice at home. These bursts of activity are very beneficial. Moreover, studies show that exercising after breakfast makes the activity after lunch and dinner even more powerful in keeping the blood sugar under control. If you have angina (chest pain), caution is indicated. Patients with angina should not walk after meals if it brings on chest pains. Instead, they should wait for a few hours to get in their exercise.

Long-Term Sensitiviy

Clearly, the most beneficial effect of an exercise program is the long-term increase in insulin sensitivity. Insulin insensitivity is the culprit in the type 2 diabetic condition, representing 90 percent of the cases of type 2. Therefore, exercise is clearly indicated in helping these patients.

One method of estimating insulin sensitivity is to measure the binding of insulin to various cells in the body. Dr. Oluf Pedersen of the Department of Internal Medicine at County Hospital in Aarhus, Denmark, found that exercise increased the binding of insulin to certain blood cells by 30 percent. He also found that the increased binding, and thus increased sensitivity, was dependent on the degree of exercise conditioning. ("Increased Insulin Receptors After Exercise in Patients with Insulin-Dependent Diabetes Mellitus," *New England Journal of Medicine, 302*:886–892, 1980.)

Dr. Philip Felig, professor of medicine at Yale University School of Medicine, measured insulin sensitivity in six nonobese, but sedentary volunteers who did not have diabetes. In the *Journal of the American Medical Association,* he reported that one hour of exercise a day, four days a week, increased insulin sensitivity in these subjects by 30 percent (*242*:1591, 1979). Like Dr. Pedersen, Dr. Felig found that the amount of exercise determined the degree of increase in insulin binding and insulin sensitivity. Given the fact that maturity-onset (type 2) diabetes is a situation in which there is low insulin binding and reduced tissue sensitivity, he notes that "we would anticipate that exercise would have an effect in improving the diabetic beyond that attributable to weight reduction and specifically related to enhanced insulin sensitivity and binding" (*JAMA 242*:1591, 1979).

Exercise Thins the Blood, May Help Prevent Eye Problems

The blood functions best when it is fluid rather than viscous, flowing easily through the capillaries. One measure of the fluidity of the blood is the "stickiness" of the platelets, small sand-like particles that are important for the normal formation of a blood clot after a cut. Despite their usefulness in stopping bleeding, platelets can be a hazard if they precipitate a clot in the blood vessels, since such a clot, or *thrombus*, can cause a stroke or heart attack, by blocking one of the large vessels going to the brain or heart. In addition, small clots formed by platelets can block the tiny vessels that nourish the eyes and the kidneys. This kind of blockage is thought to be one of the major causes of blindness and kidney failure so common in diabetic individuals.

Greg Peterson, a research assistant to Peter Forsham, M.D., at the University of California–San Francisco School of Medicine, measured the effect of exercise on platelet stickiness in six insulin-dependent diabetic patients. He did this by passing a blood sample through a tube of glass beads and measuring the percentage that stuck. Before exercise, the platelet stickiness was high; 74 percent of the platelets stuck to the beads, but 30 minutes on the treadmill or bicycle reduced the percentage to 53 percentage.

Exercise, by keeping the blood fluid, could help prevent damage to the eyes and kidneys in the insulin-dependent diabetic. However, diabetic patients should be careful not to exercise too strenuously. Intense exertion could possibly cause rupture of the small vessels of the eyes and other organs. This is particularly dangerous in the diabetic individuals who are "out of shape."

General Benefits Are True for Diabetics as Well

Exercise is particularly beneficial for the diabetic person, but the general benefits of vigorous activity are more than enough reason for anyone—with or without diabetes—to start an exercise program.

If you were looking at two men of the same body build and weight, it would be difficult to tell which one was active and well conditioned. However, the changes that can be measured on the inside are astounding. Exercise has a beneficial effect on every system in the body!

Exercise and Mood

Every day, joggers, bicyclists, and walkers come out by the millions in this country. Ever wonder why? Are they diabetics trying to lower their blood sugar level? Are they trying to prevent or treat heart disease? No. For most, exercise is used as a "pepper-upper"—a tonic. It's not that those chugging around the track felt bad, it's that exercise makes them feel better.

This is common knowledge. Who has not felt his mood lift with a brisk walk? Who hasn't cleared her mind and solved some problem while engaged in physical activity?

The salubrious effect of exercise on our psyche results from the elevation of certain hormones in the brain. Exercise promotes an increase in beta-endorphins, very potent mood elevators. In fact, it is their effect on the beta-endorphin system that allows the drugs morphine and Demerol to relieve pain and create a feeling of euphoria.

With exercise, the endorphins go up naturally: Mood is elevated, thinking is clearer, life is just "better"—sometimes a lot better. Numerous studies have found that exercise alone is better than psychotherapy at eliminating depression.

Oxygen Utilization

When you exercise, you flood your system with oxygen. If the exercise is vigorous enough, your uptake of oxygen can go up 1000 percent. One of the first signs of conditioning is the body's improved utilization of oxygen, both during exercise and at rest. The well-conditioned body simply extracts oxygen from the blood more efficiently, benefitting every system in your body.

One of the signs of ageing is decreased ability to use oxygen during exercise. For instance, during maximum exercise, a man of 50 will use less oxygen than a man of 25 under the same conditions. However, this is one measurement of ageing that you can stop—even reverse. The maximum uptake of oxygen can be increased in anyone at any age with regular exercise, and some well-conditioned men and women of 50 match 25-year-olds on this score.

Exercise Elevates HDL Cholesterol

The level of cholesterol in the blood is highly predictive of an impending heart attack. As the level of cholesterol in the blood goes up, the chances of having a heart attack or stroke increase. This is as true for the diabetic person as it is for the nondiabetic population, only more so. However, researchers have found that the form of cholesterol called high-density lipoprotein (HDL) cholesterol is beneficial in preventing heart attacks.

All cholesterol molecules are carried in the blood attached to complexes of fat and protein. The dangerous form of cholesterol is called low density lipoprotein (LDL) cholesterol because it is attached to light, fluffy complexes that are mostly fat and thus are very light. When a sample of blood is centrifuged (spun very rapidly), LDL complexes come to the top. These cholesterol complexes plug up the arteries and cause strokes and heart attacks.

HDL cholesterol is attached to carriers made up mostly of protein, which is denser than fat. They are heavier than the LDL fraction and gravitate to the bottom when the blood is centrifuged. These are the good complexes; they do not stick to the walls of the arteries.

In fact, the HDL cholesterol mobilizes cholesterol attached to the arteries, transporting it to the liver where it can be turned into bile, excreted into the intestinal tract, and eliminated from the body.

Exercise has been shown to elevate the HDL cholesterol level. It seems to burn up the fatty complexes that make up the dangerous LDL fractions, replacing them with the beneficial HDL variety. This action helps prevent artery plugging, thus protecting against heart attacks and strokes.

Exercise Lowers Triglycerides

Triglycerides in the blood are molecules of neutral fat. Many type 2 diabetics have elevated triglycerides levels. We have already discussed how elevated fat levels in the blood lead to insulin insensitivity, bringing on a diabetic condition in the first place.

Regular exercise lowers triglyceride levels and helps the body burn fats more efficiently. In patients with high triglyceride levels—250 to 350 mg/dl—exercise may bring the level down to 100 in less than a week. In addition, regular exercise is almost essential for successful and sustained weight loss.

Exercise Strengthens the Normal Heart

The heart of a well-conditioned individual is so much stronger and efficient than the unconditioned heart that it has a special name: *the athletic heart*. The characteristics of an athletic heart are:

• *A slower resting pulse rate*. The normal resting heart rate is between 60 and 90 beats per minutes. However, after a few weeks of conditioning exercise, the resting pulse rate of the conditioned heart will fall to about 45 to 60 beats per minute. Because it is stronger, the conditioned heart pumps more blood in each beat, thus needing fewer beats to pump the same amount of blood.

• *A higher exercise pulse rate*. The well-conditioned heart develops the capacity to beat faster in response to exercise than the unconditioned heart. During exercise, when the call for more blood goes out, the athletic heart can deliver a higher pulse rate if necessary.

• *A larger stroke volume*. The well-conditioned heart delivers more blood per beat. Each stroke is stronger, and the amount of blood delivered with each stroke is increased with exercise training. This makes the heart much more efficient.

• Like the rest of the body, the heart muscle itself improves its ability to extract oxygen from blood with exercise training. This is particularly important if there are blockages that have reduced the amount of blood flow, for the heart can extract more oxygen from less blood.

Exercise Strengthens the Diseased Heart

Everyone can and should be on an exercise program, *tailored to his or her special condition.* Even patients with very severe heart disease can benefit from some form of regular exercise carefully tailored to their capacities with professional supervision.

Doctors make terrible mistakes when they decide that a patient is too ill to start a mild exercise program. True, those who have suffered heart damage and are severely disabled must start with only mild activity. For example, they may try riding a stationary bicycle with no resistance for 5 minutes or so a day. Activity can then be gradually increased from this low level, allowing the heart to increase its strength.

In his book *Cardiovascular Rehabilitation: A Comprehensive Approach* (Macmillan, 1983), Dr. Lyle Peterson, director of the Comprehensive Rehabilitation Center in Houston, Texas, reported quite remarkable results with a mild exercise program in 12 severely ill heart patients who were waiting to undergo a heart transplant operation.

These patients, all registered and waiting for a donor heart for transplantation, were referred to Dr. Peterson's center for evaluation and for mild exercise conditioning in order to strengthen them for surgery. They were all very ill and had to be closely monitored during any physical activity.

Much to the surprise of Dr. Peterson and his staff, 6 of the 12 improved so much that they were taken off the heart donor list and went home to live essentially normal lives. One patient has maintained his improvement for over five years, and he continues to exercise regularly on an exercise bicycle.

Dr. Peterson's results indicate that the power of exercise to rehabilitate damaged hearts extends even to those who have almost surely been told by their physician not to exercise. Obviously, when patients are this ill, the exercise needs to be carefully prescribed and monitored. Nevertheless, it is a powerful tool, the only tool to strengthen a weakened heart.

Exercise Builds "Collaterals" If Needed

When arteries to the heart muscle start to fill with fatty deposits, the body's normal defense is to build additional blood vessels around the artery to ensure continued blood flow. These new vessels are part of a *collateral circulation*. Many times a heart artery will close completely, but a heart attack is avoided because collateral arteries have developed around the blockage.

The dread condition of atherosclerosis of the heart arteries is like a race: The major arteries are being plugged by fat and cholesterol and the body is building collateral blood vessels to prevent the impending heart attack. Who wins? The artery plugging or the collateral circulation?

Hedge your bet. Like poisonous snakes, heart attacks are something you want to stay as far away from as possible. Regular exercise helps distance you from this disease.

You can slow, perhaps even reverse the process of atherosclerosis with this program. Second, you can speed up the development of collateral circulation by exercise, and exercise is the only activity that can do this.

If Only It Were a Pill

If all the benefits of exercise were available in a prescription drug, it would be the world's most widely prescribed medication. Everyone would be on it, diabetic or not! The resistance to using exercise on the part of both doctors and patients is innately human—exercise requires effort, and the search for some miracle pill to obviate the need for effort is neverending. However, the effort need not be unpleasant. For patients who successfully start an exercise program and persevere until it becomes established in their daily lives, the effort becomes more joyful release than drudgery!

The Hardest Part Is Getting Started

Getting an exercise program firmly implanted in your daily life is like an airplane ride. The hardest part is getting off the ground and up to cruising altitude. Once there, it is easy and fun staying there.

The Stress Test: A Vital Precaution

Any exercise program prescribed for a diabetic should be based on an exercise stress test. During a stress test, the patient exercises on a treadmill or a stationary bicycle while an electrocardiograph (EKG) machine monitors the activity of the patient's heart. The patient exercises at gradually increasing work levels, and as the heart rate increases, the EKG monitor shows any abnormalities that occur during the activity. For example certain EKG patterns indicate that the arteries may be blocked. When this blockage occurs the heart fails to get enough blood at certain levels of exertion. If the blood flow to the heart is severe enough, a heart attack can occur.

Continous EKG monitoring also will show any tendency toward arrythmia, or skipped beats, brought on by exertion.

The stress test is indeed a useful tool for picking up any abnormalities in the heart that are present only when the heart is working hard. Not only that, but the stress test can be life-saving in preventing heart attacks from *sudden* overexertion by a person who was previously inactive.

Another important reason for the stress test is that it contains the information for writing the exercise prescription. An exercise prescription clearly states how *much* you are to exercise, *when* you are to do it, and what your heart rate should be during the activity. You should treat your exercise prescription with the same respect and discipline you treat prescriptions for drugs. For the diabetic, exercise is more than a wholesome idea that you will get around to one of these days. It is absolutely essential for optimal control of your condition. Diabetics who are experiencing proliferation or bleeding in the eyes, should exercise with caution following their doctor's advice.

The Exercise Pulse Rate

When you exercise, your pulse rate increases as the heart beats faster to pump more blood to the working muscles. The more you exercise, the faster the heart beats until finally your heart reaches the *maximum pulse rate* (MPR).

As we age, the maximum pulse rate brought on by exercise declines. You can estimate your MPR by subtracting your age from 220. For instance, a 20-year-old could be expected at maximum exercise to have a pulse rate of 220 minus 20, or 200 beats per minute. A 65-year-old would be expected to have a pulse rate of 155 beats per minutes (220 minus 65).

During the stress test, while under EKG monitoring, the function of the heart in response to exercise is accurately determined. Usually, the goal of this test is to exercise the patient to a pulse rate of 85 percent of that person's maximum calculated pulse rate. At this level of exertion, most abnormalities of consequence will appear.

Then, depending on how the patient responds to the test, an exercise prescription can be written that includes his or her exercise pulse or *training pulse* rate: the rate to strive for during walking or bicycling sessions. Usually the training rate is about 75 percent of the maximum calculated pulse rate, but the actual MPR can vary substantially. Having done thousands of exercise stress tests on patients, I know that the test serves only as a guideline. Exercise training, as already mentioned, will *increase* the maximum heart rate that can be achieved by maximum exercise.

At age 35, I remember recording a pulse of 216, which was far above my calculated maximum pulse of 185. My wife and I were in San Francisco and we had a race. I was at a slight disadvantage as she was in a car and I was on foot. The race was straight up the steep Scott Street hill starting at the Marina Green. It was a little over a mile. Even if you have never been to San Francisco, you surely can appreciate the steep hills of this city that are often portrayed on television shows. The Scott Street hill is so steep that if you turn your car to face the curb, you are afraid that it will turn over and roll down to the bay.

Since my wife had the car, I got a two-minute head start. About one-and-a-half blocks from the top of the hill, I looked over my shoulder; much to my dismay, I saw her rapidly closing the gap. I won the race and my pulse went to 216 in the process. I do not advise this sort of nonsense for anyone.

The Frequency of Exercise

Most training programs should be at least four days per week and at most six days, with rest days spaced in between. Many of my patients exercise every day, and this is acceptable if they are used to it and the exercise is not too vigorous. For instance, a walking program of 30 to 40 minutes per day can be done every day, but vigorous jogging sessions of 45 to 60 minutes should best be done five or six times per week with a day or two of rest in there.

Vigorous exercise programs deplete the muscles of a stored carbohydrate called glycogen, the primary muscle fuel. It is the glycogen stores that must be replenished with occasional rest days, otherwise exercise becomes very difficult, not to mention unpleasant.

Types of Exercise

Your choice of exercise should be worked out after a stress test, as already mentioned, and with professional advice. The only type of exercise I prescribe as a treatment for diabetes or heart disease is aerobic conditioning exercise designed to elevate the heart rate and sustain that elevation for 20 to 40 minutes. Types of aerobic exercise are walking, bicycling, swimming, slow jogging, or any other exercise that moves the body through space at a rate that permits a sustained elevated pulse rate.

Aerobic exercise must be differentiated from weight lifting or the stretching exercises of Yoga. Also, many patients feel that their daily activities are already filled with beneficial exercise, particularly housewives who "walk all over the house, up and down stairs" or gardeners who "work hard for hours digging and planting." Many also feel that their work provides more than enough exercise, particularly if they "walk all over the job site." Unfortunately, these forms of activity, though better than just sitting at a desk, almost never are enough to accomplish aerobic conditioning and should not be counted as part of your exercise program.

In addition, most exercise received while playing tennis, golf, softball, bowling, or other recreational sports should not count either. What is missing is a *sustained* elevation of pulse rate.

There is no way around it. If you want the enormous benefits of aerobic conditioning, an exercise program must be added to the day. It must be—demands to be—made a priority. Don't kid yourself.

How to Get Started

After a stress test has determined your exercise pulse rate, and after your doctor has written your exercise prescription, you and your doctor need to sit down and work out the "what," "when," and the "where" of your program.

What will it be? Walking? Stationary bicycling? Swimming?

When will you be doing it? This is very important! The program will not start until you have designated some time during the day for the activity. Though this seems obvious, I have had many patients who kept putting it off because they just could not "find the time."

Where is all this activity going to take place? In sections of the country where the weather does not permit year-round outdoor activity, the exercise program must continue either in a closed shopping mall, an indoor swimming pool, a heated gym or athletic club, or in the home on a treadmill or exercise bicycle.

Having worked out exercise programs for thousands of patients, I know the importance of discussing each of these things so that the patient understands exactly what is to be done. This discussion also underscores the importance your doctor should be putting on the need to exercise.

I do want to emphasize again that everyone, *before* starting an exercise program, should get checked out by a physician. Ease into your program slowly, probably with walking only. This is the only safe and effective way to do it.

6

Vitamin and Mineral Supplementation

Surely some controversy will be aroused by my recommendation that diabetic patients take vitamin and mineral supplements. Actually, vitamins and minerals are chemical agents that, if used rationally and in a balanced manner, can have a positive effect on the metabolism of diabetics and normals alike. Nevertheless, there is a strong bias in medicine against using nutritional supplements unless a classic deficiency exists. In fact, it is often considered "unprofessional" to recommend a nutritional supplement to anyone unless a gross nutritional deficiency is obvious.

Why is there so much negative bias among physicians against nutrition in general and nutritional supplements in particular?

Most Physicians Are
Ignorant About Nutrition

One obvious reason for negative bias of physicians toward nutrition in general and nutritional supplements in particular is ignorance. Clinical nutrition is given scant attention in medical school. Usually, nutrition is dismissed with a few lectures on the general digestion and breakdown of fats, carbohydrates, and proteins, while vitamins and minerals are covered in simplistic lectures that only describe their most basic normal function and the effects of gross deficiency.

What is never broached in any systematic way is how nutritional patterns may be associated with the development of degenerative conditions like diabetes, heart disease, cancer, or multiple sclerosis, and how these patterns can be altered to prevent and treat disease. Consequently, physicians graduate from intensive and grueling programs with no inkling that what people eat has a profound effect on their health and that altering nutritional patterns is an extremely powerful tool.

When one considers the hundreds of millions of people who seek help from physicians for forms of heart disease and diabetes that are purely the results of faulty nutrition, it is alarming that so little clinical nutrition is covered in medical school.

Arthur M. Sackler, M.D., International Publisher of the Medical Tribune, in an editorial entitled "On the Nonsense of Official Recommended Daily Allowances (RDAs)," writes:

> The contrast between advances made in such areas as diagnostic technologies, cardiovascular surgery, genetics, and recombinant DNA and the backwater in which real nutrition research and practice are stagnating is staggering. The reasons are multiple. Doctors are taught little if anything about nutrition in medical school. (*Medical Tribune,* September 18, 1985, p. 46.)

Where there is ignorance, there must be bias.

Ironically, I believe that another source of physician bias is the presence of "official standards."

THE RECOMMENDED DIETARY ALLOWANCES

Just what are RDAs? The purpose of the Recommended Dietary Allowances (RDAs) established by the Food and Nutrition Board of the National Academy of Sciences is "to set levels of intake of the essential nutrients considered, in the judgment of the Food and Nutrition Board on the basis of available scientific knowledge, to be adequate to meet the known nutritional needs of practically all healthy persons."

In general, they state that healthy individuals who are

consuming food containing the RDAs of the essential nutrients have not been known to develop any nutritional deficiency diseases related to the nutrients. The Food and Drug Administration also has a set of RDAs and these are often referred to as USRDAs.

Well, just who is healthy? As Dr. Sackler points out, in this country there are:

Alcoholics	10,000,000
Allergics	35,300,000
Arthritics and rheumatics	27,238,000
Diabetics	12,000,000
Hypertensives	25,524,000

Just from A to H, we have a total of 110 million. Of course, there are overlaps among the patients but most are adults in a total population of 161,864,000 over 21 years of age. If to these you now add the gross deviations between individuals' needs of even the "healthy," one must ask for how many Americans the RDAs are truly applicable. (*Medical Tribune,* September 18, 1985, p. 46.)

Even if you are "healthy," the RDAs are designed to *prevent deficiency*, not to insure optimal health. The amount necessary for optimal function could be several times the amount necessary to prevent deficiency.

Furthermore, the RDAs do not take into account the fact that most nutrients play several roles in metabolism depending upon the amount available. For instance, only 5 to 10 milligrams of vitamin C daily will prevent scurvy, the vitamin C deficiency disease. The RDA is 60 mg. However, several studies have shown that 2000 to 3000 milligrams of vitamin C per day can enhance the function of the body's white blood cells and increase production of several immunoglobulins (substances produced by the body to increase resistance and fight disease). Both these effects would be beneficial to the body's immunity.

Second, the RDAs do not take into account individual

differences. The obvious differences among people in such characteristics as weight, hair color, temperament, athletic ability, musical talent, and intelligence are minor when compared to the tremendous variations that exist under the skin. For instance, the gastric juice of one "normal" man may contain 400 percent more pepsin than his equally "normal" neighbor. There are numerous items for which differences between "normal" individuals are not 25 to 50 percent but rather 500 to 1000 percent.

Many of the vitamins and minerals are involved in enzyme production, and the levels and proportions of enzymes that are circulating in the blood of normal individuals vary remarkably. These variations suggest a similar variation in vitamin or mineral requirements at any given time. For example, what may be an optimal amount of pantothenic acid for one individual may be completely inadequate for another.

Also, the optimal vitamin or mineral intake for any individual may vary with time and circumstance. For instance, many researchers suggest that stress dramatically increases the need for vitamin C and other nutrients as well. The thinking behind the RDAs simply ignores the possibility that individuals are different with, most likely, different requirements for certain nutrients and that time and circumstances therefore are likely to alter the amount of nutrients an individual needs.

Third, the RDAs tend to assume that everyone eats a "balanced" diet, which is just not true. Most Americans get their calories from steam tables, processed and precooked dinners, and fast food outlets. Much of the food eaten by Americans consists of high fat processed carbohydrate combinations often lacking the nutrients necessary to metabolize these foods adequately.

In short, there is no evidence that I know of indicating that the existence of the RDA guidelines has done anything to improve the nutritional health of the nation or even to improve our understanding of nutrition. One has to wonder what goes through the minds of those who actually believe the RDAs, as they are currently formulated, are true indicators of nutritional requirements for all healthy people, much less the ill.

However, the presence of the guidelines may, in subtle ways, make matters worse.

The RDAs and Physican Mindset

The very existence of the Recommended Dietary Allowances of vitamins and minerals thwarts the use of nutritional supplements by physicians. These recommendations have created a mindset among physicians that any amount of a nutrient above the "recommended level" is unwarranted and only creates "expensive urine."

What is overshadowed by the presence of the RDAs is the fact that many vitamins or minerals at larger doses than the RDA can act beneficially in certain conditions, usually with less toxicity than most prescription drugs.

For instance, the RDA for pantothenic acid (calcium pantothenate), a water soluble member of the B complex, is 10 milligrams (mg) per day. However, when it is used in much larger doses, pantothenic acid has been shown to have beneficial results on rheumatoid arthritis. The General Practitioner Research Group found in a controlled study that up to 2000 mg. of this inexpensive and nontoxic vitamin had "highly significant effects . . . in reducing the duration of morning stiffness, degree of disability, and severity of pain" in patients with rheumatoid arthritis (*Practitioner 224*:208, 1980).

Many physicians are unaware of this potential for calcium pantothenate and would be hesitant to use 200 times the RDA to treat the symptoms of their arthritic patients, even though there has been no demonstration of toxicity of the vitamin at this dosage.

Another example is vitamin B_3 (niacin), for which the RDA is 20 mg a day. However, if 2000 to 6000 mg of niacin are used, it becomes a drug capable of markedly lowering the cholesterol and triglyceride levels in the blood and can save lives as a result. At this dosage, niacin does have side effects, but the side effects are less dangerous than those of the prescription drug Atromid-S, which is designed to do the same thing. The existence of an RDA for this vitamin acts as a barrier for many physicians in considering it for therapeutic use in larger doses. (In diabetics, dosages of niacin over 100 mg a day should not be used, as it has the tendency to elevate the blood sugar.)

In summary, Arthur M. Sackler, M.D., concludes:

The nutrition ignorance which breeds nutrient arrogance is beginning to be modified by a public whose nutrient interests and insights are outstripping what should have been the leadership and knowledge of the medical profession.

One of the fallacies involved in the RDA approach to nutrition is one that was brilliantly addressed 120 years ago by the father of experimental medicine when he challenged the use of statistical averages as confusing and distorting. "Averages," Claude Bernard said, "are applicable only to reducing very slightly varying numerical data about clearly defined and absolutely simple cases." Nutrient requirements, intake, and preparation are neither "slightly varying," "clearly defined," nor "absolutely simple."

To further complicate matters, in addressing our total population we do not address the "average" healthy person, because tens of millions have complicating conditions. Their needs are neither "slightly varying," nor "clearly defined," nor "absolutely simple."

The common belief that RDAs are generally applicable to all sectors of our population as a standard is a misleading chimera. As standards, they are more often fallacies than facts. (*Medical Tribune*, September 18, 1985, p. 62)

Nutritional Quackery

The negative bias of physicians is certainly not helped by the nutrition quackery that abounds in our culture. Claims are made that this or that vitamin will cure heart disease, grow hair, improve sex, improve athletic performance, stop aging, and make you smarter in the process.

These claims may be based on some real but less dramatic benefits of the vitamin in question, but the outlandish nature of the claim is so offensive to most physicians that it makes the whole nutritional supplement field stink. When this is the case, the vitamin huckster does everyone a disservice by alienating all but the most gullible.

This chicanery creates "guilt by association" for anyone who advises or uses vitamins or minerals in treating diseases. Thus most physicians, to protect their integrity, shun the use of all nutritional supplements and react with predictable scorn anytime their patients raise questions about a claim relating to a certain vitamin or mineral.

Though understandable, this backlash is tantamount to throwing the baby out with the wash.

What Do Vitamins and Minerals Do?

Most vitamins and minerals have multiple roles in the body's metabolism, but their major function is in the role of enzyme production, in which they function as coenzymes.

Enzymes are the essence of metabolism. They are usually made by the body by the combination of an apoenzyme, which is produced in the body, and a coenzyme, usually a vitamin or mineral. The apoenzyme is produced according to genetic programming and varies considerably from person to person. The apoenzymes join with a coenzyme to produce the enzyme.

Nutrient Deficiency Results in Enzyme Deficiency

When vitamins or minerals are deficient, the result is usually a reduced enzyme production. Herein lies the problem in determining the optimal level of vitamin and mineral nutrition. A small amount of a nutrient that functions as a coenzyme will eliminate the obvious signs of deficiency disease, but larger amounts may be optimal, as the larger amount will allow enzyme production to increase to the maximal amount or the limits of the genetic programming of the individual.

Nutrients Function Independently, as Hormones

In addition to functioning as coenzymes, many nutrients function independently to alter metabolism. For instance, vitamin D acts like a hormone in controlling the body's calcium metabolism. A deficiency of vitamin D would have a significant effect on the body's use of the mineral. Some nutrients function both as coenzymes and as independent affecters of metabolism as well.

Toxicity and Fat Soluble Vitamins

The major danger with toxicity of nutritional supplements rests with the fat soluble vitamins, A, D, and E.

Unlike its precursor, beta carotene, preformed **vitamin A** is highly toxic in large doses. The toxic dose varies in different individuals. Toxic reactions include hair loss, ulceration of the skin, and blurred vision. Vitamin A toxicity may produce a symptom complex called pseudotumor of the brain. The headache, blurred vision, incoordination, and other signs and symptoms of increased pressure in the brain are similar to symptoms that often occur with brain tumor. If vitamin A toxicity is the cause, however, the symptoms disappear when use of the vitamin is discontinued. Most people can tolerate up to 10,000 units of preformed vitamin A without developing toxicity.

However, there may be no reason to take *any* preformed vitamin A. Research has shown that beta carotene, the immediate precursor of vitamin A, is essentially nontoxic even in high doses. It seems to confer the same benefits as preformed vitamin A. At least, that is the current state of knowledge.

Vitamin D is responsible for maintaining calcium and phosphorus balance and controlling the absorption of these two minerals when they are mobilized from the bones. This vitamin can be obtained in the diet or is produced by the body in response to sunlight when it directly strikes the skin. Therefore, deficiencies would only be expected in areas of low sunlight (those with long winters in the higher latitudes) or in people whose jobs prevent exposure to the sun and who also have a deficient intake of the vitamin. Nutritional sources of Vitamin D are rare. The best source is oily fish, but most people receive vitamin D from fortified milk products. The best source, however, is the sun.

This fat soluble vitamin is stored in the liver, and toxicity can occur with excessive intake. Toxic reactions to vitamin D usually cause excessive calcium to be mobilized from the bones. This calcium is then deposited in the soft tissue of the body such as the blood vessels, liver, kidneys, heart, and lungs. Toxicity does not occur if vitamin D is produced by exposure to sunshine, because the body regulates how much is produced and stored.

Vitamin E toxicity apparently does not occur with daily dosages of 600 units or less. I have found no research on this vitamin that suggests any benefit from taking more than 600 units, so toxicity should not be a problem.

With dosages higher than 600, some toxicity has been reported, but these reports have usually consisted of anecdotal observations rather than controlled studies. Hyman J. Roberts, M.D., of the Palm Beach Institute for Medical Research in Palm Beach, Florida, reported that he found dosages of vitamin E in excess of 800 units per day to be associated with blood clots in the legs, breast enlargement, and fatigue states ("Perspective on Vitamin E as Therapy," *Journal of the American Medical Association 256*:129, 1981). However, controlled studies have not substantiated that vitamin E causes these symptoms.

Since very large doses of vitamin E is a new phenomenon in our culture, it is impossible to know what effect truly massive doses will have over a long time. This vitamin is beneficial in dosages up to 600 units, however, and supplementation up to this point is a good idea.

Toxicity and Water Soluble Vitamins

The water soluble vitamins (the B complex and vitamin C) have much less potential for toxicity than fat soluble vitamins do, because an excess can be readily excreted in the urine. Since water soluble vitamins are not stored by the body, the purpose of giving supplements of these vitamins is to saturate the metabolic systems that require them. Saturation may require dosages of the vitamin that exceed that amount necessary for the vitamin to show up in the urine.

Many physicians conclude that if the vitamin is being excreted in the urine, the dosage being taken is more than is needed for a beneficial effect. This is just not accurate. Many water soluble vitamins continue to have a metabolic effect even though the threshold for urinary excretion has been exceeded. This phenomenon occurs with many prescription drugs as well.

Vitamin B$_6$ has been found toxic in dosages of 2000 mg or more per day. Women sometimes take such high dosages of vitamin B$_6$ in the hope that it will function as a diuretic to eliminate water retention associated with the menstrual cycle. Several such women have developed a toxic reaction effecting the nerves. They became unstable, experienced numbness in their feet and hands, and became clumsy with their hand movements. No other cause of the nerve toxicity could be found, and the symptoms regressed with termination of the vitamin. (Herbert Schaumburg, M.D., "Sensory Neuropathy from Pyridoxine Abuse," *New England Journal Medicine 309*:445–1448, 1983.)

In an editorial accompanying Dr. Schaumburg's report, Daniel Rudman, M.D., of Emory University School of Medicine pointed out that the toxicity experienced by these patients could have been brought on by the metabolic derangements of such a large dose of B$_6$ or even by the impurities contained in such a large amount of the vitamin preparation. Regardless, this was the first report of a major toxic reaction associated with water soluble vitamin supplementation. (*New England Journal of Medicine 309*:488, 1983.)

However, this dose was "irrationally high." These reports should not cloud the issue that the water soluble B vitamins in physiologic dosages of 50 to 150 mg and vitamin C in dosages of up to 2000 mg have not been shown to have any significant toxicity.

Vitamin B$_3$ in doses over 100 mg will often cause a "niacin flush" experienced as tingling and redness of the skin, usually around the face and ears. At large doses, there can be discoloration of the skin, elevation of the liver enzymes, elevation of uric acid concentration, and elevation of the blood sugar level. Large doses of niacin can lead to an irregular heart rhythm. These changes are considered to be temporary and stop when the vitamin is stopped.

These reactions to niacin are well known, for niacin has been used for many years as an agent to lower the blood levels of cholesterol and triglycerides. Even with these side effects, niacin is still one of the safest and certainly one of the most effective cholesterol-lowering agents. Vitamin B$_3$ does not have a place in therapy for the diabetic patient, however, because of its effect on the blood sugar level.

Vitamin C in doses larger than 1 gram can cause diarrhea and has been suggested to precipitate some types of kidney stones in those at risk. There may be more serious specific health risks for a few individuals who are missing one of the enzymes required for the degradation of ascorbic acid.

Minerals and Trace Elements

Nutritionally important minerals are inorganic substances that are essential for optimum metabolism. They are quite different from vitamins. Vitamins are organic, always contain carbon, and are manufactured by plants and animals. Generally, food that contains vitamins will have about the same amount of the vitamin regardless of the soil where the food comes from. Of course, processing, cooking, and storage affect the vitamin content of foods.

Minerals, on the other hand, are not manufactured by organisms and must come from the soil and be incorporated into plants. The potential for mineral deficiency is much higher than the potential for vitamin deficiency, because the amount of minerals in the soil varies greatly from region to region.

In China, for instance, one area has excessive selenium in the soil. In another, the selenium content is very low. In these two sections of the same country, people suffer with either selenium toxicity or deficiency, depending on where they live.

In nutritional terms, essential minerals are called minerals if they are required in the diet in amounts greater than 100 mg per day. The minerals include calcium, magnesium, phosphorus, sulfur, sodium, and potassium. Minerals required in smaller amounts are called trace elements. These include iron, chromium, selenium, manganese, zinc, iodine, and copper. For the diabetic, the most important trace element is chromium.

Vitamins, Minerals, Trace Elements, and Diabetes

The diabetic condition imposes requirements for vitamins and minerals that are different from those of people who do not have the condition. Therefore, supplementation is even more reasonable than it is for the general healthy population (whoever they may be). Some of the special needs of the diabetic are: chromium, beta carotene, vitamin B_6, and magnesium. Garlic and fish oils also have useful functions.

Poor healing of tissue damaged by injury or surgery is a well-known problem in the diabetic condition. Researchers at Albert Einstein College in New York found that **vitamin A** accelerated wound healing in animals and improved the function of the immune system. The researchers concluded that "just as supplemental vitamin A improves immune responses of traumatized animals and surgical patients, it will be especially useful in preventing wound infection and promoting wound healing in surgical diabetic patients" (*Annals of Surgery, 194*:42, 1981). Although this study focused on vitamin A, its precursor beta carotene can be supplemented continuously with less chance of toxicity.

Certain forms of diabetes seem to be related to deficiencies of **vitamin B_6.** This vitamin is necessary for the normal metabolism of the amino acid tryptophan. Abnormal metabolism of this amino acid has been shown to cause a form of diabetes. When B_6 is supplemented, diabetes in some improves significantly. Moderate amounts of B_6 supplementation may reverse some forms of diabetes that are associated with pregnancy.

Chromium

As early as 1854, it was reported that brewer's yeast improved the diabetic condition. Later, researchers found that the active ingredient in brewer's yeast is a complex of chromium and several amino acids that has become known as the Glucose Tolerance Factor (GTF). When Dr. Walter Mertz gave chromium supplements to six diabetics, three of them demonstrated improved control ("Effects and Metabolism of Glucose Tolerance Factor," *Nutrition Review 33:*1929, 1975). GTF chromium does not act like insulin but rather seems to enhance insulin sensitivity. Dr. Mertz has noted that chromium concentration in tissues of Americans declines with age and that this may be a reason for the significant increase in diabetes as we get older. He also has noted that chromium supplementation can sometimes take two to three months before any beneficial changes are noted.

The general multiple vitamin and mineral supplement we use with almost all patients enrolled in the Institute contains 400 micrograms of chromium.

Magnesium

Almost every patient at the Institute receives a series of injections of magnesium sulfate. One milliliter of a 50 percent solution of magnesium sulfate is mixed with 1 ml of heparin 1:1000 solution and injected intramuscularly, six times over a period of twelve days. On leaving the Institute, many diabetic patients leave with a prescription for one or two of these injections per month, in addition to the oral magnesium as contained in the multiple vitamin and mineral formula that is prescribed for them.

Low magnesium levels seem to be a common factor among people with the diabetic condition. H.M. Mather of the Department of Medicine, St. George's Hospital, London, measured the blood magnesium level in 582 consecutive diabetic patients visiting the hospital's outpatient clinic. He also measured the magnesium levels of 140 nondiabetic subjects. He found that the diabetics had a significantly lower blood magnesium level. In fact, 25 percent of the diabetics tested had lower levels than all of the controls except one.

The diabetic condition itself may cause reduction in magnesium levels. Elevated blood sugars stimulate excessive urination, which can wash essential minerals and trace elements out of the body. Therefore, the diabetic condition predisposes the patient to numerous deficiencies, yet the potential of these deficiencies is rarely addressed.

In addition, when insulin-dependent diabetics go out of

control and into ketoacidosis (insulin coma) there is marked mineral depletion. These minerals need to be replaced over a prolonged period.

Many diabetics are taking hypertensive medication and/or diuretics. Diuretics are notorious wasters of all minerals, yet potassium is the only mineral that is routinely replaced.

As Dr. Mather pointed out, magnesium has a fundamental role in carbohydrate metabolism in general, and a very specific role in the efficient action of insulin itself. A low level of magnesium can certainly contribute to poor control of the diabetic condition. He also concluded "that it is at least conceivable that the hypomagnesaemia occurring in diabetic patients may predispose to their markedly increased incidence and morbidity of ischemic heart disease" ("Hypomagnesaemia in Diabetes," *Acta Clinica Chemica 95*: 235–242, 1979).

In 1981, Dr. Takeo Takemura of the Department of Internal Medicine, Osaka City University, Japan, reported to the Japan Diabetic Society that low magnesium levels were associated with an increased incidence of diabetic retinopathy—damage to the eyes that leads to blindness, a major complication of diabetes. He studied 68 diabetic patients and compared their magnesium levels to those of 32 healthy nondiabetics. He found that the diabetic group had magnesium levels of 1.59 mEq/L (millequivalents per liter) compared to a control value of 1.65 mEq/L. He also found that the diabetics had elevated magnesium in their urine, which measured an average of 5.59 mEq/L, compared to 4.01 mEq/L for the controls.

Dr. Takemura reported that in the diabetics as a whole, those whose blood sugar was above 250 had the greatest degree of magnesium reduction in the blood and the highest level of magnesium in the urine. Probably this was due to the diuretic effect of elevated blood sugars.

In addition, in those with the greatest degree of retinopathy, the magnesium value in the blood was significantly lower than either the diabetic group as a whole or the control group. In the blood of these patients with eye problems, the magnesium level measured 1.49 mEq/L compared to the 1.65 of the controls.

Magnesium should be balanced with calcium so that the ratio of calcium to magnesium intake is roughly 2 to 1. However, the magnesium injections may be helpful intermittently to insure that the magnesium stores do not become depleted.

Garlic

The oils found in onion and garlic, particularly garlic, have been found in numerous studies to confer benefit. They have been shown to significantly aid in lowering the blood levels of both cholesterol and triglycerides. They also have a tendency to thin the blood, and in some ways seem to enhance the immune system, perhaps by their nontoxic antibacterial mechanism.

For years I have tried to find convenient ways to increase my patients' consumption of garlic. The garlic capsules are convenient, but often the deodorized variety have eliminated the essential elements that confer benefit.

I recently have been using the "garlic cocktail," which consists of six ounces of unsweetened grapefruit juice or unsalted tomato juice, one whole glove of fresh garlic, and two sprigs of parsley blended together. The resulting concoction is only 60 percent as offensive as it sounds! In fact, it is tolerated quite well, as the juices do wonders to mask the odor and taste of the garlic. One clove of garlic does not seem to be enough to create chronic offensive breath odor, but many patients, to avoid this, drink the garlic cocktail at night.

Here at the Institute, most patients consume one garlic cocktail per day and are instructed to continue this practice at home. What is valuable about this method of garlic supplementation is that it is easy to do, and therefore can regularly supply a modest amount indefinitely. The regularity of any supplement program is key to its benefits.

What Is Optimal?

It is beyond the scope of this book to discuss each vitamin or mineral that can have beneficial results if supplementation is used to insure optimum level. This subject has been discussed in two readable, well-referenced books that I highly recommend: *The Complete Guide of Anti-Aging Nutrients,* by Sheldon Saul Hendler, M.D., Ph.D. (Simon & Schuster, 1985) and *The People's Guide to Vitamins and Minerals* by Dominic Bosco (Contemporary Books, 1980).

INDICATIONS: For supplementation of vitamin and mineral deficiencies.

Each eight tablets contain:		%U.S RDA
Vitamin A (as Beta Carotene)	25,000i.u.	500
Vitamin A (as Retinyl Palmitate)	5,000i.u.	100
Vitamin D$_3$ (Cholecalciferol)	400i.u.	100
Vitamin E (d-Alpha Tocopheryl)	400i.u.	1333
Vitamin C (Ascorbic Acid)	2,000mg	3333
Folic Acid	400mcg	100
Thiamine (Vitamin B$_1$)	50mg	3333
Riboflavin (Vitamin B$_2$)	10mg	588
Niacinamide (Vitamin B$_3$)	80mg	400
Niacin (Vitamin B$_3$)	20mg	100
Vitamin B$_6$ (Pyridoxine)	75mg	3750
Vitamin B$_{12}$ (Cyanocobalamin)	40mcg	666
Biotin	300mcg	100
Calcium Pantothenate (Pantothenic Acid)	50mg	500
Choline	250mg	†
**Calcium	1,000mg	100
Iodine (Kelp)	150mcg	100
*Iron Chelate	18mg	100
***Magnesium	500mg	125
*Copper Chelate	3mg	150
*Zinc Chelate	30mg	200
****Potassium	300mg	†
*Manganese Chelate	10mg	†
*Chromium Chelate	400mcg	††
Selenium Chelate	200mcg	††
Molybdenum Chelate	150mg	††
Silicon Chelate	20mg	††
Rutin	200mg	††
Bioflavonoids	100mg	††
Hesperidin	50mg	††
Inositol	40mg	††

*Each tablet contains a Mineral Protein Chelate made with specially isolated soy protein.

**Derived from Calcium Chelate, Carbonate and Gluconate

***Derived from Magnesium Chelate, Oxide and Gluconate

****Derived from Potassium Chelate and Chloride

†The need in human nutrition has been established, but no U.S. RDA has been determined.

††The need in human nutrition has not been established.

U.S. RDA—United States Recommended Daily Allowance

Figure 9 Vitamin/mineral supplement formula currently used at the Institute. The formulas are continually being revised in response to research and individual needs.

The use of the RDAs as a tool to prevent deficiency is on shaky grounds. It is even more difficult to propose levels of vitamin and mineral intake that would be optimal for the healthy or diabetic individual. Therefore, the regimen we use here at the Institute is more like an insurance policy, designed to provide insurance against any deficiency and to approach the level that may be optimal without risking significant toxicity. We reviewed an enormous amount of research on vitamins and minerals in deriving this formula. It is in no way written in stone, as it is altered and changed as more information becomes available.

The multiple vitamin and mineral formula shown in Figure 9 is used here at the Institute with almost every patient. For more information about this formula, and how to obtain it, please contact the Institute.

MaxEPA Fish Oil

In addition, every patient is given supplements of fish oil called MaxEPA to lower blood fat levels and prevent blood clots, thereby helping to ward off heart attacks and strokes. Over the last several years, the oils found in cold-water fish have received a lot of attention. They seem to have considerable health benefits.

It all started several years ago when it was noted that the Eskimos, who consume a high-fat diet in which the fat comes from fish, had far less heart disease than inhabitants of other countries where meat was the staple food. The reason: fat from marine mammals and fish does not lead to heart attacks, it prevents them.

The oil found in fish, unlike the fat of land-based animals, is unsaturated and therefore more like a vegetable oil. Fish oil, however, differs from vegetable oils in that it belongs to the Omega 3 class of oils, meaning that the first unsaturated bond occurs at the third carbon atom. Most vegetable oils are in the Omega 6 class of oils, with the first unsaturated bond occurring at the sixth carbon atom.

Unsaturated oils are the precursors to powerful hormone-like substances called prostaglandins that effect many systems in the body. Omega 3 and Omega 6 oils stimulate the production of different prostaglandins. Fish oil stimulates prostaglandin production that dramatically lowers the blood cholesterol level.

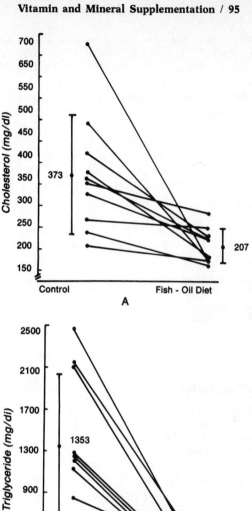

Figure 10 The effect of dietary fish oil in ten patients with elevated cholesterol and triglyceride levels. Reprinted, by permission of *The New England Journal of Medicine, 312*:1210–16, 1985.

Dr. William Connor and his group at the Department of Medicine, Oregon Health Sciences University, gave ten patients with dangerously high levels of cholesterol and triglyceride, supplementary fish oil for four weeks. The average cholesterol level dropped from 373 milligrams per deciliter, to 207, a drop of 166 mg/dl or 46 percent. The triglyceride level fell even more dramatically from 1353 mg/dl to 281—a drop of 1072 mg/dl (Phillipson, B.E., Rothrock, D.W., and Connor, W.E., et al. "Reduction of Plasma Lipids, Lipoproteins, and Apoproteins by Dietary Fish Oils in Patients with Hypertriglyceridemia," *New England Journal of Medicine 312*:1210–16, 1985.)

Fish Oil, a Blood Thinner

Second, fish oil acts as a safe blood thinner by reducing the production of a substance known as thromboxane A_2. This hormone, increased by animal fats in the diet, causes the blood cells, particularly the small particles in the blood called platelets, to stick together, forming dangerous clots that cause heart attacks or strokes.

Howard R. Knapp, M.D., and his coworkers at Vanderbilt University in Nashville, Tennessee, studied 13 men with severe atherosclerosis of the leg arteries. They found that five capsules of MaxEPA fish oil a day for four weeks significantly reduced production of thromboxane A_2, and at the same time increased the production of another substance, prostaglandin I_3, which is a natural blood thinner.

For several years now, patients with heart disease or tendencies toward stroke have been advised to take a single aspirin per day as a blood thinner. Aspirin works like fish oil by reducing thromboxan A_2, but it may also halt production of the beneficial prostaglandin I_3.

Fish oil may be superior to aspirin as a blood thinner, as it not only reduces the "bad" elements that cause clots but also increases the "good" elements that prevent them.

The one, two punch of blood-fat control and blood-thinning properties makes fish oil a real plus in treating patients with heart disease, or in trying to prevent it. This would be particularly important to the diabetic patient, who has an increased tendency toward atherosclerosis and heart disease.

Fish Oil Reduces Inflammation and Aids Arthritics

At the 1986 meeting of the American Rheumatism Association in New Orleans, two studies demonstrated that fish oil significantly reduces the pain of rheumatoid arthritis.

Dr. Joel M. Kremer of Albany Medical College in New York found that 15 capsules of MaxEPA substantially relieved the joint pain in 20 arthritis patients compared to 20 taking a placebo. Dr. Richard I. Sperling, an Associate Professor at Harvard University, had similar results with 12 arthritis patients given 20 capsules of MaxEPA per day. (*Medical World News*, July 14, 1986, p. 9.)

Fish oil seems to reduce production of a potent inflammatory agent called leukotriene B_4 and increases the production of the benign leukotriene B_5.

Fish Oil, an Essential Nutrient?

The benefits of fish oil have caused many researchers to now consider it an essential nutrient. Since Americans eat comparatively little fish, increasing consumption of fish to about two meals per week would be advised or taking supplements of fish oil on a daily basis makes sense. I have some concerns about consuming more fish as the source of fish oil, since doing so would keep the level of protein elevated. Excessive protein poses a potential problem for us all, particularly the diabetic who is prone to kidney damage.

Supplements of fish oil called MaxEPA are available without a prescription. *However, if you have any heart or blood vessel disorder, are allergic to fish, or are on medication, you should see your doctor before taking them.* The optimum dose of fish oil depends on the initial levels of the cholesterol and triglyceride in the blood as well as the individual's health history. At this writing, other brands of fish oil supplements are making their way into the marketplace. Some of these are coming from pharmaceutical companies. At present we use MaxEPA at the Institute.

PART III
Problems of Too-Aggressive Treatment

7

Insulin:
The Dangers of Excess

In a book about diabetes treatment, it is difficult not to pay homage to insulin and what it has meant to hundreds of millions of diabetics worldwide. But you know that. Without insulin, many diabetic patients would live only a short time.

However, considering all those with diabetes, insulin is essential for only about 10 percent. For the majority, the diabetic condition can and should be controlled with diet, exercise, and weight control following the principles outlined in this book.

Like most medical therapeutics, insulin is a double-edged sword. Inappropriate use of it can cause more problems than benefits.

Hypoglycemia

One of the most common problems of insulin therapy is episodes of hypoglycemia (dangerously low blood sugar) from too large a dose. People who take insulin are warned that hypoglycemia may occur and told to keep some rapidly absorbed carbohydrate available at all times (fruit juice, sugar). Hypoglycemia occurs most frequently in thin diabetics, as they are much more sensitive to insulin than are those who are overweight.

Hypoglycemia is clearly the most common and by far the

most dangerous complication of insulin therapy. In several studies documenting the frequency of the condition, it was found that over 90 percent of diabetics on insulin claimed to have had hypoglycemic episodes. Up to 60 percent reported having an attack at least once a month. Each year about 25 percent of insulin users will have a severe reaction—severe being defined as requiring assistance from another person or requiring hospitalization.

In another study of 100 patients, 55 percent had become comatose from severe hypoglycemic reactions. This complication of insulin therapy accounts for about 3 to 7 percent of deaths in the insulin-treated diabetic, and it surely has led to brain damage in a much higher percentage. Hypoglycemia is the rule, not the exception, in insulin-treated diabetics, and it represents a serious threat. (Philip E. Cryer, M.D., "Glucose Counterregulation, Hypoglycemia, and Intensive Insulin Therapy in Diabetes Mellitus," *New England Journal of Medicine, 313*:232–241, 1985.)

For some reason, many physicians are less worried about the dangers of hypoglycemic attacks than about the consequences of elevated blood sugar levels. Often patients are "expected" to have hypoglycemic attacks, as indication of good control.

I find this attitude hard to understand and certainly do not agree with it. As we shall see, hypoglycemia brought on by too much insulin is not only a clear and present danger for the diabetic but is also a major cause of poor control as it causes a rebound hyperglycemia (elevated blood sugar levels).

In addition, we are still trying to delineate how important it is to maintain insulin-dependent diabetics in "tight control" as compared with "loose control." *Tight control* is defined as keeping the fasting blood sugar as close as possible to the levels found in nondiabetic people—generally in the 80 to 130 range. Loose control allows the blood sugar levels to drift higher, to the 150 to 200 range, thus avoiding frequent hypoglycemic attacks. Most physicians strive for the tightest possible control and accept the increased frequency of hypoglycemia as necessary.

However, to date there is no significant evidence that tight control actually lowers the complication rate of insulin-dependent diabetics when compared to more loose control. Diabetics who are frequently "out of control" are a different matter. These patients often have blood sugar levels in the 300 to 400 range and need a program to improve these levels.

On the other hand, a severe hypoglycemic attack can be fatal. In a celebrated attempted murder trial in Massachusetts, Claus von Bulow was accused of trying to kill his wife with insulin injections. (He was acquitted.) Hypoglycemia is especially damaging to the brain; it kills brain cells. This damage is permanent because unlike other body cells, dead brain cells are not replaced by new cells.

I therefore find it difficult to justify the belief that tight control is best. First, tight control *automatically* increases the frequency of hypoglycemic reactions, which are a known danger. Second, there is *so little evidence* that tight control is any more effective than loose control in reducing the major complications of the diabetic condition.

If you are taking insulin and are about to start this diet program, I suggest that you consult with your physician about reducing your insulin dosage about 25 to 30 percent. This is done routinely for all insulin-dependent patients who enter the Institute. By making the patient more sensitive to insulin, this diet reduces the insulin requirement. Therefore, it sets the stage for hypoglycemia unless the insulin dosage is reduced. If the blood sugar rises, more insulin can be added back to the regimen. It is always safer to reestablish control of blood sugars that are moderately too high rather than trying to raise levels that are too low.

Types of Insulin

Most insulin preparations used today use insulin extracted from the pancreas of cattle or hogs. Insulin is a protein, which means it is composed of amino acids hooked together to form chains. The human insulin molecule contains 51 amino acids. The amino acid composition of insulin varies from species to species. The importance of these differences lies in the fact that insulin is injected into the body, and thus the protein is intimately exposed to the body's immune system.

If there is a significant difference in amino acid structure, the body will synthesize antigens to a "foreign" protein, and the individual will become *allergic*. This means that each time that individual comes into contact with that substance, antigens will attach to it and cause an allergic reaction. This reaction may take the form of a rash or a more severe reaction called an anaphylactic reaction may occur. An anaphylactic reaction can be fatal. (Fortunately this is rare with insulin therapy.)

For patients who do need insulin, I regularly prescribe pork insulin because it is more like human insulin than beef. It differs from human insulin by only one amino acid, while beef insulin differs in three amino acids. Consequently, pork insulin is less likely to provoke allergic reactions than beef insulin.

Human insulin is now available. It is synthesized in the laboratory and has the identical amino acid sequence of the insulin synthesized in the normal human pancreas. Many research programs are now under way to determine whether human insulin (called Humulin) is superior to purified pork insulin products. A form of "human" insulin is derived by chemically altering pork insulin.

At present, human insulin does not seem to offer significant benefits over purified pork, but the jury is still out.

Long- and Short-Acting Preparations

Insulin that has not been altered to extend its time of action is called Regular insulin. After injection, it begins to lower the blood sugar in about 30 minutes. It reaches its peak action in about two hours and will have an effect for about six hours.

Certain proteins or zinc may be added to the insulin preparation to slow down the absorption rate. The most commonly used preparations are called NPH and Lente. They start to work after 2 to 3 hours, have a peak action between 8 and 10 hours, and will work for about 24 hours.

Regular and NPH are the most commonly used insulin preparations, but there are two others. Semi-Lente acts a little more slowly than Regular and Ultra Lente, a very slow acting insulin that will work up to 36 hours.

Dosage Schedules

Both the amount and the schedule of injections must be individually prescribed for each patient. It is important for patients to be aware of the time the insulin they use reaches its peak activity, as this is the time they are most likely to have a hypoglycemic reaction. For instance, when NPH is used in the morning around 8:00 A.M., its peak action occurs at 4:00 P.M., which is the most likely time for the blood sugar to fall below normal. If Regular insulin is used at 8:00 A.M., the peak action starts in midmorning.

Patients most often use combinations of NPH and Regular given in the morning. Some take a second dose in the late afternoon. Most diabetics follow one of two schedules: a single injection of NPH and Regular in the morning, or an injection in the morning followed by an injection, again using a mixture of NPH and Regular, in the late afternoon, usually around 4:30 or 5:00 before the evening meal. Generally the evening dose of insulin is much lower than the morning one to avoid the possibility of hypoglycemic reactions in the early morning while sleeping. If the hypoglycemia goes unnoticed, it can be very dangerous.

Patients who are monitoring their blood sugar levels at home (and this is almost a must for those using insulin) and who are using a mixture of NPH and Regular in a single dose, should regularly check their blood sugar level fasting, when they first get up, again right before lunch, and again at four in the afternoon. These blood sugar levels should be recorded in a diary so that the physician can get an idea of how much control the patient is achieving.

Also, patients are taught to alter their insulin dosage according to the recorded blood sugar levels. Again, these adjustments are individualized. The records may show fluctuations, with blood sugar levels that are too high or too low at certain times of the day. For instance, a patient's records may show that for several days in a row, he has run high blood sugar levels around noon. That patient's Regular insulin may be increased by about 2 units a day until the blood sugar is brought under better control. If the blood sugar level is consistently high in the afternoon, around 4:00 P.M., the patient may be instructed to increase the NPH insulin given in the morning by 1 or 2 units. Again, these adjustments vary for different patients and should be made under a physician's supervision.

It is important that the insulin dosage be increased in only very small increments to avert the deleterious effects of too much insulin, which I believe is one of the biggest problems of diabetic therapy today. Also, only one change at a time should be made. Excessive use of insulin starts a vicious cycle of hypoglycemia, followed by hyperglycemia, followed by more insulin followed by rapid deterioration known as:

The Somogyi Effect

Dr. Michael Somogyi is another clear-thinking, sound researcher who made significant contributions between the mid 1930s and the early 1960s. He is best known for describing how large doses of insulin are a major factor in the poor control that classifies the "brittle" diabetic.

Too much insulin causes hypoglycemia, and the body responds by releasing insulin antagonists: cortisol and epinephrine (adrenaline) from the adrenal gland, growth hormone from the pituitary gland, and glucagon from the pancreas. Epinephrine and glucagon are the most powerful hormones for elevating the blood glucose level. Glucagon works exclusively on the liver, while epinephrine works on both the liver and the muscle tissue.

Glucagon, a powerful insulin antagonist, is made in the alpha cells of the pancreas which are located in the Isles of Langerhans, right next to the beta cells that produce insulin! Epinephrine not only elevates the blood sugar but also is responsible for the racing heart and the "cold clammy" reaction of hypoglycemia.

These hormones are rapid and extremely powerful elevators of blood sugar and will almost always cause an overshoot with the blood sugar level going too high, spilling into the urine.

These high readings are then treated with *more* insulin, which causes an even deeper plunge of the blood sugar, a higher compensatory response, and possibly even larger doses of insulin. This rebound effect of excessive doses of insulin is internationally known as the *Somogyi Effect*.

Dr. Somogyi felt that most diabetics can and should be controlled on very low doses of insulin. He stated:

No diabetic patient is adequately "regulated" with insulin until his daily requirement is 20 units or less, or, in exceptional cases, between 20 and 30 units. The large doses generally used in insulin therapy result from unawareness of the diabetogenic effect of hypoglycemia. Excess insulin, which causes hypoglycemia, aggravates diabetes, and the damage done by too much insulin is then combated with still more insulin. This leads to a vicious circle, with an unmanageable diabetes as its product. (*Bulletin of the St. Louis Jewish Hospital Medical Staff*, October 1949.)

Working as a lone voice, Dr. Somogyi spent a good deal of his time rehabilitating diabetics who came to the St. Louis Jewish Hospital out of control because of excessive use of insulin. His experience with these patients led him to conclude

that insulin therapy in its present way of application serves not so much the treatment of the common, spontaneous diabetes of the patient, but the greater part of the insulin doses administered are consumed in arduous attempts to check and control the new adreno-pituitary diabetes which has been superimposed by the effects of insulin doses that caused hypoglycemia in the course of the treatment. (*Bulletin of the St. Louis Jewish Hospital Medical Staff*, May 1951.)

Michael Somogyi was no doubt a most original thinker and surely antagonized some of the "experts" of his era. In the same publication cited above, he stated that:

The central subject of our work was the physiology and pharmacology of insulin action. . . . Theories, interpretations, that are neither supported by unequivocal experimental evidence, nor usable as working hypotheses, were strictly banned from the picture; they were disregarded, irrespective of the prestige or authority of their sources.

Not surprisingly, Dr. Somogyi was very familiar with the work of Himsworth and others of that time who had clearly shown the benefits of a high-carbohydrate diet. While other diabetic centers were forbidding liberal carbohydrates for diabetics, a high-carbohydrate diet was routine for the fortunate patients treated at St. Louis Jewish Hospital where Michael Somogyi practiced.

The Dawn Phenomenon

Dr. Peter Campbell and his associates from the Mayo Clinic in Rochester, Minnesota, have documented that most insulin-dependent diabetics have early morning surges of growth hormone, an insulin antagonist that regularly causes elevated blood sugar readings in the morning ("Pathogenesis of the Dawn Phenomenon in Patients with Insulin-Dependent Diabetes Mellitus," *New England Journal of Medicine 312*:1473–79, 1985).

This phenomenon creates a problem because the early morning blood sugar level is the level most commonly used to establish the amount of insulin used that day. Second, if this level is high, there is a tendency to try to bring it down aggressively with larger insulin dosages in the afternoon or evening. This approach only worsens the problem by creating hypoglycemia that would elevate the early morning sugar even more.

The bottom line is that we should be less concerned with blood sugars that are elevated (150 to 250) in the morning unless there is consistent elevation throughout the day.

Excessive Insulin and Increased Eye Damage

One of the major disasters of diabetes is the progressive damage to the retina that often occurs and can progress to total blindness.

It has been assumed throughout history that if the blood sugar level in diabetics could be brought down to the normal level of nondiabetics with oral medication or with insulin, the complications would not occur.

However, just the opposite occurs. Aggressive treatment with insulin in some patients actually *increases* the rate of eye damage leading to blindness, especially if tight control is achieved very rapidly. It is thought by some that the rapid drop in the blood sugar level may cause thinning of the blood and leakage from the vessels.

Drs. Mara Lorenzi and Michael Goldman of the University of California at San Diego reported the case of a 27-year-old male type 1 diabetic (let's call him Mike) who had been on insulin since age 6 ("Improved Diabetic Control and Retinopathy," *New England Journal of Medicine 308*:1600, 1983). He had been taking 35 to 42 units of NPH in a single injection for many years and did not check his blood sugars at home.

When studied he was in very poor control: his average blood sugar readings were 303 mg/dL, ranging from 217 to 381. A study of his eyes revealed only a small amount of retinal damage, and no acute areas of damage were noted. He was not doing badly, even though he had maintained 300 plus blood sugars for years.

He was referred to the university to undergo a more aggressive use of insulin to improve his blood sugar control and was trained in home monitoring techniques. He was put on two insulin injections a day (the total daily dosage of insulin was not given in this communication), and nine months later he was in much better control: his blood sugars were lowered to an average of 124 with a range of 75 to 200.

However, with the much "tighter control" his eyes began to deteriorate rapidly, and he required numerous laser treatments to control the damage.

Almost unbelievably, 21 years of once-a-day insulin shots with decidedly poor glucose control had produced only mild damage to his retina, but only nine months of two shots a day and much better control of the blood sugar had caused rapid deterioration of his eyes almost to total blindness.

The Cause: Insulin Like Growth Factor 1??

It is possible that increased use of insulin is associated with retinal damage because it promotes the increased secretion of a pituitary growth hormone called Insulin Like Growth Factor 1. (This hormone has also been called somatomedin-C, but I like the newer name better.) Blood levels of Insulin Like Growth Factor 1 rise when more insulin is used or when the patient's diabetic condition is brought under better control.

When Mike was in poor control with an average blood sugar of over 300, his blood levels of Insulin Like Growth Factor 1 on two separate measurements were found to be 52 and 98 ng/ml. With two injections of insulin per day, his blood sugar was lowered to an average of 124, but levels of the hormone increased to 144 and 150 on two measurements. Concurrently, destruction of the retinas in both his eyes accelerated significantly.

Several large-scale studies comparing "tight control" of the blood sugar in diabetics with more loose control have shown that retinopathy is increased in the tight-control group. In one study 70 diabetic patients all taking insulin and all with mild development of retinal damage were divided randomly. Half the patients were given continuous insulin through a pump. The other half were treated in the conventional manner with insulin injections. Those receiving the pump therapy had very significant improvements in their blood sugar control, but the condition of their eyes unexpectedly worsened in comparison with those on conventional therapy. In fact, in those on the insulin pump with improved blood glucose control, there was worsening in 40 percent of those in whom eye damage had already been established. ("Blood Glucose Control and the Evolution of Diabetic Retinopathy and Albuminuria: The Kroc Collaborative Study Group." *New England Journal of Medicine 311*:365–372, 1984.)

In another study reported at the 1983 meeting of the American Diabetes Association Meeting, Dr. John Dupree of the University of Western Ontario, reported a comparison of 35 patients on the insulin pump with 34 patients receiving conventional treatment. Again, those on the pump had much tighter blood glucose control, but their eyes got worse over a ten-month period, compared with those on conventional treatment with less than optimal blood glucose control. (John Dupree, M.D., "Near Normal Glycemic Control Does Not Slow Progression of Mild Diabetic Retinopathy," 1983.)

At the same ADA meeting, Torsten Lauritzen and his colleagues at the Steno Memorial Hospital and the Department of Ophthalmology at Gentofte Hospital in Denmark reported that they followed 30 diabetic patients for one year. Half were treated intensively with the insulin pump. The researchers found that retinal deterioration continued in both groups, but "the frequency of deterioration was highest in the pump group, especially among the 10 patients with the best blood glucose control." These findings were disappointing to the researchers, who offered the following explanations:

1. With marked lowering of the blood sugar, there may be a reduction in blood flow to sections of the retina thus causing an increase in acute damage.

2. Secondly, tight control alters other hormones, and in particular elevates Insulin Like Growth Factor 1, as was noted by Dr. Mara Lorenzi (above).

The elevation of Insulin Like Growth Factor 1 may be particularly important: Thomas Merrimee, M.D., and his colleagues at the University of Florida studied 80 diabetic patients and found that those with rapidly deteriorating retinopathy all had markedly increased levels of Insulin Like Growth Factor 1 compared with diabetics not experiencing retinal damage ("Insulin Like Growth Factors, Studies in Diabetics With and Without Retinopathy," *New England Journal of Medicine 309*:527–530, 1983).

It is too early to say why the very tight control that is characteristic of the insulin pump therapy using multiple shots of insulin causes a worsening in eye problems. This is a very serious observation. It has been shown over time that high blood glucoses cause microvascular complications in diabetes in laboratory animals.

As bleak as these initial studies are, updates on the ongoing studies are slightly encouraging. Dr. Torsten Lauritzen, head of the Steno Study Group which found that one year of insulin pump therapy had accelerated the degree of eye damage in those who had already some damage, reported that after two years of intensive insulin therapy, those on the pump had about the same degree of eye damage as those following conventional insulin therapy with less tight control ("Two-Year Experience with Continuous Subcutaneous Insulin Infusion in Relation to Retinopathy and Neuropathy," *Diabetes*, v. 34 [Suppl. 3]:74–79, 1985). It may be that the accelerated damage occurs only after initiation of tighter control, and slows down considerably after the control is established, while those on looser control experience a continuous damage to the retina.

This is also the observation of the Kroc study group, sighted above. Dr. William Tamborlane, Professor of Pediatric Endocrinology at Yale University School of Medicine, is one of the investigating physicians with this ongoing study. In a recent telephone conversation, Dr. Tamborlane confirmed that their observations were similar to the Steno Group study in that two years of intensive insulin therapy was not associated with greater eye damage than conventional insulin therapy. The rate of damage that was experienced by those on the intensive therapy slows considerably while those on conventional therapy "catch up."

It is certainly too early to tell whether intensive insulin therapy will ultimately be found better than looser control, but at two years, it has at least been partially indicated as a significant hazard to the eyes. The conflicting data concerning the effects of intensive insulin therapy and eye damage has led to some inside joking on the part of diabetic specialists. When the physician is successful in bringing down the blood sugar level, fine; when he fails, "it is to protect the eyes."

Dr. Tamborlane also pointed out that aggressive use of insulin either by the pump or multiple injections blunts the body's defense mechanism for combating hypoglycemia. As already discussed, in the diabetic who has just started insulin injections, a falling blood sugar stimulates release of epinephrine and other insulin antagonists that act to elevate the blood sugar level. These insulin antagonists also cause a "cold, clammy" feeling, which is a clear signal to the diabetic to eat something.

In patients on aggressive insulin therapy, they seem to "get used to" the swings of lower blood sugar levels and the warning signals do not activate until the blood sugar has already reached a dangerously low level. This increases the risk that these patients will become disoriented or slip into insulin shock and coma before they have time to eat something.

This blunting of the warning system intensifies the dangers of aggressive insulin therapy as hypoglycemic attacks become much more frequent and severe.

We do need to find out very soon if the benefits of the insulin pump or intensive insulin therapy outweighs its considerable risk. The National Institutes of Health has just started a long range study to determine if tight control of the blood sugar will alter the complication rate compared to patients that are receiving what is generally standard treatment with less tightly controlled blood sugar measurements. Those in the tight control group will be more closely monitored and many of them will be using the insulin pump.

The efforts on the part of the patients who are to be in the tight control group are considerable and represent a stumbling block to attracting volunteers for the study. Even though the patients will receive free insulin and medical care, patients are not rushing to the study. According to a recent report:

> The potential risks of tight control . . . aren't eliminating as many applicants as is the degree of compliance required. Participation requires agreeing to "almost an hour-to-hour effort on the part of patients" who are randomized to intensive therapy, noted Dr. John Malone, principal investigator for the trial at the University of South Florida in Tampa and co-director of the medical college's diabetes center. Tight control can mean severe dietary limitations, insulin injections at least three times daily, finger pricking at least four times daily (though some participants will be randomized to insulin pumps), and constant attention to exercise (*Medical World News*, "Tight Control Trial Needs More Diabetics," pg. 6, Feb. 23, 1987).

An interim report on 278 patients (146 are in the tight control group) already enrolled in the study showed that 95% of those seeking closer control had lower blood glucose readings and glycosylated hemoglobin measurements than those followed on conventional insulin therapy. However, the intensive control group had a threefold increase in severe hypoglycemia and a twofold increase in coma, though none suffered permanent damage that could be identified. It noted that two thirds of the hypoglycemic episodes occurred in 12 of the 146 patients in the intensive insulin therapy group, which may mean that certain patients may have an increased risk of hypoglycemia when intensive insulin therapy is used.

What continues to plague those of us who treat diabetic patients is that the complications of this disease have never been shown to be significantly reduced by improved control of the glucose either with insulin or with the oral drugs. For some reason, we insist on putting all our eggs in one basket, concentrating almost exclusively on the blood sugar level and trying continuously to improve upon the *delivery* of insulin.

What is lacking is significant appreciation of the role the insulin antagonists play in the development of the complications—the very thing many researchers like Himsworth, Somogyi, and others have been pointing out for years. Yet in the minds of so many researchers and physicians, the problem is only the lack of insulin. We have been whipping this horse for so long that it is tired and bleeding. Insulin can only do so much, but we continue to expect it single-handedly to lead us to the promised land.

The Insulin Pump: Is It Really an Improvement?

The last ten years have produced a new era in the administration of insulin. The development of small paper strips that give immediate, reliable estimates of the blood glucose level from a finger stick has made it possible to fine-tune insulin dosages in the home on a daily, even hourly basis.

It is now feasible for diabetic patients using fast-acting insulin to keep their blood sugar levels close to those of the nondiabetic population. In addition, continuous infusion pumps that the patient wears can deliver a small amount of insulin constantly, with the patient self-administering additional boluses of insulin before meals. In one sense, this capability would seem to solve all the problems experienced by diabetic patients. Does it? No.

The big advance is not the insulin pump but the techniques that permit measurement of the blood sugar level by the patient at home. With this capability, intensive insulin therapy can be instituted with dramatic reductions in the blood sugar level using *conventional* methods of insulin injections.

The continuous insulin pump does not seem to improve upon the blood sugar levels achieved with frequent injections. Donald R. Coustan, M.D., of Brown University in Providence, Rhode Island, divided a group of 22 pregnant diabetic patients at random, with 11 using the pump and 11 using conventional methods but with frequent injections ("A Randomized Clinical Trial of the Insulin Pump vs Intensive Conventional Therapy in Diabetic Pregnancies," *Journal of the American Medical Association* 255:631–636, 1986). He found no difference in blood sugar levels or other measurements of diabetic control. The keys to success are education and motivation.

The pump, on the other hand, has problems both because it is a mechanical device and because it is invasive—that is, installed in the body. One of the most frequent complications is infection at the infusion site. Another potential complication would be severe hypoglycemia, particularly at night, but then hypoglycemia is a danger with any intensive insulin therapy program.

In short, the insulin pump does not seem to have any significant advantages over regular insulin injections with close monitoring of the blood glucose level. But it certainly has a lot of disadvantages, both physical and psychological.

> Mrs. G.M. had been on the insulin pump about two years when she arrived at the Institute for treatment with our methods of more aggressive use of diet and exercise. She was not an insulin-dependent diabetic, but she was started on the pump because it was hoped that it would help prevent the complications down the line.
>
> Following our diet and exercise program, we were able to stop the pump and use only small doses of insulin to cover the occasional peak elevations of her blood sugar.
>
> She was happy to give up the pump, and it was clear that with the improved diet and exercise, it was not necessary. She then told me something that had not occurred to me.
>
> The pump was a constant reminder to her of her disease. She could never "get away" from her problem.

So often in medicine, we vigorously treat "the disease" and forget what the treatment does to the patient. The fact that the pump was, to Mrs. G.M., a constant and unpleasant reminder of her illness surely never entered the mind of the physician who prescribed the pump. It had never occurred to me until she had mentioned it, but I now consider it to be a strong argument against the use of the insulin pump.

The real question is whether a more aggressive use of insulin benefits the diabetic patient—particularly the type 2 diabetic—when compared with the less aggressive approach of diet, weight control, and exercise.

Insulin in the Non-Insulin Dependent Diabetic

It seems like a contradiction that insulin would be used in a "non-insulin dependent" diabetic, but it often is. The overwhelming majority of diabetic patients (around 90%) have non-insulin dependent, or type 2, diabetes.

As discussed earlier, type 2 diabetics may have blood sugars that can go quite high, up to 200 or even 300 mg/dL, but they are not prone to the condition called ketoacidosis, which leads to diabetic coma. This serious complication happens only in the insulin-dependent type 1 diabetic patient.

Also, this more benign form of diabetes is generally not related to a lack of insulin but to high-fat, low-carbohydrate nutrition, obesity, and lack of exercise that render the tissues insensitive to insulin produced by the pancreas. As pointed out in Chapters 2 and 3, insulin is often produced in this form of diabetes, but the body has become insensitive to it. What is needed for these patients is not insulin, but low-fat, high-carbohydrate diet, weight loss, and exercise—the essence of this book.

Though type 2 patients do have diabetes, their main problems are the complications of this condition. The most serious of these is accelerated atherosclerosis (plugging of the arteries with fat and cholesterol) that leads to heart attacks and poor circulation in the legs. The question then arises, Will the use of insulin reduce the complication rate in this form of diabetic patient?

In order to find out, a long-term, randomized, prospective study, The University Group Diabetes Program (UGDP), was funded by the National Institutes of Health. It was carried out in 12 diabetic centers across the country.

Begun in the years 1961 to 1965, this study was done to determine the effectiveness of the various agents that lower the blood sugar level in the non-insulin dependent diabetic. One part of the study, the effectiveness of the oral hypoglycemic agents to reduce the complication rate, is discussed in the following chapter. As you will see, this is the most controversial aspect of the study.

However, and equally important, part of the UGDP attempted to determine whether insulin, in dosages that would significantly lower the blood sugar in the non-insulin dependent diabetic, slows down the rate of complications *as it is believed to do.* To find out, 619 non-insulin dependent diabetics were put in one of three groups.

• *Group 1, insulin variable* (204 patients): In this group, the dosage of insulin used was altered to achieve blood sugar levels as near normal as possible.

• *Group 2, insulin fixed* (210 patients): In this group, a fixed dose of insulin was used calculated on the basis of body weight and height, and this dosage was not altered for the entire length of the study, even if the blood sugar went up.

• *Group 3, placebo* (205 patients): Only dietary restrictions were used.

All the patients were followed for a minimum of 9 years, and 460 of them (74%) were followed for 11 years or more.

We cannot overestimate the importance of this study, for it gives a long-term picture of what happens to type 2 diabetics when insulin is used to lower the blood sugar level. (Genell L. Knatterud, Ph.D., Christian R. Klimt, M.D., et al., "Effects of Hypoglycemic Agents on Vascular Complications in Patients with Adult-Onset Diabetes," *Journal of the American Medical Association* 240:37–42, 1978.)

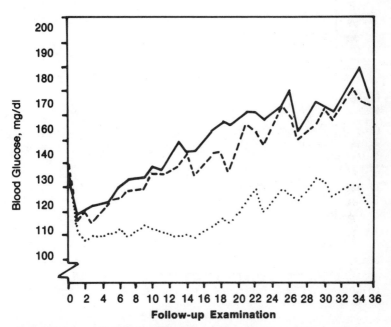

Figure 11 Average fasting blood glucose levels at the start of the experiment and at each follow-up examination from 1961 to 1974. *Solid line* represents placebo; *broken line,* insulin in a fixed dose; and *dotted line,* insulin in a variable dose. From "Effects of Hypoglycemic Agents on Vascular Complications in Patients with Adult-Onset Diabetes," *Journal of the American Medical Association* 240:38, July 7, 1978. Copyright © 1978, American Medical Association. Used by permission.

Insulin Definitely Lowered the Blood Sugar

Over the nine years of the study, the insulin-variable group (group 1) had a significant reduction in their blood sugar levels. Those in the insulin-fixed group (group 2) and the placebo group (group 3) had gradual increases in the blood sugar level with time (see Figure 11).

As Figure 11 shows, those taking insulin in a variable dose had very significant reductions in their blood sugar compared with those taking insulin in fixed dose or those taking no insulin at

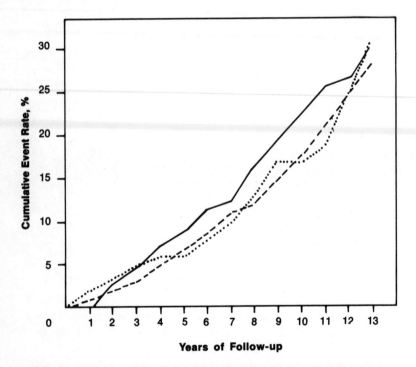

Figure 12 Cumulative death rate for all causes per 100 population by year of follow-up. *Solid line* represents placebo treatment; *broken line,* insulin fixed-dose group, and *dotted line,* insulin variable-dose group. From "Effects of Hypoglycemic Agents on Vascular Complications in Patients with Adult-Onset Diabetes," *Journal of the American Medical Association* 240:39, July 7, 1978. Copyright © 1978, American Medical Association. Used by permission.

all. Despite the marked difference in the blood sugar levels, however, *there were no significant differences between the three groups in either the death rate or the complication rate* (see Figure 12).

The researchers concluded:

> In contrast to the findings for glucose [those on the variable dose of insulin definitely had better glucose control], only small differences were observed in mortality. . . . As of Dec. 31, 1974, a total of 151 deaths had been reported: 54 deaths in the placebo treatment group, 48 in the insulin standard [fixed-dose] group, and 49 in the insulin variable-treatment group. Almost the same number of cardiovascular deaths was observed in each group.

There also were no differences in the nonfatal complications of diabetes in any of the three groups. Table 5 shows the percentage of those who developed complications in each group.

TABLE 5
Comparison of Complication Rates
in the Three UGDP Groups

	Placebo %	Insulin-fixed %	Insulin-variable %
Eye complications			
Reduction in visual acuity	11.2	11.7	11.4
Acute damage to the retina	9.2	10.6	11.6
Kidney examination			
Presence of protein in the urine	4.2	2.1	5.8
Serum creatinine $\geq$ 1.5 mg/dL	16.2	8.3	9.1
Blood vessel complications			
Calcification in the leg arteries	29.6	28.8	28.4
Development of painful walking "claudication"	17.6	19.4	16.0
Amputation	1.5	0.5	1.6

Except for slight differences in the development of elevated creatinine levels in the placebo group, indicating the possibility of very slightly increased kidney damage, the researchers found no significant area where insulin in either a fixed dose (loose control) or a variable dose (tighter control) had any beneficial result on the non-insulin dependent diabetic when compared to placebo. Bear in mind that this form of diabetes accounts for *90 percent* of the diabetic population. The researchers concluded:

> Thus, over the time period studied with an average follow-up of 12 years, insulin used in a fixed dosage or used in a variable dosage to normalize glucose levels was no better than diet alone in prolonging life or in preventing the vascular complications considered in this report in the adult-onset, non-ketosis-prone diabetic.
>
> The UGDP findings provide no evidence that insulin or any other drug lowering blood glucose levels will alter the course of vascular complications in the type of diabetes that is most common, adult-onset diabetes. Weight reduction has been shown to be feasible and effective in lowering blood glucose, thus dietary management deserves greater emphasis in this type of diabetes than it has received to date, as others have suggested. In any case, the UGDP results suggest that the use of any other additional therapeutic agent must be justified on grounds other than the prevention of macrovascular complications.

Sometimes it is very difficult for physicians to accept and act upon scientific studies that contradict commonly held beliefs. In 1986, most non-insulin dependent diabetics are still treated aggressively with the oral drugs (discussed in the next chapter) or with insulin. This is done in the belief that the complications of the condition will be lessened if the blood sugar levels are lowered by the oral medications or insulin. The dangers of these two agents are usually ignored or are considered "necessary evils." The patient, out of fear of his or her "disease" and its complications, willingly accepts the risk of the therapies. This behavior contradicts the results of major scientific studies.

It makes one wonder why studies are done in the first place.

8

The Oral Drugs

In 1978, Rebecca Warmer, Sydney Wolf, M.D., and Rebecca Rich, working for the Public Citizens' Health Group of Washington, D.C., published a 121-page book provocatively titled *Off Diabetes Pills, A Diabetic's Guide to Longer Life.* The book began:

. Are you taking tolbutamide (Orinase), tolazamide (Tolinase), chlorpropamide (Diabinese), or acetohexamide (Dymelor)? These pills could cost you your life. This booklet is written for you, to explain why you must do three things:

Warning: Antidiabetic Pills Are Dangerous to Your Health
Stop taking antidiabetic pills as soon as you can;
Go on a diet and lose weight;
Stop seeing your present doctor unless he or she genuinely tries to help you lose weight and agrees to switch you to insulin if you still have diabetic symptoms at or below your ideal body weight.

These steps could mean the difference between life and death.

The book was published as a public service and is available from the group in Washington, D.C., or from us here at the Whitaker Wellness Institute.*

*The Whitaker Wellness Institute, 4400 MacArthur Blvd., Suite 630, Newport Beach, CA 92660 (714) 851-1550

As you might imagine, the book stimulated considerable controversy, but no more than the issue of the pills themselves and their role in the treatment of non-insulin dependent (type 2) diabetics.

The Pills

The oral hypoglycemic pills were developed in the 1950s and were shown to lower the blood sugar level in diabetic patients. However, their effectiveness is limited to only a small percentage of the patients who are currently taking the drugs. They act by stimulating the pancreas to increase its secretion of insulin. To a lesser extent, they seem to enhance the peripheral sensitivity to insulin.

Since the overwhelming majority of diabetics do not need insulin, these drugs were rapidly embraced, worldwide, before any studies were done to see whether they would reduce the long-term complications of diabetes.

It was "assumed" that any drug that lowered the blood sugar level would reduce the complication rate, particularly the worst complication of diabetes, which is heart disease. The incidence of heart attacks and death from heart disease among diabetics is about twice that of nondiabetics.

Acceptance of the Drugs Before Proof of Benefit

It is not difficult to understand why these drugs were so rapidly accepted before any long-term studies had been done to prove their efficacy.

First, the requirement of insulin injections is never a joyful experience for either physician or patient. A pill that could be used instead of a needle to lower blood sugar would be eagerly welcomed.

Second, the pills represented something for the non-insulin dependent patient that would replace the need for diet treatment. It became the "answer," the magic bullet, that relieved the responsibility of both doctor and patient to alter diet or exercise patterns.

Third, the rapid and widespread acceptance of the oral drugs reflects the tunnel vision of many physicians who assume that all diabetic complications will be eliminated if the blood sugar level can be reduced by any means, regardless of other effects the drug has on the body.

A Landmark Study

The University Group Diabetes Program (UGDP) set out to determine the benefit of these drugs. The study was funded with 14 separate grants from the Public Health Service of the U.S. government. Its purpose was clear from the onset: It was to determine whether control of the blood sugar with either the oral drugs or insulin in the adult-onset, type 2, non-insulin dependent diabetic reduced the incidence of heart disease or other major vascular complications associated with diabetes. (We discussed the results of the study with insulin in the previous chapter.)

In 1961, 1027 type 2 diabetic patients were enrolled in the study and were followed in 12 clinics in the United States and Puerto Rico. Each patient was put on the diabetic diet, which at the time was about 35 to 40 percent fat calories, and was randomly assigned to one of the five treatment groups:

• *Group 1: Placebo.* Each patient took a pill that looked like either Orinase (the generic name for this drug is tolbutamide) or DBI (generic name, phenformin).

• *Group 2: Orinase.* This is a sulfonylurea drug. The trade names of similar drugs include Diabinese, Dymelor, and Tolinase. The newer and more powerful drugs are called DiaBeta and Glucotrol (glyburide) or Micronase (glipizide). Since they all have similar actions, the studies on Orinase implicate all of them as dangerous agents, and they all carry a strongly worded, mandatory warning about their dangers.

• *Group 3: DBI.* This is another form of oral hypoglycemic drug that has since been taken off the market.

• *Group 4: Insulin in a fixed dose.* This means that a single dosage of insulin was calculated on the basis of body size and then given unchanged for the duration of the study.

• *Group 5: Insulin in a variable dose.* This means that the dosage of insulin was varied in order to obtain and maintain as near normal blood sugar as possible.

Except for those on insulin, neither the patient nor the physician were aware of who was taking what.

The test on Orinase was intended to run until 1971, but the researchers stopped it in 1969 because the rate of death from heart disease was so high that they considered it unethical to continue the study further. Over the eight-year period of the study there were *250% more deaths* from heart disease in the group taking Orinase than in the placebo group.

The group taking phenformin fared even worse. The death rates for all causes of death were 62 percent higher than in the placebo group, and the deaths from cardiovascular disease were increased by 300 percent.

Statistical analysis showed that these differences could not have occurred just by chance. Therefore, unless there is some other explanation, the increased death rate had to be related to the drugs themselves, Orinase and DBI.

Very careful analysis of all other factors was carried out to see if something had been overlooked in assigning the patients to the various groups, yet nothing could be found that would explain why those taking the drug had a *higher* death rate from heart disease than those on placebo. The UGDP published the results and summarized their findings:

All UGDP investigators are agreed that the findings of this study indicate that the combination of diet and tolbutamide (Orinase) therapy is no more effective than diet alone or than diet and insulin in prolonging life. Moreover, the findings suggest that tolbutamide and diet may be less effective than diet alone or than diet and insulin at least insofar as cardiovascular mortality is concerned. For this reason, use of tolbutamide has been discontinued in the UGDP. Patients originally assigned to the tolbutamide treatment group . . . are no longer being treated with tolbutamide. ("University Group Diabetes

Program: A Study of the Effects of Hypoglycemic Agents on Vascular Complications in Patients with Adult-Onset Diabetes. 11. Mortality Results." *Diabetes* 19 [Suppl]: 814, 1970.)

In an additional publication the researchers further stated:

Until it is possible to find a cause or combination of causes or to discern a subgroup predisposed to this risk, this drug (Orinase) must be considered hazardous for long-term use. (UGDP, *Journal of the American Medicial Association 218:* 1400–1410, 1971.)

Then the rebuttals started. What seemed clear suddenly became muddy. It is not difficult to understand why: Drug interests and physician assumptions and pride are often major obstacles to accepting scientific reality if that reality runs counter to vested interests or strongly held assumptions and beliefs.

The Drug Interests

When the UGDP results became public, tens of millions of dollars were being spent on the oral diabetic medications. If primary care physicians across the country were immediately to stop prescribing the oral drugs and intensify efforts of diet and exercise instead, the drug companies sharing in the revenues generated by the oral diabetic drugs would be severely crippled. It is not surprising that the drug companies went to work immediately to cast as much doubt as they could on the conclusions of the UGDP study. They were unbelievably successful. Physicians have never stopped using the drugs. Even today, 15 years later, they are still prescribing these drugs that might be associated with several thousand unnecessary deaths a year in the diabetic population.

Today, most physicians honestly believe that the UGDP results were inaccurate. No fault in the design or conduct of the study can be found to support these beliefs. It is not unreasonable to credit them to the campaign waged against the study by the drug companies and by physicians who simply *would not* accept the results.

The Attack

Physician attitudes and beliefs are strongly influenced by the drug companies, more so than most physicians care to admit. One powerful tool of influence used by drug interests are journals called "throwaways" or "medical tabloids" that are sent to every physician without charge.

For instance, I receive, without charge, about 15 to 20 weekly medical journals or newspapers. They contain little if any original scientific material. Instead they serve almost exclusively as a vehicle for opinions of some of the experts in the field. The drug companies advertise heavily in these publications. More important, they exert considerable influence on what is written.

Dr. Roger Palmer, former head of the Department of Pharmacology at the University of Miami School of Medicine, points out that many prominent physicians become unwitting spokesmen for drug interests. They are approached by the editor of a "throwaway" and asked to write, for a fee, about a drug that they favor.

This opinion is then published alongside numerous advertisements for the drug. Since most physicians are just too busy to read the original research, their opinions are often shaped by this obviously biased material. They are left with the assumption that a specific drug is the only reasonable treatment for a given condition. This is great for the drug interests, but not so good for patients who might possibly do just as well or even better without the drug that was discussed.

The results of the UGDP study caught everybody by surprise! The drugs already enjoyed universal acceptance and widespread use. Immediately following the publication of the UGDP results, and before the implications of these results had been discussed in legitimate scientific literature, the drug interests utilized their throwaways to discredit the study and challenge the validity of the results. Since the drugs were already trusted, it was not difficult to discredit a study that would shatter that trust.

By calling on physicians who were deeply critical of the study and publishing only their opinions, even when their appraisals were grossly inaccurate, these publications created the belief that the design of the study was so flawed the results could not be accepted.

Dr. Thaddeus Prout, Associate Professor of Medicine at Johns Hopkins School of Medicine, Baltimore, Maryland, one of the primary researchers and spokesman for the UGDP, said in a phone interview that the drug companies "got there first." Using their sophisticated avenues of communication with the medical community, they biased the nation's physicians against the results of the study before the researchers had time to clarify the importance of their findings.

Physician Pride

A second reason for the resistance to the UGDP findings and the conclusions was that physicians had been using the drugs with confidence for years. In the university centers where young physicians are trained in the treatment of diabetic patients, the oral drugs were an integral part of treatment protocols. The results of the UGDP called upon the heads of these respected departments to seriously rethink the role that the drugs had been given for so long at their medical centers. Most of them just could not do this. It was too uncomfortable. The drugs were just too popular and the original assumptions about their benefit had turned into belief.

In private practice, where most diabetics are treated by their own physicians, the drugs were even more popular. They could be given to the diabetic patient with the feeling that something positive was being done. The drugs are easy to take, while the alternative—vigorous diet changes with or without insulin—requires work.

The study and its conclusions just had to go, and in the minds of most physicians, that is exactly what has happened.

Just How Dangerous Are the Drugs?

The results of the UGDP study showed that the oral hypoglycemic agents increase the death rate from heart disease of diabetics by 1 percent per year. This means that each year one additional death would be expected in a group of 100 diabetics taking the oral drugs compared with a group of 100 treated with diet alone. Over a ten-year period one could expect about 10 more deaths to occur in the 100 patients taking the pill compared to those treated with diet alone.

This is both a small and enormous number—at the same time.

A 1 Percent Annual Increase in Death Is Small

An increase of 1 percent annually is too small for any physician or clinic to pick out as a part of their clinical experience or expertise. After all, *some* diabetic patients in a physician's practice are likely to die of heart disease in any given year—especially if the doctor's practice includes many diabetic patients. One additional death is unlikely to make the physician suspect that something is wrong. It is still less likely to make him or her think that the prescribed therapy is related to that death.

Physicians characteristically feel certain that they are providing the best for their patients' well-being. Ironically, if a diabetic patient dies while taking oral drugs, the death may even stimulate the physician to increase the use of the drugs with other patients. The physician's thinking would be that deaths are occurring because the blood sugar is not controlled rigidly enough, hence more drugs would be warranted.

It is virtually impossible for even the most expert of physicians to "see" the toxicity of a popular remedy without the benefit of a long-term controlled study designed to uncover that toxicity objectively. Therefore, relying on "personal expertise and clinical experience" alone is foolish and extremely dangerous.

However, that is exactly what many of the critics of the UGDP did. Dr. Joseph Goodman, in a letter to the *Cleveland Plain Dealer,* stated:

> Oral antidiabetic drugs have been extensively used by the medical profession for approximately 20 years. Doctors have considered these drugs to be effective in the treatment of diabetic patients without any fear of harmful effects and with

few or no side effects. . . . The UGDP report of a higher rate
of cardiovascular disease in persons taking antidiabetic drugs is
purely statistical in a small segment of patients as opposed to
the greater and longer experience of the medical profession at
large (February 18, 1975).

Dr. Goodman's assessment is confusing—even irrational. To
state that the findings of an eight-year study were "purely
statistical" doesn't make any sense. We physicians would like to
have the opportunity to use pure statistics, not unscientific
"personal experience," to guide our judgment whenever a drug is
used for treatment of any condition.

Second, that "small segment" of patients was carefully se-
lected and randomized to accurately represent the greater number of patients that were being treated and would be treated by
doctors who believed the drugs to be safe and beneficial. As a
representative of the very large number of diabetic patients, that
small segment demonstrated that in the large population of
diabetics, the loss of thousands of lives each year may be directly
related to use of oral antidiabetic medication.

A 1 Percent Increase in Death Is Enormous

If 3,000,000 diabetic patients suffer an increase in death rate of 1
additional death per 100 patients because of the drug, that equals
30,000 additional deaths per year, 300,000 more deaths in 10
years! This magnitude of increased death can be established only
by a study the size and length of the UGDP in which a therapy is
compared to a placebo and both groups are followed long enough
to establish a difference in outcome. It could never be recognized
by anyone without the aid of comparing the drug to a placebo
control group.

This situation is what makes medicine so dangerous.
Throughout history, physicans have rendered considerable harm
to patients with remedies that both physician and patient believed
to be safe and effective.

Countering Dr. Goodman's assessment of the UGDP, Dr. J.R.
Carter and four other diabetic specialists wrote:

For every 100 middle-aged patients treated with tolbutamide, there would be per year about 2 deaths from cardiovascular disease as compared to about one death in 100 patients treated with insulin or diet alone. We find it impossible to believe a physician in the midst of a busy practice would be aware of one extra death per year in 100 patients whom he never originally isolated in his mind or in his records for study. (*Cleveland Plain Dealer,* April 10, 1975.)

How Do the Drugs Harm the Heart?

An explanation of the increased death rate from heart disease associated with the oral drugs was discovered and reported by Dr. Gerald Levey and Dr. Roger Palmer, Chairman of the Department of Pharmacology at the University of Miami School of Medicine. Dr. Palmer found that tolbutamide (Orinase) increases the level of the enzyme adenyl cyclase in the heart muscle fibers. This enzyme increases the oxygen demand of the heart muscle, increasing the work of the heart and thereby putting more strain on it. In addition, this increased activity in the heart brought on by the high adenyl cyclase level may also increase the tendency toward irregular heart rhythms, a particularly dangerous side effect in people who have any degree of heart disease. Dr. Palmer and his colleagues concluded:

Therefore, any positive inotropic effects [stimulating to the heart] of tolbutamide might increase myocardial work and oxygen consumption and increase the extent of myocardial injury in human beings. These findings could explain the increased incidence of cardiovascular death reported in the University Group Diabetes Program study. Increasing oxygen demand would be particularly disadvantageous in diabetics, a patient population known to have an increased incidence of coronary artery disease. . . . It would [also] be expected that in addition to the demonstrated inotropic effect, a chronotropic or arrhythmogenic effect of tolbutamide could also be produced which might increase the incidence of cardiac arrythmias.

(Gerald S. Levey, M.D., and Roger F. Palmer, M.D., "Effect of Tolbutamide on Adenyl Cyclase in Rabbit and Human Heart and Contractility of Isolated Rabbit Atria," *Journal of Clinical Endocrinology, 33*: 317–334, 1971.)

In addition, the oral hypoglycemics seem to lower the HDL fraction of cholesterol in the blood. This fraction of cholesterol is the "good" cholesterol, meaning that when this fraction is elevated, the risk of heart attack is lessened. When it is lowered, the risk of heart attack is increased.

Dr. G.D. Calvert at the Flinders Medical Centre in Bedford Park, South Australia, found that diabetics on the oral drugs had significantly lower HDL levels than diabetics treated with insulin or diet alone (*Medical World News,* January 8, 1979, p. 56).

Stimulated by the adverse findings of the UGDP, researchers from around the world went back and reviewed some of their records:

Dr. D.R. Hadden reviewed the records of 670 female adult-onset (type 2) diabetics treated in a diabetic clinic in Belfast, Northern Ireland, from 1958 until 1970. Those taking the oral drugs had twice as many heart attacks as diabetics treated by diet alone (*Lancet 1*: 335–338, 1972).

There is some evidence that the death rate of maturity-onset diabetics has increased and that life expectancy has decreased since the institution of the oral agents. This decline in life expectancy has been reported in England and Wales, Japan, Germany, and Israel (Rebecca Warner, Sydney Wolf, M.D., and Rebecca Rich, *Off Diabetes Pills*, Public Citizens' Health Research Group, 1978). Dr. I. Kessler from Johns Hopkins University observed an increase in mortality rate in diabetics diagnosed at the Joslin Clinic, a well-known center for diabetes treatment. From 1950 until the late 1960s there was a 110 percent increase in the death rate in men and an 88 percent increase in the death rate for woman diabetics compared to the general population of the same age and sex (Presented at the 9th Annual Meeting of the Society for Epidemiological Research, Toronto, Canada, June 16–18, 1976).

Other Dangerous Side Effects

Besides being associated with an increased rate of death from heart disease, these drugs are loaded with other side effects. In some patients they cause significant hypoglycemia that can become prolonged and is particularly dangerous in the elderly. That the drugs will have this effect in some and not in others probably reflects differences in rates of excretion of the drug.

Also, other drugs that are commonly used to treat high blood pressure, heart disease, and infections will at times enhance the action of the diabetic drugs, making them more likely to cause severe hypoglycemia. Hypoglycemic reactions can cause irreversible brain damage and can even be fatal.

What makes this complication particularly dangerous is the lack of physician awareness that it can occur. All physicians are aware of the hypoglycemic reactions that occur with insulin, but the oral drugs are not perceived as powerful enough to have this side effect. Often, when the elderly suffer from this drug-induced hypoglycemia, they are thought to have suffered a stroke or to be senile.

One of the most commonly used drugs in this country, chlorpropamide (Diabinese) is more likely to cause hypoglycemic reactions because it stays in the blood much longer than tolbutamide (Orinase). Also, the newer agents, which are called the "second generation" drugs, are much more powerful and therefore more likely to have hypoglycemia as a serious side effect.

Like all prescription drugs, the oral hypoglycemic agents have a long list of side effects that have occurred to some patients. They have been known to cause hypothyroidism, skin rashes, severe allergic reactions, opacities in the cornea of the eye, water retention, elevated blood pressure, and increased stomach acid secretion.

However, the most damning evidence against them remains the significantly increased death rate from heart disease. Yet this observation has yet to be appreciated by most physicians despite evidence that the drugs may be causing mayhem on a worldwide scale. Dr. John K. Davidson, Professor of Medicine, Emory University School of Medicine, and head of the Diabetic Unit at Grady Hospital, Atlanta, Georgia, wrote in 1975:

There has been a striking increase in death rate and decrease in life expectancy in maturity-onset diabetics in America, Europe, Asia, Africa, and Australia during the last 20 years. These changes have paralleled the increasingly widespread neglect of diet therapy and the almost unbridled enthusiasm among many physicians and patients for the use of sulfonylureas and phenformin as treatments of choice.

If a drug is to be considered "safe," it should not shorten life expectancy nor be associated with fatal side effects or with severe drug reactions. The increased number of cardiovascular deaths in the UGDP study, the not uncommon occurrences of irreversible hypoglycemic brain damage and death with sulfonylureas and fatal lactic acidosis with phenformin, and the previously noted decreased life expectancy of the maturity-onset diabetic population throughout the world are the dramatic consequences of unrestricted use of oral hypoglycemic drugs. ("The FDA and Hypoglycemic Drugs," *Journal of the American Medical Association 232*: 854, 1975.)

Despite the overwhelming evidence to the contrary these drugs are still considered to be safe and are used extensively in this country and abroad. Why?

What Was Wrong With the UGDP Study? Why Are the Results Still Ignored?

The UGDP simply exploded into everyone's face. Everyone—the researchers, the drug companies, and the nation's physicians—fully expected the study to show that the drugs *reduced* deaths from heart disease. Only those who trusted the scientific method and were able to put numerical realities above empirical beliefs could adjust accordingly.

The physicians who registered the harshest criticisms about the study did so from an extremely biased position. Since they could not or would not believe the results, they reasoned that something had to be wrong with the study! As pointed out, it was these critics who, with the aid of the drug companies, received the widest exposure in the ensuing controversy.

Most of the critics felt that the excess cardiovascular deaths found in those taking Orinase occurred because the study was not truly randomized; that those taking Orinase had more heart disease at the beginning of the study and would be expected to have more heart attacks anyway.

This implies that the drug group had "bad luck at the draw." Stanley Schor, M.D., of the Department of Biometrics, Temple University Medical School in Philadelphia, summarized these and other criticisms in the *Journal of the American Medical Association* ("The University Group Diabetes Program, A Statistician Looks at the Mortality Results," *JAMA 217*: 1671–75, 1971). In the same edition of the *Journal* (pages 1676–1687), Jerome Cornfield of the Department of Biostatistics, Graduate School of Public Health, University of Pittsburgh, answered the criticisms leveled by Dr. Schor and, using the factual data of the study, discounted, for the most part, each one.

For instance, Dr. Schor pointed out that it was not known what percentage of each group were smokers. If the group taking the tolbutamide contained more smokers than the placebo group, they would have more heart deaths as a result. Since it was not known what percentage of each group were smokers, the results were therefore questionable.

However, the purpose of randomization, as Dr. Cornfield stated, is to distribute *all factors* both known and unknown equally into the various groups. In the case of the smokers verses non smokers, there would be only 1 chance in 50,000 that a significantly higher percentage of smokers would, by chance, wind up in the group taking the drug. Even if this did occur, it would result in only a 16 percent increase in cardiovascular deaths!

Dr. Schor felt uneasy with the fact that some of the patients did not take the drugs as they were supposed to or were transferred out of that group because of side effects. He suggested that this could alter the results. This happens in every study of this kind, but Dr. Schor criticized the investigators and questioned the results: "The investigators stated that the transfer problem took place in too few patients to have an effect on the mortality. This is simply not true. There seem to be many more transfers than there are deaths."

However, Dr. Cornfield pointed out, the investigators *did* record the results for the patients that adhered strictly to the drug regimen. It was found that those who took the Orinase exactly as they were supposed to had an even *higher* death rate. At five years, those who adhered to the Orinase regimen strictly had a 400 percent increase in death rate compared to the recorded 250 percent increase of the group as a whole. At 8 years the strict adherers had a 600 percent increase in death. On this issue, Dr. Cornfield concluded: "The analysis suggested by Dr. Schor, difficult to interpret though it is, does nothing to weaken the UGDP finding and in fact tends to strengthen it."

Dr. Schor thought it was "deplorable" that the researchers stopped the study when it became obvious that Orinase was causing a large increase in heart deaths. He felt that if the study had been continued and the increased death rate continued, no one would have argued with the results.

However, the study was not done to see whether Orinase killed people, it was done to determine whether it helped them! At the time the study was stopped there was *no possibility* that Orinase would turn out to be beneficial. As Dr. Cornfield justifiably asked, why would anyone want to sacrifice more lives just to see how deadly the drug was?

In looking at these two summary critics appearing side by side in the same journal, it is striking that Dr. Schor rarely referred to the published data in an effort to substantiate his criticisms in a factual manner. On the other hand, Dr. Cornfield extensively drew on the published material to rebut Dr. Schor's criticisms, citing page numbers and tabular information. In several instances, it appeared as if Dr. Schor's reading of the data was sketchy, if not inaccurate. Dr. Cornfield concluded that:

> none of the possible errors suggested so far do in fact account for the UGDP findings. Although further investigation, particularly if undertaken in a nonadversary framework, may still be useful, it seems likely that a point of diminishing returns may not be far off, and that continued analysis of the UGDP, in the hope of finding errors which alter the conclusions, will become increasingly unrewarding.

An Independent Review

Both of these summaries appeared in 1971, yet the controversy was just heating up, and the use of the oral drugs for the treatment of diabetes actually increased! The controversy was fierce; the study was attacked from every angle.

As a result, Dr. Robert Marston, then director of the National Institutes of Health, contracted an independent committee from the Biometric Society, an international group of experts, to evaluate all the data generated by the study. In Feburary of 1975 they reported:

> On the question of cardiovascular mortality due to tolbutamide and phenformin, we consider that the UGDP trial has raised suspicions that cannot be dismissed on the basis of other evidence presently available. . . . [We] consider that in the light of the UGDP findings, it remains with the proponents of the oral hypoglycemics to conduct scientifically adequate studies to justify the continued use of such agents. ("Report of the Committee for Assessment of Biometric Aspects of Controlled Trials of the Hypoglycemic Agents," *Journal of the American Medical Association 231:* 583–608, 1975.)

In an editorial published along with this report, Thomas C. Chalmers, M.D., of Mount Sinai Medical Center in New York stated:

> The probability that oral hypoglycemic agents cause premature deaths from cardiovascular disease remains valid.
>
> There are even more important questions to be asked as a result of the controversy over the UGDP study than how a particular diabetic patient should be managed. Assuming that the hypoglycemic drugs are actually dangerous, why have their sales continued to expand steadily in the past 15 years, with only a slight dip for one year after the UGDP report?
>
> One explanation is the strong desire of both physicians and patients for a way to treat diabetes that does not involve injections, and this has resulted in a natural reluctance to accept any possibility that the drugs might be harmful. This has

been fostered by one-sided presentations of the controversy by one or more of the so-called throw-away medical journals so widely read by physicians. . . .

Undoubtedly, the situation will improve now that not only has the UGDP study been found to be valid by the Biometric Society group, but also there has been parallel confirmation in well-done retrospective studies, analyses of deaths in coronary care units, disturbing increases in worldwide death rates among older diabetics, and a pharmacologic explanation for the potential lethality of cardiovascular events.

DBI Is Banned in the United States

A year after the publication of the results on Orinase the results on DBI were published. They were worse. They were associated with a 300 percent increase in heart-related deaths, were found to increase the blood pressure, probably contributing to the heart death increase, and had the unique characteristic of causing lactic acid to increase to fatal levels in the blood in some diabetics.

DBI is quite different from Orinase with a different mode of action. We still do not know how the drug lowers the blood sugar, but the toxicity of this agent uncovered by the UGDP was not challenged nearly as vehemently as that of Orinase. It was as if the shock and bitterness of the Orinase controversy were all the empiricists (those refusing to have their opinions altered by controlled trials) could handle at the time. In addition, the FDA began to move more rapidly because the tendency of the drug to cause fatal lactic acidosis was difficult to argue. They moved to ban the drug.

At this juncture, a group of doctors, with the support of the drug companies, formed the Committee for the Care of Diabetics with the purpose of blocking the FDA's intention of taking DBI off the market and the intention of putting warning labels on Orinase and other similar diabetic drugs. With DBI, they failed.

In 1977, in an unprecedented move, the FDA removed DBI from the market on the grounds that it was deemed "an imminent hazard." At that time, 336,000 diabetics were taking the drug.

Strong Labels Finally Appear

In March of 1984, the FDA finally succeeded in its attempts to put strong warning labels on all oral hypoglycemic drugs. The warning for the drug Diabinese reads:

Warnings: SPECIAL WARNING ON INCREASED RISK OF CARDIOVASCULAR MORTALITY

The administration of oral hypoglycemic drugs has been reported to be associated with increased cardiovascular mortality as compared to treatment with diet alone or diet plus insulin. This warning is based on the study conducted by the University Group Diabetes Program (UGDP), a long-term prospective clinical trial designed to evaluate the effectiveness of glucose-lowering drugs in preventing or delaying vascular complications in patients with non-insulin-dependent diabetes. The study involved 823 patients who were randomly assigned to one of four treatment groups (*Diabetes, 19* [supp. 2]: 747–830, 1970).

UGDP reported that patients treated for 5 to 8 years with diet plus a fixed dose of Orinase (1.5 grams per day) had a rate of cardiovascular mortality approximately 2½ times that of patients treated with diet alone. A significant increase in total mortality was not observed, but the use of Orinase was discontinued based on the increase in cardiovascular mortality, thus limiting the opportunity for the study to show an increase in over-all mortality. Despite controversy regarding the interpretation of these results, the findings of the UGDP study provide an adequate basis for this warning. The patient should be informed of the potential risks and advantages of DIABINESE and of alternative modes of therapy.

Although only one drug in the sulfonylurea class (Orinase) was included in this study, it is prudent from a safety standpoint to consider that this warning may also apply to other oral hypoglycemic drugs in this class, in view of their close similarities in mode of action and chemical structure.

For emphasis, the text of this warning is set in bold face type. As stated, the basis for the labeling was the UGDP studies, and plans for the labeling were made soon after the results were published. However, the Committee for the Care of Diabetics was successful in delaying this action by the FDA for almost 13 years!

At present, many physicians feel comfortable prescribing these drugs which are clearly labeled as being associated with an increased risk of death from cardiovascular disease, even though that is the very fate that both patient and physician fear most.

If ever there is an example of empiricism winning over science in the practice of medicine it is the continued use of the oral hypoglycemic.

The Diet Alternative

Leading the charge for discontinuing use of the oral drugs has been John K. Davidson, M.D., Professor of Medicine and Head of the Diabetes Unit at Grady Hospital, Emory University Medical School, in Atlanta. Following the publication of the UGDP studies and his careful reading of them, he took 1500 diabetic patients off the oral medication and put greater emphasis on diet and weight control. Eighteen months later, he found that 60 percent of those patients experienced no increase in the blood sugar levels when the drugs were stopped and diet therapy alone was used. In addition, he suspended the use of insulin in all patients who were above ideal body weight using diet and weight control only (*International Diabetic Foundation Bulletin, 20* (19): 99–108).

It should be pointed out that this discussion of the oral drugs is based primarily on the UGDP studies and the direct aftermath and discussion of those studies, findings, and conclusions. Though there has been no other long-term controlled study of these agents, and though the FDA is quite explicit in the wording of the warning concerning these agents, there are many physicians who do use them in certain varieties of non-insulin dependent diabetes along with a diet and exercise program. However, most do agree that these agents should never be used in the place of an appropriate diet and exercise regimen.

The New Generation Oral Drugs

The first generation sulfonylurea drugs include Orinase, Diabinese, Tolinase, and Dymelor. These drugs are very similar to Orinase and thus are incriminated by association with the negative findings of Orinase.

In addition, there are several new generation sulfonylurea drugs that became available in the late seventies and early eighties long after the UGDP studies were complete. These drugs are similar to the older generation drugs, but may have less of the negative side effects. These drugs are glyburide which is marketed by the name of DiaBeta, or Micronase, and glipizide, marketed by the name Glucotrol.

These drugs have the same mechanism of action as the older drugs and therefore should be suspect of also causing an increase in heart attack rates. Indeed they carry the same warning label about the potential increased risk of heart attack that is required of Orinase and Diabinese. However, they have not been studied in the long-term controlled manner that was afforded Orinase, and some shorter term studies indicate that with respect to increased heart attack rate, they may be safer than the older drugs if used in patients who have already obtained optimal weight, and are following a good diet and exercise program.

Micronase and diaBeta (glyburide), like Diabinese, has a long duration of action and thus has an increased potential of creating severe and prolonged hypoglycemic reactions. This is particularly important if the drug is used in the elderly, as the symptoms of hypoglycemia could be thought to be senility, or a stroke. For this reason, this drug is particularly dangerous for patients over 65.

Many of the known complications of the standard drugs Orinase and Diabinese do not seem to be a problem with these newer drugs. For instance the older drugs, Diabinese and Orinase, have the tendency to elevate the uric acid level and to lower the sodium level in the blood. This does not seem to be a problem with the newer drugs.

The current use of any of the oral drugs represents to some extent laziness and lack of understanding of the problem at hand with most of the non-insulin dependent diabetics. If used correctly in patients who are on the appropriate diet and exercise program and are approaching optimal weight, some of the new generation drugs have a specific and beneficial place. As succinctly put by Dr. Michael Berger, M.S., Professor of Medicine, Department of Medicine, Dusseldorf University, Dusseldorf, West Germany:

> Unfortunately the use of sulfonylurea drugs has become entrenched as the "treatment of laziness," both on the part of the physician and the patient. How much easier it is to prescribe or swallow a pill than to explain or observe a weight-reducing diet in combination with increase in caloric expenditure [exercise]. The central problem of the syndrome for which Sims had coined the term "diabesity" (representing more than 90% of the patients with NIDDM in the industrialized world) is insulin resistant due to hyperinsulinemia [excessive insulin secretion by the pancreas] associated with obesity/hyperphagia [overeating] and immobilization. Any rational attempt to treat this disorder should be based upon attempts to decrease, rather than increase, insulinemia in order to improve sensitivity to endogenous insulin. Thus, hypocaloric dieting and increased physical activity must remain the basis for therapy for overweight patients with non-insulin dependent diabetes mellitus. Only if patients are still hyperglycemic despite significant weight loss of several weeks or if they are already of normal weight and reasonably physically active, is the use of sulfonylurea drugs justified, and in a high percentage of patients, will prove successful. ("Oral Agents in the Treatment of Diabetes Mellitus," found in *Clinical Diabetes Mellitus, A Problem Oriented Approach*, edited by John K. Davidson, M.D., Ph.D., Thieme Inc., New York, 1986, page 268.)

9

Additional Drugs in the Diabetic Patient

Unfortunately, diabetics have long been known to have higher than average rates of high blood pressure (hypertension) and arteriosclerosis (cholesterol deposits to the arteries). These conditions lead to high rates of heart attack and amputation. These additional problems respond to the same diet and exercise program used here at the Institute for better diabetes control.

In many patients with these conditions, the drugs used to treat these associated problems may worsen the diabetic condition. They may also subject the diabetic patient to the complications related to the drug itself. Needless to say, drugs for blood pressure control are beneficial when all the nondrug methods have been exhausted. However, when drugs are used before any attempt is made to use diet and exercise, they often do more harm than good.

The MRFIT Study

The National Institutes of Health funded a large study to determine whether aggressive treatment of hypertension and the other risk factors of heart disease would reduce the death rate from heart attack. This project, known as the MRFIT study, involved 250 researchers from 28 institutions at a cost of $115 million.

Twelve thousand male subjects were recruited—a huge sample. Half were give Special Intervention (SI) meaning that all the risk factors of heart disease were aggressively approached. Those who smoked were told to stop or cut down. Those who had high cholesterol levels were told to reduce their fat intake from 40 percent of their calories to 35 percent. This was a step in the right direction, but a little half-hearted. A better goal would have been reduction of fat intake to 25 percent of the caloric intake. Those with high blood pressure received more aggressive treatment to lower the blood pressure.

The other half received Usual Care (U.C.), meaning that they were treated at their doctors' discretion.

The final analysis was like a bomb explosion! Those who received the Special Intervention were no better off overall, and for some, the death rate was increased by the more aggressive therapy.

Those in the SI group who had high blood pressure and abnormalities on their electrocardiograms and were given diuretics fared worse! In this group there was a 65 percent increased death. Further research suggests that this increase may have been related to the thiazide diuretics used to lower the blood pressure. In the Special Intervention group, more diuretics were used, and the patients usually took higher doses than those in the Usual Care group.

This was an alarming finding. Why should diuretic therapy be associated with such adverse effects? This question has been the source of much research and controversy since the publication of the study. We now appear to have at least a partial explanation. In order to understand it, we must first take a look at high blood pressure and what effects it has on the body.

High Blood Pressure: What Is It?

The heart pumps blood through the arteries by generating a considerable amount of pressure. Blood pressure as we know it is the measurement of two levels of pressure and is stated in two numbers—for example, 120/80. These numbers refer to millimeters of mercury (mm Hg) in the familiar glass tube of the measuring device. The first measurement is called the *systolic* blood pressure. It reflects the pressure the heart generates when it contracts, sending a spurt of blood shooting through the arteries. The second number reflects the pressure that remains in the arterial system when the heart relaxes, making ready for the next beat.

The arteries are muscular tubes that expand and contract with each heartbeat. If the muscle fibers contract, the resistance of blood flow is increased and the blood pressure goes up. If the arteries relax, the blood pressure drops.

Certain hormones and nerves stimulate the heart to beat faster and more strongly, raising the blood pressure. Others signal the arteries to contract, also elevating the blood pressure. In addition, eating excessive amounts of salt causes water retention (edema) that increases the amount of fluid in the systems. Again, the blood pressure goes up.

The Consequences of High Blood Pressure

Obviously, pressure is needed to pump blood through the system. Also, the blood pressure rises with exertion and falls with rest. Ordinarily, the resting pressure is used for diagnosis. If this pressure is higher than is needed, it causes increased strain on the heart and blood vessels and leads to heart attack, strokes, and kidney failure. It is generally considered that resting blood pressure readings below 140/90 are safe and higher levels risky. The higher the level, the greater the risk. However, recent studies have shown that the lower the blood pressure, the better, as long as it is stable and not caused by another problem. This means that a blood pressure of 105/60 is safer than 125/85.

How High Blood Pressure Is Treated

Knowing that elevations of blood pressure are dangerous, physicians for years have been using drugs to bring it down. For patients who have very high levels, 180/115 for example, there is no debate that controlling the pressure with drugs prevents disasters. However, there is considerable debate about the benefits of using drugs to treat mild or moderate elevations in the range of 150/100 or lower, because the drugs themselves have side effects that could cancel out the benefits of the drug-induced lower pressures.

Of all the agents used to lower the blood pressure, the thiazide diuretics have come under the most attack. This is alarming, because this type of diuretic is *the most frequently prescribed agent* for blood pressure control! There is now considerable evidence that patients taking thiazide diuretics experience an increased death rate despite the effectiveness of the diuretic in lowering the blood pressure. Commonly used thiazides include Dyazide, Hydrochlorothiazide, Diuril, Hygroton, Moduretic, Aldactazide, Maxzide, and others. In many instances, a thiazide diuretic is added to another drug for convenience. Such preparations include Inderide, Corzide, Timolide, and others.

Increased Death in the MRFIT Study

As mentioned, the death rate for patients in the MRFIT study who had high blood pressure and an abnormal EKG was 65 percent higher among those given the thiazide diuretics than it was for those not given the drugs. The key to the mystery was found in the changes in the EKG, the tracings of electrical activity of the heart.

High Blood Pressure, Heart Size,
Irregular Rhythm, and Sudden Death

Sustained high blood pressure causes the heart to work harder, and the heart muscle begins to enlarge. Body builders strive for large muscles, but when this happens to the heart, the result is danger. Numerous studies have shown that any *abnormal* enlargement of the heart either from high blood pressure or other forms of heart disease increases the risk of *sudden* death, usually by arrhythmias (abnormal heartbeat). The EKG changes that were associated with the increased death rate in those taking diuretics were usually the changes that one sees when the heart has enlarged.

Potassium, Magnesium, Diuretics,
and Irregular Rhythms

The rhythm of the heart depends on balanced levels of potassium, magnesium, calcium, and sodium. The thiazide diuretics have long been known to be associated with wasting of both potassium and magnesium. They are also associated with increased rate of arrhythmias. In the SI group, those receiving more aggressive treatment of hypertension, blood potassium levels were lower than those in the UC group. In fact, there were three times as many in the SI group with potassium levels of 3.5 mEq/dL or lower (3.5 mEq/dL is the lower limit of what is considered normal) compared with the UC group. Serum magnesium levels are not routinely measured by physicians and were measured only in two clinics during the latter years of the trial. It was found that those taking the diuretics had lower overall magnesium levels than those not taking them, and 15 percent of the diuretic takers had magnesium levels below what is considered normal.

Almost as one would expect, the risk of developing an arrhythmia was 20 percent higher among those taking diuretics than those not taking them.

The Stress Potassium Sudden Death Connection

At the moment of heart attack, the body, sensing danger, floods the bloodstream with the "flight or fight" hormone called epinephrine (adrenaline). These powerful hormones increase the heart rate and constrict the blood vessels, making you ready to either run or fight in response to danger.

But with a heart attack, the danger is within, not without, and the flight or fight hormones put additional strain on the already damaged heart muscle. Recently, it has been demonstrated that these same hormones cause a drop in the potassium level and increase the risk of sudden irregular heart rhythms. Dr. W. D. Cooper has demonstrated that the frequency of irregular heart rhythms immediately after a heart attack was inversely proportional to the level of serum potassium at the time of the attack. ("Cardiac Arrhythmias Following Acute Myocardial Infarction: Associations with the Serum Potassium Level and Prior Diuretic Therapy," *European Heart Journal* 5:464, 1984.)

In patients who are taking the thiazide diuretics, the stress of the heart attack is even more dangerous. First, these patients may well have a reduced level of potassium to begin with. In addition, Dr. A. D. Struthers has demonstrated that the thiazide diuretics are associated with an even greater drop of the potassium level in response to epinephrine. He gave six healthy men a thiazide diuretic for seven days and compared them to controls. The diuretic caused the potassium to drop to 3.4 mEq/dL compared to 3.8 in the controls. He then infused epinephrine. The subjects receiving the diuretic experienced a further drop to 2.7 (a very dangerous level) compared to 3.1 for the controls ("Prior Thiazide Diuretic Treatment Increases Adrenaline-Induced Hypokalemia," *Lancet* 1 (1985): 1358).

So, What Happened in the MRFIT Study??

The researchers have pieced together the negative results of increased death in those taking thiazide diuretics in this way.

• High blood pressure leads to gradual thickening and enlargement of the heart muscle, which leads in turn to increased risk of sudden death, probably by arrhythmia. These changes in the heart muscle are reflected in EKG tracings.

• Diuretics are often given to patients with elevated blood pressure. Even though they lower the blood pressure, use of the diuretics also may lead to very significant reductions in both potassium and magnesium, which results in an increased risk of developing arrhythmia.

• At the moment of a heart attack, the body is flooded with epinephrine which lowers the potassium level and can initiate sudden fatal cardiac arrhythmias. The thiazide diuretics have been shown to enhance the negative effect of epinephrine on the blood level of potassium.

• Therefore, for many hypertensive patients taking the diuretics, the risk of death from the drug could be greater than the risk of death from the disease itself.

An excellent review of the potential problems posed by diuretic therapy was recently published by Lewis H. Kuller, M.D. ("Unexpected Effects of Treating Hypertension in Men with Electrocardiographic Abnormalities: A Critical Analysis," *Circulation 73*: 114–123, 1986).

Other Studies Show the Dangers of Diuretics

Dr. T. O. Morgan randomly assigned 172 men with mild high blood pressure (diastolic levels or 95 to 109 mm Hg) to four groups. One group received no therapy at all, the second received a low-salt diet, the third received chlorothiazide (a thiazide diuretic) without potassium supplementation, and the fourth group received Inderal, a beta blocker medication that lowers the blood pressure by blocking the heart's response to epinephrine. In the three groups that were not taking the diuretics, the mortality rates were similar and were about the same as one would predict from life expectancy tables.

Those taking the diuretics fared much worse than the other three groups, with a marked increase in fatal heart attacks and sudden death. In the group of 55 taking the diuretics, there were 13 deaths, while there were only 13 deaths in 117 patients in the other three groups. Because of the variability of time the patients were followed, the death rates were calculated in terms of risk of death per 100,000 days of exposure to the drug. The numbers were:

Risk of Death per 100,000 Days of Therapy

No therapy	9.25
Low-salt diet	8.00
Inderal	7.66
Thiazide	19.23

The authors concluded that "the possibility must exist that thiazide therapy was the factor which influenced the increase in the mortality rate." ("Failure of Therapy to Improve Prognosis in Elderly Males with Hypertension," *Australia Medical Journal, 2*: 27, 1980.)

Diuretics in the Diabetic Patient

It has long been known that the thiazide diuretics may cause a worsening of the diabetic condition. This phenomenon is most likely related to potassium wastage, since low potassium levels impair the natural release of insulin by the pancreas. Another potential danger of the thiazides is their tendency to cause magnesium loss. As discussed in Chapter 6, low magnesium levels are associated with poorly controlled diabetes and an increased tendency toward eye complications. When thiazide diuretics are used, efforts are usually made to replace potassium, but rarely if ever is magnesium replaced. The long-term use of diuretics has been shown to be associated with progressive worsening of the diabetic condition.

In addition, thiazide diuretics have been associated with elevations in both cholesterol and triglycerides levels. This simply adds to the diabetic's already increased risk of heart disease.

Beta Blockers and the Diabetic Patient

A class of drugs known as beta blockers are commonly used for the treatment of high blood pressure and therefore are often given to diabetic patients. Beta blockers include Inderal, Corgard, Lopressor, and Tenormin. These drugs block the body's response to epinephrine (adrenaline) and characteristically lower the blood pressure and the heart rate.

In the diabetic, beta blockers have been shown to cause a worsening of the diabetic condition, primarily by inhibiting the release of insulin by the pancreas. In addition they pose a danger to the diabetic on insulin because they block the body's normal response to hypoglycemia. When the blood sugar falls, the body releases epinephrine that elevates the blood pressure and heart rate and mobilizes glucose from the liver stores of glycogen. These compensatory reactions are blocked by the beta blocker drugs, and this increases the danger of hypoglycemic attacks. They also block the "warning signs" of a hypoglycemic attack, thus increasing the danger.

These deleterious effects of the beta blockers are most pronounced with the "nonselective" drugs, Inderal and Corgard, which block the response to epinephrine almost totally. Lopressor and Tenormin are more "cardioselective." That is, they seem to concentrate their blocking activity primarily on the heart and blood vessels. They do not affect the release of insulin by the pancreas or the body's response to hypoglycemia to any great extent. Writing in *Clinical Diabetes Mellitus, A Problem-Oriented Approach,* edited by Dr. John Davidson, Dr. W. Dallas Hall states: "It seems only rational to choose only cardioselective beta-blockers in diabetic patients [with high blood pressure or heart disease], particularly those who are insulin-dependent" (p. 457).

Needless to say, the diabetic condition makes the use of drugs for high blood pressure much more complicated and dangerous. Therefore, every effort should be made to control the blood pressure with a strict diet and exercise program. This is particularly true for obese diabetics who almost always have a form of high blood pressure that would disappear, along with their diabetes, if a strict diet and exercise regimen were instituted.

However, physicians often turn to drugs for other problems

associated with diabetes besides hypertension. The increased danger of the commonly used drugs in the diabetic patient is not generally recognized. Dr. Mary E. Callsen, internal medical resident at Brooke Army Medical Center in San Antonio, Texas, did a small but very informative pilot study on the use of nondiabetic drugs in 122 subjects who had type 2, non-insulin dependent diabetes. Of the 122, fifty were being treated with oral drugs (see Chapter 7), 47 were treated with insulin (even though they were non-insulin dependent), and 25 were receiving diet therapy alone.

Dr. Callsen found that 96 percent of the study group (117 out of 122) were receiving drugs for medical problems other than diabetes. The most common additional problems for which medications were prescribed were hypertension (occurring in the majority of all three groups) and atherosclerotic heart disease. Additional problems included rheumatoid arthritis, gout, and gastrointestinal disorders.

The patients who were being treated with diet alone for their diabetes were taking an average of 3.3 drugs for other problems. Those on the oral pills were receiving an average of 3.8 additional drugs. Those being treated with insulin were using an average of 4.4 additional medications. In the whole group, 85 percent (104 of the 122) were taking other medications known to cause deterioration of diabetic control, yet physician awareness of this was low.

For example, 68 percent of the entire group of diabetic patients were taking thiazide diuretics. However, only a little more than half of the physicians prescribing the thiazides were aware that diuretics may have negative effects on diabetic control. Over 20 percent of the patients were taking beta blockers, even though these drugs are associated with worsening of diabetic control.

Dr. Callsen found that the more drugs a diabetic patient was taking, the worse the diabetic control. The rare patients being treated only for diabetes were found to be in the best diabetic control. (Presented at the 44th Annual Meeting of the American Diabetes Association with a synopsis in *Cardiovascular News,* Feburary 1985.)

Blood Pressure Control and Quality of Life

Often the quality of life is not considered when hypertensive medications are prescribed. Sexual performance routinely deteriorates with drug control of hypertension. In addition, patients report poor concentration, decreased work performance, and significant reductions in energy. The medications thought necessary for blood pressure control make it difficult to use exercise to lower the blood pressure because patients taking the medications have neither the energy nor the inclination to become more active. Even when diuretics alone are prescribed in cases of mild elevation, patients often state that they "just don't feel well."

Dr. Gordon Williams, chief of endocrinology/hypertension at Brigham and Women's Hospital in Boston, recalled his experience with a 32-year-old truck driver referred to him for treatment of high blood pressure (170/115 mm Hg):

> When he came to me, he felt perfectly all right. He was strong and virile and he could bench press 300 pounds. He didn't think anything was wrong with him, and then his physician told him (after a routine checkup) that he had hypertension. Well, one year and five medications later, he came back to the office. Now his blood pressure was normal. But he was a fatigued, impotent wimp. Somehow, the fact that my patient had a normal blood pressure but a markedly deteriorated quality of life doesn't constitute a success. (*Medical Tribune*, September 17, 1986, p. 8.)

His awareness brought on by this case led Dr. Williams and seven other investigators to study the alteration in quality of life associated with three commonly used medications, Aldomet, Inderal, and Capotan. They found that Capotan had the least effect on work and sexual performance. This particular medication can be quite dangerous in diabetic patients who have protein in their urine—a sign of kidney disease. Otherwise, it can be used judicially when necessary.

Diet Therapy and Quality of Life

Lying dormant in the archives of every medical library is the work of Dr. Walter Kempner of Duke University, who demonstrated that a diet of primarily rice and fruit, which is high in potassium and low in sodium, is quite effective in lowering the blood pressure even in the most difficult cases of hypertension ("Treatment of Hypertension Vascular Disease with Rice Diet," *American Journal of Medicine 4*:545–577, 1948). When diet is used to replace drugs, the quality of life is enhanced, not decreased. All that is necessary is for the physician and the patient to give vigorous diet therapy a chance. Medications can then be added if necessary.

The following case illustrates how temporary use of a rice and fruit diet can be helpful in both hypertension and diabetes as well. Mrs. G.M. came to our Institute with a 15-year history of non-insulin dependent (type 2) diabetes, high blood pressure, and the more recent development of heart disease with angina pectoris (chest pain). She had been treated with drug therapy exclusively. She had developed angina pectoris about two years previously and had recently had an angiogram that showed significant blockages in her coronary arteries. One cardiologist had enthusiastically recommended bypass surgery. Another had been much less enthusiastic. Therefore, she chose a conservative route and enrolled in our Institute to see if vigorous diet therapy could help. Until this time she had not altered her diet a great deal and had been following the pre-1979 recommendations of the American Diabetes Association that contained about 40 percent fat calories. When she arrived she was taking Capotan (50 mg a day), hydrochlorothiazide (50 mg a day), Tenormin (50 mg a day), and Procardia (10 mg four times a day). She wore a nitroglycerine patch, delivering 10 mg a day, and had been directed to use a nitroglycerine sublingual (under-the-tongue) spray when needed for chest pain. She was receiving insulin by a continuous infusion pump. The pump delivered one unit every hour (24 units), and she gave herself an additional 42 units divided between three meals and bedtime snack. This was a lot of insulin (64 units a day) considering that she weighed only 152 pounds.

We put Mrs. G.M. on a diet or rice and fruit to lower her blood pressure rapidly and reduce the need of so much medication. After 10 days she was shifted to the regular diet program outlined in this book. Her insulin pump was stopped because the change in diet would have almost insured her having significant hypoglycemia reactions. She was put on doses of 5 to 10 units of insulin before each meal. Her hypertensive medications were gradually reduced and then discontinued without significant elevation in the blood pressure. In addition, the frequency of her angina attacks was reduced from three to four times per day to one a day. This attack occurred while she was mildly exercising, which she had not been doing before arrival. In fact, she had been totally inactive for the last eight months. At the end of two weeks she was taking only Procardia (10 mg three times a day) and insulin 20 units in divided doses before meals. She wore a nitroglycerin patch delivering 5 mg a day and used a nitroglycerine spray when needed. Her laboratory values on admission and after 12 days were:

	9/10/86	9/23/86
Weight	151.75lb	152
Blood pressure	110/62	136/72
Cholesterol	233	188
HDL cholesterol	51	55
Cholesterol:HDL ratio	4.3	3.4
Fasting glucose (FBS)	193	125
Uric acid	7.9	5.8
Triglycerides	145	112
BUN	20	11
Glycohemoglobin	7.7	7.5

More dramatic was the rapid transformation in the way she felt. On arrival she was despondent to the point of hopelessness. At the end of only 12 days she was hopeful and had experienced a dramatic increase in her energy level and was walking 5½ miles a day as a part of her exercise regimen.

The positive experience of Mrs. G.M. is not uncommon for the many diabetic patients who go through the Institute. The dietary regimen we utilize is outlined in the following pages. We obviously put a high priority on nutrition, exercise, and vitamins and minerals. When this is done, often patients simply lose the requirement for medication.

About the Institute

The Whitaker Wellness Institute is not a hospital and is not designed to look or feel like one. It is located in a resort hotel next to the Pacific Ocean. What is accomplished in this environment could not be accomplished in the usual hospital setting.

Hospitals deal with crisis intervention and use the tools necessary to rescue patients from disaster. As such, they are quite impersonal and often uncomfortable places charged with fear.

This Institute deals with creating health. As such, at the Institute the environment is comfortable, personal, pleasant, and charged with hope and enthusiasm.

The Institute was founded on the concept of nutrition which, though not all of the program, is the most important aspect of the treatment. The food here is unprocessed, whole, natural, loaded with fiber, low in cholesterol and fat. It is designed to create health. In order to get a feel of how the Institute functions, it might be helpful for me to describe a typical day.

A Typical Day at the Institute

It starts early—8:00 A.M. for "vitals." Patients weigh in, have their blood pressure and pulse recorded, and give a history of the day before—how far each walked, the pulse rate attained during exercise, and a rundown of any symptoms experienced. These daily reports help us evaluate progress and alter medication dosage.

8:30 A.M. Breakfast, which could be almond oatmeal, pancakes, French toast (egg whites only), or cold cereal with the ever-present oatmeal muffins, fresh fruit, and vitamin supplements.

9:15 A.M. to 10:00 A.M. Three times weekly each patient is individually evaluated. Medications are changed—insulin is almost always reduced in a gradual manner, as are the numerous heart and blood pressure drugs used by so many patients prior to entering the Institute. The drug modification always depends upon how each patient is doing. Also, the patient's individual laboratory tests are discussed as are all aspects of each particular case. We believe that patient education and open discussion about all aspects of the treatment are essential to the practice of medicine.

10:00 A.M. to 10:45 A.M. Scheduled exercise. Most patients exercise throughout the day, but each morning at 10:00 A.M. the group exercises together and each patient is monitored by the staff. During this time we can determine if patients are taking their pulse accurately, are exercising at an appropriate level, and whether they should decrease or increase their activity. Symptoms are also checked "in the field," which gives the staff a good sense of how each patient is doing.

12:00 noon. Lunch. It could be Mexican burritos, Chinese vegetables with rice, corn chowder with salad and bread, non-fat pizza or a host of other pleasing and healthy dishes, plus vitamin supplements.

1:30 P.M. to 2:30 P.M. Seminar. Each day a specific subject is discussed, which includes heart disease, the bypass operation, diabetes, the reversal of atherosclerosis, the cholesterol controversy, etc. It is during these seminar sessions that patients begin to understand their problem as well as the role the diet and exercise program plays in their improvement. These seminars inform and motivate patients to follow the program at home. Some of the session deals with food preparation for the family so that, in addition to printed recipes and menus, patients clearly understand the mechanics of following this program at home. These sessions are the backbone of this program. Each session has also been recorded on tape and every patient is given the complete series. This provides reinforcement and program recall after they return home. Because friends of former patients have heard these tapes and have requested copies from the Institute, these tapes are now available to anyone wishing to have a personal copy of the series.

4:00 P.M. Relaxation time. Patients gather to undergo a special relaxation session. Each lies on a foam rubber mat and is guided in progressive relaxation using biofeedback techniques. The purpose is to train patients in relaxation techniques to help overcome stress and to guide them in "health visualization," which is actually visualizing oneself as healthy, active, thin, without pain or medication. We realize that stress plays a role in disease, and these relaxation visualization sessions are useful in controlling the contribution stress makes to disease. Patients enjoy this peaceful interlude at the end of the day.

5:30 P.M. Dinner. This is a time to enjoy the end of a day of accomplishment. Dinner is served in the main dining room. The delicious healthful meal is enjoyed with good fellowship and leisurely conversation. Since the evenings are free, some patients stay to enjoy the music and dancing in the dining room after dinner.

Many patients, particularly diabetic patients, have such poor circulation in their legs that open ulcers develop. This often leads to amputation. To heal the ulcers and avoid this complication patients spend at least one hour daily with their legs in a pressurized oxygen tank. The tank fills with 100 percent oxygen under pressure and releases the pressure every fifteen seconds. The oxygen, which is humidified, is forced by the pressure into the open ulcer, which rapidly begins to heal. Sometimes ulcers that have been getting worse for months will heal in a matter of weeks.

Obviously, the days are full and active. For the first time, patients spend the whole day doing things to improve their health. Many accomplished and disciplined people, expert in their field, limp into the Institute riddled with heart disease, diabetes, high blood pressure, and other serious problems. For many, this is their first experience at improving their health and concentrating on the needs of their body. They quickly understand that their body is a wonderful, finely tuned miracle that must be cared for. They are eager to learn how to reverse the diseases which have taken their toll.

Observations of the Doctor

After observing about two thousand patients start and complete this program, I have seen some general changes that occur in patients while in the Institute.

First several days: Almost everyone is a little skeptical. After all, a medical clinic housed in a resort hotel does not fit the general picture. However, most are convinced that this approach makes a lot of sense and have decided before arrival to give it a try. There is a lot of testing in the first few days—complete physical examination, blood test, exercise test, etc. Patients meet the other members of the group and often talk about why they came and what they hope to get out of the program. They begin to make friends rapidly. Everyone is in the same boat, going in the same direction, with the same goal—to regain their health.

End of first week: The mood is considerably lighter. Information in the seminars convinces patients of the benefits of the more active life-style. For a few, improvements have already begun—a little less angina, more physical endurance, less insulin, etc. Friendships are becoming stronger and a group spirit begins to form. Even though each comes from a different walk of life and will return to such, they're all learning the same thing: how to alter their life-style in key areas to regain and maintain their health. This is fertile ground for camaraderie.

Start of the second week: The second week is different from the first. The routine of activities, exercise, oxygen, and relaxation has been established and patients now concentrate on improvements. During this last week many medications and symptoms are gone. Patients who had never walked a mile, and considered it impossible, are walking four or five miles without difficulty. An interim blood test generally shows improvements which would include a much lower cholesterol level and lower blood sugar. Blood pressures are down and most have lost some excess weight. Seminars continue to give more information and serve to reinforce each patient's commitment to the program. Most are already planning how to handle the business lunch, shopping, and when and how they will do their exercise. For the most part, the patients are continually surprised at how pleasant the food can be. They have experienced a wide variety of foods, many of which they had considered taboo: pancakes, waffles, spaghetti, potatoes, even potatoes baked in strips that taste like French fries.

The Institute regularly publishes a newsletter to keep patients informed on recent research. If you are interested in the newsletter or more material about the Institute, please write or call us at:

The Whitaker Wellness Institute
4400 MacArthur Blvd., Suite 630
Newport Beach, CA 92660
(714) 851-1550

PART IV
A Month of Menus: Recipes and Meal Plans

The preceding chapters have set the stage. Now the fun begins. What follows was written by Barbara Tancredi. Ms. Tancredi was the chef at our Institute for close to a year and a half. She is also a housewife, and each recipe included was tested on her family as well as being used here at the Institute.

I told her to be practical in her instructions so that the program could be followed as easily as possible. She is very detailed in describing exactly what is needed, down to the kitchen utensils and the shopping requirements.

At first glance, this diet change appears to be a burden. However, with time and practice it becomes easier. With any kind of change you make in your life, practice and experience eliminate the rough points.

Each menu has a nutritional scoreboard so you'll know what you are eating and will get used to thinking in terms of caloric composition.

Each day's menu provides approximately 1800 calories. Obviously, you may have to go up or down on the calories depending upon requirements for weight loss or activity.

Generally, I'm a little less concerned with calorie intake, within certain limits of course, than I am with the composition of foods.

I do hope this book helps you in overcoming diabetes. We would certainly like to hear from you.

We publish a newsletter from the Institute which is our way of updating our patients on new aspects of the program. If you are interested, give us a call.

The recipe nutrient totals were calculated using the computer software "Datadiet Nutrient Analysis System" developed by:

IPC Datadiet
5 Town and Country Village
Suite 747
San Jose, CA 95128

A Month of Menus

Our Purpose

The purpose of this section is to help you succeed in preparing a healthy dietary regimen from readily available, common foods, using uncomplicated recipes to produce familiar dishes (nothing unrecognizable) that contain approximately 1800 calories per day per person, with high fiber, low fat, no salt or sugar, and with approximately 70 percent of the calories coming from complex carbohydrates.

You can do it! Just follow these pages as though they were step-by-step instructions. Don't skip anything. For example, with kitchen equipment, if you neglect to obtain a blender you will find yourself frustrated when trying to whip up many recipes! You'll be defeated before you even begin. We have deliberately kept the required equipment and pantry stock down to a minimum. You'll be relieved to know that you don't have to own every spice and herb known to man to succeed with these recipes!

The recipes in this section have been fully kitchen tested. Each and every one of them has been prepared in our kitchen to conform to the requirements not only of health but especially of taste! Too many recipes exist boasting no fat, no sugar, no salt, and frankly, we find most have no taste, either. So we insisted that our recipes undergo strict taste tests, because if they don't taste good we may find you in the closet with a salt shaker!

STEP ONE: Obtaining the Necessities

Start out your new dietary regimen by obtaining the necessities. When your kitchen is fully and properly equipped with cookware, baking and condiment supplies, food staples, and serving and storage dishes, you will be ready to begin. Then, when you start to prepare that first recipe and find that every ingredient is at your fingertips—success! When your griddle and bakeware don't cling to the batter—success! All because you took the time to prepare.

Use our lists like a shopping guide (you probably have most of the items already). Some of what you don't have you might obtain from a friend or relative to cut costs, or you may find secondhand supplies in a thrift store. However, as you will see, you don't need that many items to begin with. Also, what you *do* need isn't expensive compared to a microwave oven, which you don't need, or a food processor, which you also don't need.

So take the time to stock up. Plan to begin your new regimen after your cupboards and pantry are stocked with the items on our lists. It will be well worth the effort and any delay.

Vegetable-Broth Seasoning—Our New "Salt"

*If food were meant to be tasteless
We wouldn't have taste buds.*

The number-one reason why people fail in a no-salt regimen is that the foods just don't taste good. We must find a suitable replacement! Because no matter how much garlic, herbs, Tabasco, or spices you pour on a dish, nothing "grabs" you like salt. While various herbs and spices are wonderful, they need to be an addition to salt, not its replacement. So we're going to ask that you do two things: First, when you see salt in a recipe, scratch it off and write in "vegetable-broth seasoning" (except use three times as much). Second, when you see salt used for boiling pasta or baking cookies, cakes, pies, etc., scratch it off completely and leave nothing in its place. It isn't necessary.

The "vegetable-broth seasoning" can be any dehydrated vegetable powder found in your market or health-food store which has been produced from dehydrated vegetables, grains, and even fruits, but no salt. These are combined in such a way that they taste salty owing to the combination of ingredients used. They are used to season and can also be made into a broth. While most are acceptable (you will need to experiment to find which ones you like), we recommend Dr. Jensen's Broth or Seasoning very highly. It's the best we've found so far. It has a superior taste without the aftertaste that some vegetable seasonings have (especially those that contain grains that may have turned slightly rancid). In fact, as far as we're concerned, we don't miss salt one iota when we use this seasoning.

Taste is so important in the success of a healthy diet that we feel this is something we need to emphasize. Think of your vegetable-broth seasoning in the same way you used to think of salt—a versatile, everyday kind of seasoning. Use it wherever you would use salt (except in the unnecessary places like baked goods), but more liberally. With the proper use of this seasoning, food can be truly delicious!

Condiments and Baking Staples

Specific Brands

- Dr. Bernard Jensen's Broth or Seasoning
  124 E. Cliff St.
  P.O. Box 8
  Solana Beach, CA 92075
  (619) 755-4027

As of May 1986, a 5-pound jar (which will last you 3 to 6 months) cost $36.67 plus tax and C.O.D. charges. Smaller quantities are available (for example, a 12-ounce jar costs $5.95). *They will ship anywhere in the world.* A phone call will start the process. You will receive your order with an invoice and may pay after receiving the product. Other arrangements are also available for retailers and businesses.

- Butter Buds Brand Natural Butter Flavored Mix
  Produced in Wisconsin for Butter Buds Division
  Cumberland Packing Corporation
  60 Flushing Ave.
  Brooklyn, NY 11205
  (718) 858-4200

A call in May 1986 revealed that Butter Buds is available throughout the United States, as well as in Canada.

- Pam Vegetable Cooking Spray—
  "Stops Foods from Sticking"
  Boyle-Midway, Inc.
  New York, NY 10017

A no-salt, no-cholesterol spray to take the place of oils, butter, grease, or margarine on baking pans, griddles, and waffle irons. It contains vegetable oil, alcohol, lecithin, and a propellant. There are similar sprays with the same ingredients which are also acceptable. This product is used in such a minute amount (as compared to oil or margarine) that it is insignificant in the diet. Used as directed.

- Rumford Baking Powder
  The Rumford Company
  900 Wabash Ave.
  Terre Haute, IN 47801

A double-acting baking powder that contains no aluminum. We found that those containing aluminum left a bitter aftertaste and were of questionable safety where health is concerned.

Nonbranded Products:

- Herbs and Spices. These are the ones used most often:
  Basil
  Cinnamon
  Garlic powder or fresh garlic
  Onion powder or fresh onion
  Oregano
  Pepper, black
  Pumpkin pie spice
- Extracts used most often:
  Lemon
  Orange
  Vanilla
- Dry baking ingredients:
  Arrowroot
  Baking soda
  Carob powder (unsweetened)
  Cornstarch
  Tapioca
- Flavorings:
  Mustard (a natural type)
  Olive oil
  Parmesan cheese, grated (store in refrigerator)
  Safflower oil (milder tasting than olive)
  Soy sauce, low sodium
  Vinegar (any kind except distilled)
- Sweeteners:
  Chopped dates (Make sure that they are coated in oat flour and not dextrose. You can also make your own.)
  Date sugar (dates that have been dehydrated then granulated)
  Frozen apple juice (Keep in the freezer. Use in its concentrated form for sweetening.)
  Fruit preserves
  Fruit syrup (just fruit and juices, no sugar added)
  Molasses, unsulphured
  Raisins
  Raw honey

• Other:
  Eggs (for the whites in baking and omelettes)
  Yeast ("active dry" keeps longest)

Food Staples—Always Have These on Hand

Fresh:

Eggs (for the whites)
Garlic
Onions

Dry:

Barley
Beans—Have a variety on hand, including pinto, split pea, white beans, garbanzos (if you decide not to used canned), and more.
Cold cereals—Keep several on hand that are made from whole grains and contain no added fats or sugar.
Cornmeal or corn flour
Herb teas—We like the tea bags better than the bulk; they're more convenient.
Lentils
Nuts and seeds—These are used in small quantities for flavor and texture. Stock up on sunflower seeds, sesame seeds (unhulled), walnuts, almonds, and pecans. Look for the words "raw" and "unsalted" on the package, or buy them from the bulk containers.
Oat bran—This can be found in many markets today, but if not, the health store should have it. You'll be using quite a bit, so buy several pounds at a time.
Oatmeal—Get the long-cooking type.
Pasta—The whole grain is best. You can also get whole grain to which spinach or other vegetables have been added. There are "lighter" versions like "artichoke" which are great and will be closer to what you are accustomed to. Get spaghetti, macaroni, lasagna, and rotelli.
Rice—Brown rice only. The long grain cooks up fluffy, whereas the short grain cooks up "nutty," like wild rice. Choose your favorite.

Whole-grain breads—Read the labels. Look for breads that are truly whole grain. Some breads are white flour that has been colored (usually with caramel coloring), but the label says "whole wheat." Some day there will be a law against this. Any whole grain is good. What you want to avoid in the bread are preservatives, conditioners, sugars, and added fats. There are too many great breads made without any of these. Or you can make your own!

Whole-wheat flour

Canned or Jars:

Applesauce—Unsweetened

Garbanzo beans—No sugar added. You can also stock up on other beans, but watch the label for undesirable additives. If the only addition to the bean is salt and something to retain the color, rinse the beans in cold water in your colander before using them.

Juices—Stock up on several unsweetened juices like apple, grape, pineapple, orange, and more. The sweeter ones can also be used to sweeten when you cook soups, casseroles, baked goods, and desserts.

Mushrooms—Because mushrooms add so much, and fresh ones spoil so quickly, have a can or two on hand. Rinse off the salt before using.

Pineapple—Unsweetened (They are usually packed in their own juice.)

Salsa—The ingredients should simply be tomatoes, green chiles, and onions. A little salt is fine since we use salsa in such minute quantities. However, if you can get one unsalted, do so.

Spaghetti sauce—Read the label. No salt, no sugar, and no meat. Many sauces today say "100% natural," but they are counting white sugar as natural. "Prego" made by the Campbell Soup Company is a great one without salt.

Tomatoes—Because we use so many tomatoes with our rice and pasta and bean dishes, as well as the many vegetable dishes that use them, have several cans of peeled and chopped tomatoes on hand. Fresh tomatoes are usually expensive (save them for your salads) and difficult to keep on hand at all times. Also have large cans of tomato puree on the shelf.

Tomato paste—You can make your own puree by blending the

paste with water, or you can use the paste as is, a spoonful at a time, to add a touch of flavor to a soup or casserole.

Tomato catsup—A natural kind made with honey and no salt. Your health food store carries this or can obtain it for you.

Unsalted Spaghetti Sauce Recipe

Because many of our recipes call for an unsalted spaghetti sauce, make up a pot of it and then freeze it in 1- or 2-cup portions. Remove the sauce from the freezer the night before you need to use it and keep it in the refrigerator. You may also purchase a natural, unsalted spaghetti sauce from the market or health store if you want. Either way will yield the same results.

6	cups tomato puree (2 28-ounce cans)	2	tablespoons olive oil
2	cups minced green pepper	½	cup tomato paste (approximately 1 6-ounce can)
2	cups fresh minced onion (approximately 1 medium onion)	2	tablespoons honey
		4	teaspoons oregano
8	cloves garlic, blended with ½ cup water in blender	2	tablespoons vegetable-broth seasoning

Combine all of the ingredients in a large pot and simmer slowly for 1 hour. You may add more tomato puree for thickness or more water if you desire your sauce less thick. The amount of vegetable-broth seasoning is less than for a ready-to-serve sauce because you will be adding more seasonings when using this sauce with various recipes.

Makes 8½ cups

Note: If you are using this sauce for pasta and want it to be ready to serve, add mushrooms (optional), and increase the seasoning to 4 tablespoons vegetable-broth seasoning.

UNSALTED SPAGHETTI SAUCE

4/4/9 CALORIES : 729
CAL FROM CARB : 69%
CAL FROM PRO : 12%
CAL FROM FAT : 19%

P/S RATIO .61 : 1

DATE:

GRAM WT.	1226.50	g	*RIBOFLN	.68	mg
CHOLSTRL	0.00	mg	*NIACIN	14.42	mg
CALORIES	660.80	kcal	*VIT C	503.68	mg
PROTEIN	21.00	g	*PANTO	.60	mg
*FAT	15.82	g	*B6	.73	mg
CARB	125.77	g	*FOLACIN	30.57	mcg
CALCIUM	186.02	mg	*B12	0.00	mcg
PHOS	434.41	mg	MAGNES	224.35	mg
*IRON	17.92	mg	*ZINC	1.42	mg
SODIUM	114.25	mg	SAT FAT	1.80	g
*POTAS	4602.25	mg	MONO UNS	9.90	g
*VIT A	15567.50	IU	POLY UNS	1.10	g
THIAMIN	1.05	mg	*FIBER	7.06	g

Prepackaged Cold and Hot Cereals

The criteria to use when choosing prepackaged cold and hot cereals is that they be whole grain and contain no added fats or sugar. By sugar we mean refined sugars. This includes white sugar, anything ending in -ose (glucose, fructose, maltose, dextrose, etc.), and brown sugar. Even the so-called "raw sugar" is just one step away from being white sugar. Avoid it. Good sweeteners would be honey, dates or date granules, raisins, pure maple, and we'll include barley malt. But try to use mostly just whole grains like the puffed grains, whole-wheat flakes or squares, cereals like Grape-Nuts, and of course just plain whole grains that you cook up hot. We use oatmeal, cornmeal, multigrain, whole-wheat flakes, roman meal, millet, and many others.

*Throughout this section, asterisks indicate the value may be higher due to unknown amounts for one or more foods.

Kitchen Equipment

While you truly don't need much in quantity, you do need to pay attention to the quality of what you use in the kitchen. Just one example is your waffle iron. If it doesn't have a nonstick surface, you will meet with disaster. Until we got wise we spent more than a few precious moments scraping waffles off a nonstick iron. The same goes for pancakes. They must be cooked on a nonstick griddle to succeed.

Pots and pans You will use sizes from ½ quart up to 8 quarts. The best pots and pans are stainless steel. Look for a waterless type if you want the very best. These are designed with tight-fitting lids, and have a bottom and core that allows even heat throughout the pan, creating an "oven" effect. This cooks the food evenly instead of burning the bottom without even cooking the rest. In your set you'll need a small and large skillet.

Casseroles These are either clear glass, Corning Ware, or stoneware with lids. All are good. You'll use from a 1-quart size up to 4 quarts and perhaps even larger if you cook for company or a large family.

Pyrex baking dishes These don't have lids. They are square or rectangular and are used to cook lasagna and similar dishes where you don't need a lid (although when cooking without fat, we usually cover these dishes to keep them from drying out). Your pie dish will also be in this category.

Nonstick cookware You will need one griddle. This is a square or rectangular pan that is flat and has a handle. It will be used to cook pancakes and grilled sandwiches. You need a waffle iron that has a nonstick coating. This is a self-contained appliance that plugs into a wall outlet. Your bakeware needs to be nonstick coated. This includes a bread-loaf pan, one or two muffin pans, one or two cookie sheets, and two round cake pans (usually 8½ inches round and 1½ inches deep). Lastly, you'll need a medium or large nonstick skillet. When you sauté without much fat, this skillet is a necessity.

Blender Osterizer is a good brand. Be sure that you get the 1-cup jars (usually glass or plastic). These are used for grinding dates, oats, small bits of vegetables, and fruits. You can see through the jar to monitor the progress, and using the little jar leaves the large blender jar clean for something else. Your blender will be in daily use, so keep it handy on top of the counter.

Hand mixer If you've got a large mixer, don't toss it out! But if you haven't got anything along this line, just get a small hand mixer. It is necessary for beating egg whites stiff, mixing muffin, cake, and cookie batters, and more.

Oven To be thorough, we must include the oven. But the great news is that you don't have to have a microwave. A good convection oven (the one you already have) is all you need. But if you have a microwave, use it. They're nice to warm up leftovers, and may keep you honest (you're more likely to eat what you're supposed to eat if you can quickly warm up some legal leftovers instead of succumbing to a fast-food urge elsewhere).

Colander To drain pasta; to thaw food by running hot water over it; to rinse salt off canned foods; and to rinse off berries or vegetables.

Teakettle To heat your water for herb tea.

Bowls You'll need 2-, 4-, and 6-quart bowls for serving soup, making large salads, and mixing batters. The best are stainless steel, glass, or stoneware.

Serving Dishes To be thorough, we must include the fact that you'll need plates, bowls, cups, saucers, silverware, and whatever else you use to serve the food.

Storageware Tupperware is still the best, but any good (preferably see-through) storage containers with tight-fitting lids that seal will do. Save your clear plastic date cups (if that is how they are packaged in your area) and similar containers in which food is packaged. They make good give-away containers when you send friends or family home with leftovers, or when you take food along with you to work, picnics, or on outings. They're disposable!

Knives A large serrated-edge knife is the most used. It is handy for cutting tomatoes, onions, green peppers, eggplant, and other slippery things. A butcher knife is good for chopping, and a cleaver is handy if you've got a large cutting board and a lot of chopping to do.

Utensils You'll need the following utensils:

> *Spatula*—for flipping pancakes and similar tasks. It must be made out of a material that won't scratch nonstick surfaces!
> *Wooden spoon(s)*—for stirring sauces

Ladle—for dishing up soups, sauces, and syrups. Get stainless steel.

Slotted and nonslotted spoons—these are for dishing up vegetables, casseroles, cereals, and more. The slotted spoon is for when you don't want the juice, and the nonslotted spoon is for when you do.

Tongs—for lifting things out of very hot water.

Rubber spatulas—for scraping out bowls and other dishes to get every last drop.

Measuring cups and spoons The minimum you'll want to have handy is a 1-cup measuring cup (Pyrex is best because it withstands any temperature), and a 1-teaspoon as well as a 1-tablespoon measuring spoon. But if you want to add more, have a second measuring cup (so you can have one for wet and one for dry) and the whole set of spoons from ⅛ teaspoon up to 1 tablespoon.

If you don't find it on this list, you probably don't need it. But if you've got it already, keep it. Use it if you can. Like a crockpot. It's more convenience than necessity, unless you work full time and love beans. It's great for both of these things.

STEP TWO: How to Alter a Recipe from a Standard Cookbook to Suit Your Special Needs

If you own a cookbook that contains a variety of recipes from all categories (meats, vegetables, salads, desserts, etc.), you can use it! Except for the recipes that are only meat, which obviously cannot be altered, many recipes can be changed to suit your special needs. Below are two examples of how this can be done. Basically, we are substituting something allowed for something that is not, and compensating where necessary. For example, if we substitute egg whites for whole eggs, you may need to add a little olive oil to make up for the fat you eliminated in the egg yolk.

Example:

Pink Cabbage (from *Favorite Recipes of America,* Vol. V, p. 74, 1966 P.O. Box 18324, Louisville, KY 40218)	*Altered Recipe, Pink Cabbage*
¼ cup chopped onion	¼ cup chopped onion
1 tablespoon fat	1 tablespoon olive oil
1 tablespoon flour	1 tablespoon whole-wheat flour
1 cup water	1 cup water
4 cups shredded cabbage	4 cups shredded cabbage
¼ cup sliced apples	¼ cup sliced apples
2 tablespoons vinegar	2 tablespoons vinegar
1 teaspoon salt	1 tablespoon vegetable-broth seasoning
Dash of pepper	Dash of pepper
1 teaspoon caraway seed	1 teaspoon caraway seed

Sauté the onion in fat; blend in flour until smooth. Add water; stir until thickened and clear. Add cabbage, apples, vinegar, salt, pepper, and caraway seed. Cover; cook for 1 hour or until cabbage is tender. Yield: 4 servings.

Sauté onion in olive oil; blend in the flour until smooth. Add water; stir until thickened and clear. Add cabbage, apples, vinegar, vegetable-broth seasoning, pepper, and caraway seed. Cover; cook for 1 hour or until cabbage is tender. Yield: 4 servings.

Of course, we chose a recipe that was primarily vegetable and fruit to begin with. And you will, too, when you browse through your cookbook. It would be self-defeating to try and alter a pot roast!

Example:

Carrot Cookies **(ibid., p. 292)**	*Altered Recipe,* *Carrot Cookies*
¾ cup butter or margarine	¼ cup olive oil
¾ cup sugar	¾ cup honey
1 egg, beaten	2 egg whites, beaten
1 cup mashed, cooked carrots	1 cup mashed, cooked carrots
Rind of one orange, grated	Rind of one orange, grated
3 cups sifted flour	3 cups sifted whole-wheat flour
2 tablespoons baking powder	2 tablespoons Rumford baking powder
¼ teaspoon salt	(No salt necessary)
½ teaspoon lemon flavoring	½ teaspoon lemon extract
1 teaspoon vanilla flavoring	1 teaspoon vanilla extract

Cream butter and sugar well; add egg. Beat in carrots and grated rind. Sift dry ingredients; stir into creamed mixture. Add flavorings. Drop by teaspoons on a lightly greased cookie sheet. Bake at 375° until brown. Watch closely; cookies brown easily.

"Cream" together the oil and honey. Add the egg whites. Beat in the carrots and rind. Sift dry ingredients; stir into the creamed mixture. Add the extracts. Drop by teaspoonsful onto a PAM-sprayed, nonstick cookie sheet. Bake at 375° until brown. Watch closely; cookies brown easily.

In the altered recipe, the honey adds moistness, so it partly makes up for eliminating two thirds of the fat. The two recipes would not be identical if both were baked and compared side by side. This is not our goal. Our goal is to use recipes to our advantage. We end up with carrot cookies, but a different version. A healthy, lower-fat, higher-fiber, no-salt version. And while they don't look the same or taste the same, they are both delicious. So why not choose the healthy version?

In a Nutshell: A Reminder of What Fiber Is, Why Fats Are Undesirable, and Which Carbohydrates Are Good

What Fiber Is

Fiber is found in fruits, vegetables, nuts, seeds, grains, beans, and inedible plant life. We will concern ourselves only with the edible plant life. Fiber has been found to help prevent cancer, protect against heart disease, aid in weight loss, and lessen a diabetic's need for insulin. Because this is what we are concerned with in this book, we will view fiber from this aspect alone. It lowers the blood sugar because the fibers slow down and smooth out the absorption of sugars and starches (which become sugars) from the intestine. Also, fibers of the gelatinous type literally decrease fat absorption, which aids insulin's effectiveness because fats block the action of insulin in the blood. Thus, fiber helps lower the high blood-glucose levels associated with diabetes.

Types of Fibers and Where They Are Found

- *Lignin.* The woody fiber that gives plants their structure. Found in fruits, vegetables, and grains.
- *Cellulose.* The most abundant fiber. Found in fruits, vegetables, and grains.
- *Hemicellulose.* Common to all plants.
- *Pectin.* Found primarily in the white of citrus fruits, apples, strawberries, and some vegetables.
- *Gum.* Found mostly in legumes and in some grains.

Why Fats Are Undesirable

Fats in the bloodstream block the effectiveness of insulin. That is bad enough by itself, but that's not all that fat does. "Bad" fats (mostly from animal sources like meat, lard, butter, milk, and egg yolks) also cling to artery walls, even burrowing into them, causing a blockage that leads to stroke and heart attack. A lot can be said about fat—in fact, entire books have been written about it. Let it suffice to say that we avoid fats. Except for the tiny amounts of unrefined vegetable oil that we use for cooking and flavoring—no fat is allowed.

Which Carbohydrates Are Good

The best carbohydrates (and to our way of thinking, the only carbohydrates) are "complex" carbohydrates. Simply put, this means those carbohydrates made by nature and not altered by man. All the whole grains, beans, fruits, vegetables, and even the nuts and seeds. Once you begin to refine that whole wheat into a white flour, it is no longer a complex carbohydrate, and no longer good. This applies to all foods of the vegetable kingdom. A whole raw almond is an excellent food, but grind it to a paste, roast it, then salt it, and it becomes most undesirable.

STEP THREE: How to Calculate Calories and the Percentage of Carbohydrate, Protein, and Fat

You will need your food-composition chart, a calculator (or a great head for math), and a pencil. You also need to know that carbohydrates have 4 calories per gram, proteins also have 4 calories per gram, and fat has 9 calories per gram.

APPLE PANCAKES

	Calories	Carbohydrates	Protein	Fat
½ cup whole-wheat flour	200	42.6	8	1.2
¼ cup oat bran	82.5	12.7	4.5	1.5
1 tablespoon olive oil	124	-	-	14
1 tablespoon baking soda	-	-	-	-
1 teaspoon cinnamon	6	1.8	.09	.07
2 egg whites, beaten stiff	34	.6	7.2	-
1½ cups apple juice	175.5	44.25	.3	-
½ large apple, grated	48	12	.15	.5
Totals	670	113.95	20.24	17.2

Carbohydrates are 113.95 grams × 4 (calories per gram) = 455.8 divided by 670 (total calories) to obtain the percentage of 670 that is 455.8: .68 or 68%.

Protein is 20.24 grams × 4 (calories per gram) = 80.96 divided by 670 (total calories) to obtain the percentage of 670 that is 80.96: .12 or 12%.

Fat is 17.27 grams × 9 (calories per gram) = 155.43 divided by 670 (total calories) to obtain the percentage of 670 that is 155.43: .23 or 23%.

So the apple pancakes are approximately 68% carbohydrate, 12% protein, and 23% fat. We say "approximately" because measurements (for example, "1 large apple") cannot be exact, and because numbers are often rounded off to avoid so many decimal points.

STEP FOUR: Your Calorie, Carbohydrate, Protein, Fiber, and Fat Chart

This chart is provided so that you may quickly evaluate for yourself the foods you are eating. By using this chart you can invent your own recipes, substitute equivalent foods in recipes, or even create your entire day's menu!

It is interesting to note that the foods we use *only* as condiments (oil, egg white, Parmesan cheese, and others) are both devoid of fiber and higher in protein and/or fats than we want. This lack of fiber and excess of fats and protein are, of course, why we use them in such minute quantities. If you want to investigate this further, obtain a complete list of food composition. You will readily see that meats, dairy products, and many other foods have a zero in the fiber column, and high numbers in the protein and fats column!

On the next page is an illustration of measurement equivalents to aid you in your calculations, whether they be from the chart given in this book, or on the labels of prepackaged products.

LIQUID MEASURE:

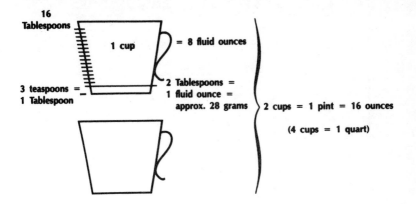

DRY MEASURE:

Weights vary due to the density of the substance. For example, 1 tablespoon of sugar equals approximately 12 grams whereas 1 tablespoon of flour equals only 8 grams.

Food-Composition Chart

This food-composition chart differs from others you will find in that it includes only those foods that are on your high-fiber, low-fat diet. Some things that you use in tiny amounts (like nuts) are included for quick reference, whereas to keep matters simple, other things that you might rarely use (like low-fat fish) are not included. The quantities listed are in the amounts you will use most, or are simplified for easy calculation (like 1 cup of flour, which can be halved easily).

Food-Composition Chart

(Taken primarily from *Nutrition Almanac*, Nutrition Search, Inc., McGraw-Hill Paperbacks, 1979 Edition.)

GRAINS

Quantity	Food	Calories	Carbohydrates	Protein	Fiber	Fat
1 cup	Barley, dry (2¾ cups cooked)	698	158	16.4	.7	2
1 cup	Barley, cooked	280	63.2	6.5	.28	.8
1 cup	Bran, wheat	121	35.4	9	5.2	2.6
1 cup	Bran, oat	330	51	18	24	6
1 slice	Bread, whole wheat	56	11	2.4	.4	.7
1 cup	Cornmeal (corn flour)	427	88	10.6	1.2	4
1 Tbsp.	Cornstarch	29	7	t	t	t
1 Tbsp.	Carob, unsweetened	14	6.5	.4	.64	t
1 cup	Whole-wheat flour	400	85.2	16	2.8	2.4
1 cup	Macaroni, cooked	151	32.2	4.8	.1	1
1 cup	Millet, whole grain, dry	746	166	22.6	7.3	6.8
1 cup	Oatmeal, dry	330	54	15	1	6
½ cup	Popcorn kernels (unpopped; approximately 9 cups popped)	486	96.3	16.2	2.7	6.3
1 cup	Rice, brown, dry	704	152	14.8	1.6	3.6
1 avg.	Shredded wheat biscuit	89	20	2.5	.5	.5

Note: t = trace, an immeasurable amount

Food	Serving					
Spaghetti, cooked	1 cup	155	32.2	4.8	.2	.6
Spaghetti (or macaroni or pastina), whole wheat, dry	4 ounces	400	80	14	2	1
Lasagna noodles, dry	12 ounces	1,260	252	42	6	6

SAUCES

Food	Serving					
Spaghetti sauce, unsalted, no sugar, no meat	1 cup	80	14	1	1	2
Salsa	2 Tbsp.	7	2	.4	.1	.08

CONDIMENTS, HERBS, SPICES

Food	Serving					
Egg white, raw	1	17	.3	3.6	0	0
Molasses	1 Tbsp.	45	11	0	0	0
Honey	1 Tbsp.	60	15	.1	0	0
Corn oil	1 Tbsp.	126	0	0	0	14
Olive oil	1 Tbsp.	124	t	t	0	14
Safflower oil	1 Tbsp.	124	0	0	0	14
Soy oil	1 Tbsp.	124	t	t	0	14
Sesame oil	1 Tbsp.	120	t	t	0	14
Sunflower seed oil	1 Tbsp.	124	t	t	0	14
Mustard	1 Tbsp.	15	.9	.9	.3	.9
Soy sauce	1 Tbsp.	12	1.7	1	0	.2
Vinegar	1 Tbsp.	2	.5	t	0	0
Allspice	1 tsp.	5	1.37	.12	.41	.17
Basil, ground	1 tsp.	4	.85	.2	.25	.06

Quantity	Food	Calories	Carbohydrates	Protein	Fiber	Fat
1 tsp.	Bay leaf, crumbled	2	.45	.05	-	.05
1 tsp.	Chili powder	8	1.42	.32	.58	.44
1 tsp.	Cinnamon, ground	6	1.84	.09	.56	.07
1 tsp.	Cloves, ground	7	1.29	.13	.2	.42
1 tsp.	Garlic powder	9	2.04	.47	.05	.02
1 tsp.	Ginger, ground	6	1.27	.16	.11	.11
1 tsp.	Marjoram, dried	2	.36	.08	.11	.04
1 tsp.	Nutmeg, ground	12	1.08	.13	.09	.8
1 tsp.	Onion powder	7	1.69	.21	.12	.02
1 tsp.	Oregano, ground	5	.97	.17	.22	.15
1 tsp.	Paprika	6	1.17	.31	.44	.27
1 Tbsp.	Parmesan, grated	23	.19	2.08	0	1.5
1 tsp.	Parsley, dry	1	.15	.07	.03	.01
1 tsp.	Pepper, black	5	1.36	.23	.28	.07
1 tsp.	Pepper, red or cayenne	6	1.02	.22	.45	.31
1 tsp.	Pumpkin pie spice	6	1.17	.1	.25	.21
1 tsp.	Rosemary, dry	4	.77	.06	.21	.18
1 tsp.	Tarragon, ground	5	.8	.36	.12	.12
1 tsp.	Thyme, ground	4	.89	.13	.26	.1
2 Tbsp.	Butter Buds (1 fl. ounce; 1 teaspoon when dry)	12	3	0	0	0
¼ cup	Date sugar	205	49.6	1.6	1.7	.3
2 Tbsp.	Fruit syrup (juice sweetened)					
1 Tbsp.	Tapioca granules	34	8.2	t	t	t

FRUIT

1 avg.	Avocado	334	12.6	4.2	3.2	32.8
1 med.	Apple, raw (with peel)	96	24	.3	1.8	1
1 cup	Apple juice, unsweetened	117	29.5	.2	.26	t
1 cup	Applesauce, unsweetened	100	26.4	.5	1.3	.5
3 avg.	Apricot, raw	55	13.7	1.1	.7	.3
1 cup	Apricot, dry	338	86.5	6.5	3.9	.7
1 avg.	Banana, raw	127	33.3	1.6	.8	.3
1 cup	Blackberries, raw	84	18.6	1.7	5.9	1.3
1 cup	Blueberries, raw	90	22.2	1	2.2	.7
1 cup	Boysenberries, unsweetened, frozen,	60	14.4	1.5	3.38	.4
1 avg.	Cantaloupe, raw	120	30	2.8	13.52	.4
1/10 avg.	Casaba melon, raw	38	9.1	1.7	1.2	t
1 cup	Cherries, sweet, raw	82	20.4	1.5	.52	.4
3.5 ounces	Currants, black, raw	54	13.1	1.7	2.4	.1
10 med.	Dates, pitted	274	72.9	2.2	2.3	.5
1 cup	Dates, dried (equals 8 Tbsps.)	505	134	4	3.6	t
2 large	Figs, raw	80	20.3	1.2	1.2	.3
1/2 med.	Grapefruit, raw	41	10.8	.5	.2	.1
1 cup	Grapes, raw	106	24	2	.9	1.5
2-inch wide slice	Honeydew melon, raw	49	11.5	1.2	.9	.5
1 Tbsp.	Lemon juice, unsweetened	4	1.2	.1	t	t
1 Tbsp.	Lemon peel, grated	t	1	.1	t	t
1 Tbsp.	Lime juice, unsweetened	4	1.4	t	t	t
1 med.	Mango, raw	152	38.8	1.6	2.7	.9

Quantity	Food	Calories	Carbohydrates	Protein	Fiber	Fat
1 avg.	Nectarine, raw	88	23.6	.8	.6	t
2 large	Olives, ripe	37	.6	.2	.3	4
1 avg.	Orange, raw	64	16	1.3	.9	.3
1 cup	Orange juice, unsweetened, fresh	112	25.8	1.7	.3	.5
1 cup	Orange juice, reconstituted	122	28.8	1.7	t	.2
½ med.	Papaya, raw	58	15	.9	1.8	.15
1 med.	Peach, raw	38	9.7	.6	.69	.1
1 avg.	Pear, raw	122	30.6	1.4	2.8	.8
1 med.	Persimmon, native	127	33.5	.8	1.5	.4
1 cup	Pineapple, raw, diced	81	21.2	.6	.5	.3
1 cup	Pineapple juice	138	33.8	1	.2	.3
¼ cup	Pineapple-Banana juice, unsweet-ened	34	8	.25	t	t
2 med.	Plums, raw	66	17.8	.5	.4	t
3 med.	Plums, prune-type	75	19.7	.8	.4	.2
1 large	Pomegranate, raw	97	25.3	.8	.5	.5
1 cup	Prunes, dehydrated	344	91.3	3.3	2.2	.5
1 cup	Prunes, softenized	411	108	3.4	1.96	1
1 cup	Prunes, unsweetened, cooked	253	66.7	2.1	2	.6
1 cup	Prune juice, unsweetened	197	48.6	1	t	.3
3.5 ounces	Quince, raw	57	15.3	.4	1.7	.1
1 cup	Raisins, packed	477	128	4.1	1.4	.3
1 cup	Raspberries, unsweetened, frozen	245	61.5	1.8	5.5	.5

Strawberries, raw	1 cup	56	12.6	1	2	.8
Tangelo, raw	1 med.	39	9.2	.5	-	.1
Tangerine, raw	1 med.	39	10	.7	.5	.2
Watermelon slice	6 x 1½ inch	156	38.4	3	1.8	1.2
Watermelon balls or cubes	1 cup	26	6.4	.5	.3	.2

NUTS AND SEEDS

Almonds	1 cup	849	27.7	26.4	3.85	77
Almond meal	1 ounce	116	8.2	11.2	.64	5.2
Brazil nuts	1 cup	916	15.3	20	4.2	93.7
Coconut, fresh-shredded (not packed)	1 cup	277	7.5	2.8	2.7	28.2
Filberts	1 cup	856	22.5	17	1.05	84.2
Peanuts, roasted	1 cup	838	29.7	37.7	3.89	70.1
Pecans	1 cup	742	15.8	9.9	2.3	76.9
Pumpkin seeds	1 cup	774	21	40.6	2.66	65.4
Sesame seeds, hulled	1 cup	873	26.4	27.3	3.6	80
Sunflower seeds, hulled	1 cup	812	28.9	34.8	5.5	68.6
Walnuts, black, chopped	1 cup	785	18.5	25.6	2.1	74.1
Walnuts, English halves	1 cup	651	15.8	14.8	2.1	64
Cashews, roasted	1 cup	785	41	24.1	1.96	64

Quantity	Food	Calories	Carbohydrates	Protein	Fiber	Fat
1 cup	Alfalfa sprouts, raw	41	6.2	5.1	1.7	.6
1 avg.	Artichoke, whole	44	9.9	2.8	2.4	.2
1 cup	Asparagus, cut pieces	35	6.8	3.4	.94	.3
1 cup	Bamboo shoots, raw	36	6.9	3.47	.93	.4
1 cup	Beans, black-eyed peas, cooked	178	29.9	13.4	-	1.3
1 cup	Beans, garbanzo, dry (approximately 3 cups cooked)	720	122	41	10	9.6
1 cup	Beans, green snap, raw	35	7.8	2.1	1.1	.2
1 cup	Beans, green snap, cooked	31	6.8	2	1.2	.3
1 cup	Beans, lentils, cooked (½ cup dry)	212	38.6	15.6	2.4	t
1 cup	Beans, limas, cooked	262	48.6	15.6	3	1.1
1 cup	Mung bean sprouts, raw	37	6.9	4	.7	.2
1 cup	Pinto beans, dry	663	121	43.5	8	2.3
1 cup	Red kidney beans, cooked	218	39.6	14.4	2.78	.9
1 cup	Soy beans, cooked	234	19.4	19.8	3	10.3
3.5 ounces	Tofu	72	2.4	7.8	.1	4.2
1 cup	Beans, yellow wax	32	7	1.9	1	.4
1 cup	Beans, white, cooked	224	40.3	14.8	3	1.1
1 cup	Beets, raw	58	13.4	2.2	1.1	1
1 cup	Beets, cooked	54	12.2	1.9	.94	.2
1 cup	Beets, canned, drained	63	15	1.7	.94	.2

3.5 ounces	Beet greens, raw	24	4.6	2.2	1.3	.3
1 cup	Beet greens, cooked	26	4.8	2.5	1.4	.3
1 piece	Broccoli (5½ inches long)	32	5.9	3.6	1.5	.3
1 cup	Broccoli, cooked	40	7	4.8	2	.5
9 med.	Brussel sprouts, raw	45	8.3	4.9	1.6	.4
1 cup	Brussel sprouts, cooked	56	9.9	6.5	2.1	.6
1 cup	Cabbage, sliced, raw	17	3.8	.9	.8	.1
1 cup	Cabbage, sliced, cooked	29	6.2	1.6	1	.3
1 cup	Cabbage, red, sliced, raw	22	4.8	1.4	1	.1
1 large	Carrot, raw	42	9.7	1.1	1	.2
1 cup	Carrots, cooked	48	11	1.4	1.5	.3
1 cup	Carrot juice	96	22.2	2.47	-	-
1 cup	Cauliflower flowerets, raw	27	5.2	2.7	1	.2
1 cup	Cauliflower, cooked	28	5.1	2.9	1.25	.3
1 cup	Celery, raw	20	4.7	1.1	.7	.1
1 cup	Celery, cooked	21	4.7	1.2	.9	.2
3.5 ounces	Chard, Swiss, raw	25	4.6	2.4	.8	.3
1 cup	Chard, cooked	26	4.8	2.6	1	.3
1 Tbsp.	Chives, chopped	3	.6	.2	.1	t
3 ounces	Collards, raw	40	7.2	3.6	.9	.7
1 cup	Collards, cooked	42	7.1	3.9	1.15	.9
1 cup	Corn, cooked	137	31	5.3	1.1	1.7
1 cup	Cucumber, unpeeled, sliced, raw	16	3.6	.9	.6	.1
3.5 ounces	Dandelion greens, raw	45	9.2	2.7	1.6	.7

Quantity	Food	Calories	Carbohydrates	Protein	Fiber	Fat
1 cup	Dandelion greens, cooked	35	6.7	2.1	1.3	.6
1 cup	Eggplant, raw (⅓ med.)	50	11.6	2.4	1.8	.4
1 cup	Eggplant, cooked	38	8.2	2	1.8	.4
1 cup	Endive, raw	10	2.1	.9	.45	.1
1 clove	Garlic, raw	4	.9	.2	t	t
1 cup	Lettuce, Boston (approximately ⅓ head)	8	1.4	.7	.25	.1
1 cup	Lettuce, romaine	10	1.9	.7	.35	.2
1 cup	Lettuce, iceberg, raw	10	2.2	.7	.35	.1
3.3 ounces	Italian-mix vegetables (3.3 ounces)	30	6	2	1.5	0
1 cup	Lettuce, loose leaf	10	1.9	.7	.35	.2
1 cup	Mixed vegetables, cooked (peas, carrots, corn, limas, green beans)	151	30	7	4.2	0
1 cup	Mushrooms, sliced, raw (4 ounces)	20	3.1	1.9	.56	.2
1 cup	Mushrooms, canned, drained	51	6.9	3.3	-	.6
3.5 ounces	Mustard greens, raw	31	5.6	3	1.1	.5
1 cup	Mustard greens, cooked	29	5	3.1	1.82	.4
¼ pound	Mung bean sprouts	49	7.4	4.3	.2	.2
1 cup	Okra, raw	36	7.6	2.4	1	.3
1 cup	Okra, cooked	46	9.6	3.2	1.5	.5
1 cup	Onions, raw (approximately 1 small)	65	14.8	2.6	1	.2
1 cup	Onions, cooked	61	13.7	2.5	1.2	.2

Measure	Food					
1 cup	Green onions, bulb and top (approximately 4 whole)	36	8.2	1.5	1	.2
1 cup	Parsley, chopped, raw	26	5.1	2.2	.9	.4
½ large	Parsnip, raw	76	17.5	1.7	2	.5
1 cup	Parsnips, cooked	102	23.1	2.3	3	.8
1 cup	Peas, raw	122	20.9	9.1	2.9	.6
¼ pound	Peas, snow, edible pods	57	13	3.6	1.2	.2
1 cup	Peas, cooked	114	19.4	8.6	3.2	.6
1 cup	Peas, split, cooked	230	41.6	16	.8	.3
1 cup	Peppers, green, sliced, raw (approximately ½ large)	18	3.8	1	1.12	.2
1 cup	Peppers, green, sliced, cooked	24	5.1	1.4	1.89	.3
1 cup	Peppers, red, sliced, raw	31	7.1	1.4	-	.3
1 large	Pickle, dill	11	2.2	.7	.5	.4
1 large	Pickle, sweet	51	12.8	.2	.5	.1
1 Tbsp.	Pimientos, canned	7.6	1.6	.25	.16	.14
1 cup	Potatoes, raw, diced	114	25.7	3.2	-	.2
1 med.	Potato, boiled in skin	76	17.1	2.1	.5	.1
1 large	Potato, baked in skin	145	32.8	4	1.2	.2
1 med.	Potato, baked in skin	100	22	2	.5	t
1 cup	Pumpkin, canned	81	19.4	2.5	3	.7
10 med.	Radish, red, raw	8	1.6	.5	.35	t
1 cup	Rutabaga, raw	64	15.4	1.5	1.4	.1
1 cup	Rutabaga, cooked	60	13.9	1.5	2	.2

Quantity	Food	Calories	Carbohydrates	Protein	Fiber	Fat
1 Tbsp.	Shallots, chopped, raw	7	1.7	.3	1	t
1 cup	Spinach, raw (approximately ⅓ head)	14	2.4	1.8	.3	.2
1 cup	Spinach, cooked	41	6.5	5.4	1	.5
1 cup	Squash, summer, cooked (approximately 2 small, e.g., zucchini)	25	5.6	1.6	.8	.2
1 cup	Squash, winter, baked	129	31.6	3.7	2.6	.8
1 avg.	Sweet potato, baked	161	37	2.4	1.8	.6
1 med.	Tomato, raw	33	7	1.6	.8	.3
1 small	Tomato, raw	25	5	1.2	.6	.2
1 cup	Tomato, canned	51	10.4	2.4	.8	.5
1 cup	Tomato juice	46	10.4	2.2	.4	.2
1 Tbsp.	Tomato paste	13.5	3.04	.5	.1	t
1 cup	Tomato purée	97	22.2	4.2	1	.5

1 cup	Turnips, raw	39	8.6	1.3	1.15	.3
1 cup	Turnips, cooked	36	7.6	1.2	1.35	.3
3.5 ounces	Turnip greens, raw	28	5	3	.8	.3
1 cup	Turnip greens, cooked	29	5.2	3.2	1	.3
4 avg.	Water chestnuts	20	4.8	.4	.2	.1
1 cup	Watercress, raw	7	1.1	.8	.35	.1
1 cup	Yams, cooked in skin (approximately 1 small)	210	48.2	4.8	1.8	.4
1 ounce	Yeast, baker's, dry	80	11	10.5	.1	.5
1 ounce	Yeast, cake, compressed	24	3.1	3.4	-	.1
1 Tbsp.	Yeast, brewer's, debittered	23	3.1	3.1	.14	.1

PREPARED FOODS

6-inch diam.	Tortilla, yellow corn	63	13.5	1.5	.3	.6
1 Tbsp.	Apple butter, unsweetened	33	8.2	.1	.2	.1

STEP FIVE: How to Use Your Menus

Read through the menus. Shop for all that you need by using the shopping guide provided. Prepare all of the menus as they are without changing anything. After you have done this for the full four weeks, you will be more familiar with how these recipes differ from what you may be used to; which foods contain fiber; how to season foods so that they taste truly great; and how 1,800 calories feels at the end of each day. After the month is over, you can pick and choose. You may end up fixing your favorites repeatedly. That's fine! There is nothing wrong with enjoying the same healthy foods again and again as long as they are within the limits you will learn. You can also repeat the month indefinitely as is or with modifications (like switching days around, or adding another ingredient to a recipe, or even making up your own meals using the information in this chapter).

The menus are designed to generate the least amount of frustration on your part. We have deliberately avoided specifying fruits, due to the unavailability of all fruit year round. When you see the following items on your menu, follow these guidelines.

• *Fruit* = A normal-size serving of fruit (for example, 1 apple, or 1 orange, or ½ of a honeydew melon, or 100 calories' worth).

• *Bread* = 1 slice of whole-grain bread, which we will assume is approximately 56 calories. Choose whole-grain breads that have no added fats or sugar (see page 170, Whole-Grain Breads).

• *Green salad* = Any mixed salad that is mostly leaf lettuce like romaine or Boston. The dressing is to be made with 1 tablespoon of oil for two people. There is no limit to the vinegar or seasonings.

• *Herb tea* = Any tea that has no caffeine. These are available in the market and health food stores. Prepare herb tea as the package directs and then add one or more of the following: apple juice, lemon, honey. If you add 1 teaspoon of honey, your tea will contain approximately 25 calories.

• *Cold cereal* = Any whole-grain cereal without added fats or sugar (see page 172). Serve cereal with apple juice. If you absolutely must, use ½ cup nonfat milk.

We specify the above so that you will be very close to the calculations you find on each day's menu.

On the menus those dishes for which there are recipes are in capital letters. If the recipe says that it serves 4, each person is to be served ¼ of the entire recipe. Of course, you may halve the recipe. We didn't always do this, because we found instances where we would have to halve an egg white. We had trouble beating 1 egg white stiff, so we knew it would be impossible to beat ½ of one—if we were able to halve it in the first place.

The Calculations

The maximum daily number of calories per person should be 1,800. For each day you will find the total calories for breakfast, lunch, and dinner to be 100, 200, or even 600 less than 1,800. These missing calories are your "evening snack" calories. You may use these at any time of day, however. You also don't have to have exactly 1,800 calories; you may have less, but no more. Therefore, you can use all or only part of your evening snack calories. This should provide you with some fun flexibility. You can use the chart provided in this book to select snacks, or you can use one of the high-fiber recipes for a dessert. If the recipe contains 800 calories and you have 200 to "spend," simply consume one fourth of the entire recipe.

The percentage of carbohydrate desirable in your diet is no less than 60% and should be between 65% and 75% at all times. The following list gives you a quick comparison and explains why we eat a lot of fruits, vegetables, nuts, seeds, and especially grains.

• *Oatmeal* (1 cup) has 330 calories, 54 grams carbohydrate, and 1 gram of fiber (which is a type of carbohydrate that is not digested). Oatmeal has 65% carbohydrate, and if you include the fiber, the total is *66%.*

• *Oat bran* (1 cup) has 330 calories, 51 grams carbohydrate, and 24 grams of fiber. Oat bran has 61% carbohydrate, and if you include the fiber, the total is *90% carbohydrate.*

• *Blueberries* (1 cup) has 90 calories, 22.2 grams carbohydrate, and 2.2 grams fiber. Blueberries have 98% carbohydrate, and if you include the fiber, the total is *100%.* (So blueberries are basically all carbohydrate except for organic water, vitamins, minerals, and enzymes.)

Compare the above to this:

• *Turkey* (4 ounces) has 199 calories, 0 carbohydrate, and 0 grams fiber. Therefore, it is *0% carbohydrate.*
• *Cottage cheese* (1 cup) has 217 calories, 5.6 grams carbohydrate, and 0 grams fiber. Cottage cheese is *10% carbohydrate.* The turkey and the cottage cheese are mostly protein and fat.

Unfortunately we cannot just comsume a cup of oat bran. But we can mix various high-carbohydrate and high-fiber foods and come up with a very high percentage of carbohydrate. Because we need to add a tiny bit of other foods to vary the texture and flavors of our food, this lowers the total percentage somewhat. But with careful planning, we can still maintain a 65% to 75% total.

Occasionally there will be foods that have less than 65% carbohydrate. In our recipes you will notice that these foods are the ones that are eaten in smaller quantities, like salads. When we average these in with the other meals, we still come up with a 65% to 75% daily carbohydrate total.

You will notice that the percentages of carbohydrate, protein, and fat do not always add up to 100% as they seemingly should. This is due to the fact that available data has been rounded off (for example 16.6 might be rounded off to 17), and when you deal with hundreds of figures that have been rounded off, the final calculations cannot be 100% accurate. But the percentages given next to each recipe title are accurate in that they illustrate which foods are very high in fiber and carbohydrates and which are not. This, of course, is the purpose of doing the calculations in the first place!

Menus

WEEK ONE SHOPPING LIST

( ) Is your pantry stocked with the baking and condiment staples?

( ) Is your pantry stocked with the food staples?
(Check for wheat flour, oat bran, brown rice, raw sunflower seeds, cornmeal, barley, lentils, and oats.)

Fresh Foods

1 small bag of Alfalfa Sprouts
Apples, Pippin or other cooking apples
1 Avocado
Bananas (used in recipes as well as eaten plain)
¼ pound of Mung Bean Sprouts
Broccoli, 1 bunch
Cabbage, 1 head
Carrots (get a 1- or 2-pound bag)
1 small bunch of Celery
Fresh Corn, 1 ear per person
Cucumber, 1
(Don't forget Eggs)
Eggplant, 2 medium
Fruit (2–3 servings per day for 7 days)
Dandelion Greens, 1 bunch
Boston Lettuce, head
Romaine Lettuce, 1 head
Mushrooms, 2¾ pounds
Onions, Yellow, 8
Green Onions, 1 large bunch
¼ pound of Snow Peas
Green Peppers, 2 large
Russet Potatoes (get a 5- or 10-pound bag)
Raisins, 1 box
Tomatoes, fresh, 10
Yams, 2 small
Zucchini, 5

Frozen Foods

Apple juice, concentrated for sweetener
1 large bag frozen Peas
1 large bag unsweetened Strawberries

Canned or Jar Foods

Apple juice, for beverage
Applesauce, unsweetened
Garbanzo Beans (several cans)
Kidney Beans (several cans)
Beets, String or julienne, 1 or 2 cans
"Mrs. Dash," extra spicy (or you can just use your pepper)
Mushrooms (if you decide you prefer canned over fresh, you'll need 3 8-oz. cans)
Pickles, dill or sweet
Pimientos, 1 2-oz. jar

Other

If you plan to prepare any of the desserts, check the recipe and list the ingredients you will need here:

You'll use the following pastas:
Vegetable Rotelli (spiral pasta)
Spaghetti
Lasagna (1 8-ounce box)
Salad Macaroni

CALORIES

_____ **Breakfast** _____

Fruit 100
OAT BRAN WAFFLES 393
Butter Buds (2 tablespoons) 12
Herb Tea (with 1 teaspoon of honey) 25

_____ **Lunch** _____

GARDEN SOUP 421
Bread 56

_____ **Dinner** _____

Green Salad 150
RICE RAFFAELE 399
Ear of fresh Corn (with 1 tablespoon Butter Buds) 106
Fresh Fruit 100
                                                      ____
                           Total   1762

                    Evening snack calories   38

Oat Bran Waffles

1 cup water	1 teaspoon baking
1 ripe banana	powder
1 egg white	1 tablespoon olive oil
	½ teaspoon vanilla
	¾ cup whole-wheat flour
	½ cup oat bran

Put all the ingredients into a blender, except for the flour and bran. Blend. While the blender is running, add the flour and bran a little at a time. Cook on a medium-hot waffle iron. Serve with Butter Buds. These waffles are naturally sweet and crunchy. No additional syrup is needed unless desired. If so, use applesauce or fruit syrup.

Serves 2

OAT BRAN WAFFLES

4/4/9 CALORIES	:	393
CAL FROM CARB.	:	66%
CAL FROM PRO.	:	13%
CAL FROM FAT	:	21%

P/S RATIO   .59 : 1

DATE:

GRAM WT.	129.37	g	RIBOFLN	.27	mg
CHOLSTRL.	0.00	mg	NIACIN	2.22	mg
CALORIES	389.86	kcal	VIT C	5.15	mg
*PROTEIN	12.80	g	*PANTO.	.40	mg
*FAT	9.23	g	*B6	.35	mg
CARB.	64.78	g	*FOLACIN	17.15	mcg
CALCIUM	143.14	mg	*B12	.01	mcg
PHOS.	417.45	mg	*MAGNES.	96.96	mg
*IRON	1.93	mg	*ZINC	.43	mg
SODIUM	28.06	mg	SAT. FAT	1.00	g
*POTAS.	717.20	mg	MONO UNSAT.	4.97	g
*VIT A	46.00	IU	POLYUNSAT.	.60	g
THIAMIN	.60	mg	*FIBER	12.46	g

*Throughout this section, asterisks indicate the value may be higher due to unknown amounts for one or more foods.

Garden Soup

5 cups water	½ cup cooked garbanzo beans
1 potato, scrubbed and diced	1 cup peas, fresh or frozen and thawed
1 carrot, scrubbed and diced	1 apple, peeled and diced
1 small tomato, diced	4 ounces vegetable rotelli (spiral pasta)
1 small yellow onion, diced	1 tablespoon olive oil
¼ small head of cabbage, chopped (approximately 1 cup)	⅛ teaspoon pepper
	1 tablespoon vegetable-broth seasoning

Start the water boiling as you prepare the vegetables. Add the vegetables to the pot one by one as they are ready. Add the pasta, cover the pot, and cook for 10 minutes. Then add the oil and seasonings and simmer 3 to 5 more minutes.

Serves 4

Rice Raffaele

3 cups cooked brown rice	2 tablespoons tomato paste
1 tablespoon olive oil	1 cup water
½ small onion, chopped	2 tablespoons mild chile salsa
8 ounces fresh mushrooms, chopped	½ teaspoon oregano
1 large green pepper, chopped (approximately 2 cups)	2 tablespoons vegetable-broth seasoning
4 small zucchini, sliced and quartered	

Sauté the onion, mushrooms, green pepper, and zucchini in the olive oil. Add tomato paste and 1 cup water and stir. Add the remaining ingredients and simmer for 15 minutes. Stir in the rice and heat through for 5 more minutes.

Serves 4

GARDEN SOUP

4/4/9 CALORIES : 421
CAL FROM CARB. : 68%
CAL FROM PRO. : 14%
CAL FROM FAT : 17%

P/S RATIO   .65 : 1

DATE:

GRAM WT.	522.04	g	RIBOFLN	.29	mg
CHOLSTRL.	0.00	mg	NIACIN	4.16	mg
CALORIES	406.65	kcal	*VIT C	63.10	mg
PROTEIN	15.00	g	*PANTO.	1.01	mg
FAT	8.12	g	*B6	.51	mg
CARB.	72.04	g	*FOLACIN	136.59	mcg
CALCIUM	107.01	mg	*B12	.00	mcg
PHOS.	274.83	mg	*MAGNES.	78.96	mg
IRON	4.87	mg	ZINC	2.12	mg
SODIUM	129.90	mg	SAT. FAT	.93	g
*POTAS.	1021.25	mg	MONO UNSAT.	4.95	g
*VIT A	4967.00	IU	POLYUNSAT.	.60	g
THIAMIN	.53	mg	FIBER	4.41	g

RICE RAFFAELE

4/4/9 CALORIES : 399
CAL FROM CARB. : 70%
CAL FROM PRO. : 11%
CAL FROM FAT : 19%

P/S RATIO   .61 : 1

DATE:

GRAM WT.	624.93	g	RIBOFLN	.49	mg
CHOLSTRL.	0.00	mg	NIACIN	6.77	mg
CALORIES	387.61	kcal	VIT C	218.25	mg
PROTEIN	10.57	g	*PANTO.	4.13	mg
FAT	8.65	g	*B6	1.69	mg
CARB.	70.02	g	*FOLACIN	62.57	mcg
CALCIUM	99.22	mg	*B12	.00	mcg
PHOS.	285.54	mg	*MAGNES.	123.63	mg
IRON	3.68	mg	*ZINC	1.97	mg
SODIUM	685.37	mg	SAT. FAT	.90	g
*POTAS.	1020.65	mg	MONO UNSAT.	4.95	g
*VIT A	1562.81	IU	POLYUNSAT.	.55	g
THIAMIN	.45	mg	FIBER	4.42	g

DAY TWO MENUS

CALORIES

_____ **Breakfast** _____

Fruit	100
APPLE PANCAKES	339
Applesauce (½ cup)	50
Herb Tea	25

_____ **Lunch** _____

Green Salad	150
EGGPLANT GINA	241
Bread (1 slice)	56
Fruit	100

_____ **Dinner** _____

CUCUMBER SALAD	293
SPAGHETTI AND BROCCOLI	208
Total	1562

Evening snack calories   238

Apple Pancakes

½	cup whole-wheat flour	1	teaspoon cinnamon
¼	cup oat bran	2	egg whites, stiffly beaten
1	tablespoon olive oil	1½	cups apple juice
1	tablespoon baking soda	½	large apple, grated

Put the liquids in a blender. While it is running, add the dry ingredients. Pour into a bowl and fold in the egg whites and the grated apple. Bake on a hot griddle sprayed with Pam. Serve with applesauce.

Serves 2

APPLE PANCAKES

			4/4/9 CALORIES	: 339
			CAL FROM CARB.	: 65%
			CAL FROM PRO.	: 12%
			CAL FROM FAT	: 23%

P/S RATIO   .67 : 1

DATE:					
GRAM WT.	287.00	g	RIBOFLN	.19	mg
CHOLSTRL.	0.00	mg	NIACIN	1.66	mg
CALORIES	328.52	kcal	VIT C	2.97	mg
PROTEIN	10.35	g	*PANTO.	.42	mg
FAT	8.62	g	*B6	.17	mg
CARB.	55.26	g	*FOLACIN	17.43	mcg
CALCIUM	41.41	mg	*B12	.02	mcg
PHOS.	231.83	mg	MAGNES.	77.94	mg
IRON	2.01	mg	ZINC	.79	mg
SODIUM	57.13	mg	*SAT. FAT	.95	g
*POTAS.	501.62	mg	*MONO UNSAT.	4.96	g
*VIT A	29.00	IU	*POLYUNSAT.	.64	g
THIAMIN	.40	mg	FIBER	7.33	g

Eggplant Gina

1   medium eggplant, sliced lengthwise into approximately 12 slices
1   small onion, chopped
1   tablespoon oregano
1   tablespoon vegetable-broth seasoning
2   tablespoons hulled sunflower seeds

16 ounces fresh mush-rooms, sliced, or 8 ounces canned, rinsed
8   ounces spaghetti sauce, unsalted
1   tablespoon vegetable-broth seasoning

Layer the ingredients in a 9 x 14-inch casserole in the order given. Cover and bake at 400° for 45 minutes.

Serves 2

Cucumber Salad

½   cucumber, peeled, sliced thin, and quartered
2   green onions, chopped
1   small tomato, chopped
½   teaspoon oregano

2   tablespoons white wine vinegar with tarragon (optional)
1   tablespoon olive oil
1   teaspoon vegetable-broth seasoning
1   cup peas, thawed

Mix all of the ingredients together and serve on a bed of lettuce.

Serves 2

EGGPLANT GINA

4/4/9 CALORIES : 241
CAL FROM CARB. : 59%
CAL FROM PRO. : 16%
CAL FROM FAT : 25%

P/S RATIO   3.91 : 1

DATE:

GRAM WT.	508.35	g	RIBOFLN	.53	mg
CHOLSTRL.	0.00	mg	NIACIN	6.23	mg
CALORIES	218.99	kcal	*VIT C	75.75	mg
PROTEIN	9.84	g	*PANTO.	2.16	mg
FAT	6.84	g	*B6	.44	mg
CARB.	35.30	g	*FOLACIN	49.74	mcg
CALCIUM	81.75	mg	*B12	.01	mcg
PHOS.	280.48	mg	MAGNES.	81.13	mg
IRON	4.99	mg	*ZINC	.42	mg
SODIUM	37.69	mg	SAT. FAT	.72	g
POTAS.	1348.31	mg	MONO UNSAT.	2.01	g
*VIT A	1890.84	IU	POLYUNSAT.	2.82	g
THIAMIN	.49	mg	FIBER	4.04	g

CUCUMBER SALAD
Each Single Serving Contains

4/4/9 CALORIES : 293
CAL FROM CARB. : 42%
CAL FROM PRO. : 14%
CAL FROM FAT : 44%

P/S RATIO   .61 : 1

DATE:

GRAM WT.	397.00	g	*RIBOFLN	.22	mg
CHOLSTRL.	0.00	mg	*NIACIN	3.60	mg
CALORIES	278.30	kcal	*VIT C	64.00	mg
*PROTEIN	10.40	g	*PANTO.	1.00	mg
FAT	14.35	g	*B6	.32	mg
CARB.	30.90	g	*FOLACIN	57.95	mcg
CALCIUM	82.52	mg	*B12	0.00	mcg
PHOS.	198.66	mg	MAGNES.	66.21	mg
IRON	4.85	mg	*ZINC	1.96	mg
SODIUM	192.81	mg	SAT. FAT	1.80	g
*POTAS.	667.50	mg	MONO UNSAT.	9.90	g
*VIT A	2910.00	IU	POLYUNSAT.	1.10	g
*THIAMIN	.52	mg	*FIBER	4.41	g

Spaghetti and Broccoli

4   ounces uncooked
    spaghetti, preferably
    whole grain
1   large head or 2 cups
    cooked broccoli
1   tablespoon olive oil

1   tablespoon vegetable-
    broth seasoning
1   clove fresh garlic,
    minced
⅛   teaspoon black pepper

Cook the spaghetti following the package directions. Toss the cooked spaghetti, broccoli, and the seasonings together. Serve hot.

Serves 2

SPAGHETTI AND BROCCOLI

			4/4/9 CALORIES	: 208
			CAL FROM CARB.	: 52%
			CAL FROM PRO.	: 15%
			CAL FROM FAT	: 33%
P/S RATIO	.61 : 1			

DATE:					
GRAM WT.	228.25	g	*RIBOFLN	.37	mg
CHOLSTRL.	0.00	mg	*NIACIN	2.10	mg
CALORIES	197.65	kcal	*VIT C	140.00	mg
PROTEIN	8.15	g	*PANTO.	1.99	mg
*FAT	7.60	g	*B6	.27	mg
CARB.	27.00	g	*FOLACIN	83.79	mcg
CALCIUM	143.51	mg	*B12	.00	mcg
PHOS.	141.58	mg	MAGNES.	50.74	mg
*IRON	1.92	mg	ZINC	.35	mg
SODIUM	17.00	mg	SAT. FAT	.90	g
*POTAS.	473.50	mg	MONO UNSAT.	4.95	g
*VIT A	3880.00	IU	POLYUNSAT.	.55	g
THIAMIN	.26	mg	FIBER	2.41	g

DAY THREE MENUS

	CALORIES

_____ **Breakfast** _____

Fruit 100
EGG-WHITE OMELETTE OVER TOAST 287
Herb Tea 25

_____ **Lunch** _____

LARGE GREEN SALAD WITH GARBANZO BEANS 218
APPLE CORN MUFFINS 226

_____ **Dinner** _____

Green Salad 150
SPINACH LASAGNA 173
Fruit 100

	Total	1279

Evening snack calories	521

Egg-White Omelette

1 teaspoon olive oil
1 small tomato, diced
½ yellow onion, chopped
1 zucchini, sliced and quartered
4 ounces fresh mushrooms, sliced
1 slice green pepper, chopped

2 tablespoons mild chile salsa
1 teaspoon vegetable-broth seasoning
⅛ teaspoon black pepper
4 egg whites
4 pieces whole-grain bread, toasted

In a nonstick skillet, sauté the tomato, onion, zucchini, mushrooms, and green pepper in the olive oil. Add the salsa, seasoning, and pepper. While the mixture simmers, beat the egg whites with a fork and pour onto the mixture, stirring while it cooks to keep it from sticking. (Use a utensil safe for nonstick surfaces.) Cook until the egg sets. Spoon over toast.

Serves 2

EGG-WHITE OMELETTE

			4/4/9 CALORIES	: 287
			CAL FROM CARB.	: 52%
			CAL FROM PRO.	: 21%
			CAL FROM FAT	: 27%

P/S RATIO .86 : 1

DATE:

GRAM WT.	343.25	g	RIBOFLN	.45	mg
CHOLSTRL.	0.00	mg	NIACIN	3.50	mg
CALORIES	274.15	kcal	*VIT C	38.00	mg
PROTEIN	14.95	g	*PANTO.	1.15	mg
FAT	8.72	g	*B6	.24	mg
CARB.	37.67	g	*FOLACIN	38.21	mcg
CALCIUM	102.88	mg	*B12	.04	mcg
PHOS.	202.83	mg	*MAGNES.	74.94	mg
IRON	2.79	mg	*ZINC	1.97	mg
SODIUM	575.75	mg	SAT. FAT	1.10	g
*POTAS.	680.50	mg	MONO UNSAT.	5.55	g
*VIT A	950.00	IU	POLYUNSAT.	.95	g
THIAMIN	.24	mg	FIBER	2.20	g

Large Green Salad with Garbanzo Beans

(5.73 grams fiber)

1	head (Boston) lettuce, washed and dried	½	cup canned garbanzo beans, rinsed
1	tomato, chopped	2	teaspoons olive oil
1	cup canned julienne beets	2	tablespoons cider vinegar
¼	cup chopped green onions	1	tablespoon vegetable-broth seasoning
½	cup canned kidney beans, rinsed		

Tear the lettuce into bite-sized pieces. Toss with the remaining ingredients. Serve on a dinner plate.

Serves 2

Apple Corn Muffins

¾ cup whole-wheat flour	2 stiffly beaten egg whites
⅓ cup yellow cornmeal	½ cup apple juice
1 tablespoon baking powder	1 tablespoon olive oil
¼ cup finely grated apple	¼ cup puréed date or date "sugar"

Sift the dry ingredients together. Add the apple, beaten egg whites, apple juice, and oil. Stir in the date purée or date "sugar." Pour into Pam-sprayed muffin pan two-thirds full and bake in preheated 375° oven for 20 minutes or until done.

Makes 8 muffins

Spinach Lasagna

8 or 9 ounces uncooked lasagna noodles	1 large bunch fresh spinach, washed and stems removed
1 small eggplant, sliced into paper-thin, round slices	1 teaspoon oregano
¾ cup unsalted spaghetti sauce	12 ounces fresh mushrooms, sliced
1 tablespoon vegetable-broth seasoning	1 small onion, chopped
	2 tablespoons Parmesan cheese

Precook the lasagna noodles. When cooked, remove immediately from the water and separate. (If you leave them in the water, they will stick together and break when you try to remove them.) Spray a 9 x 14-inch Pyrex baking dish with Pam. Layer one layer of the noodles, then one layer of eggplant. Spread this with 4 table-spoons of the spaghetti sauce. Sprinkle with 1 teaspoon of vegetable-broth seasoning. Now layer a second layer of lasagna noodles. Heap the spinach over this second layer, about 4 leaves thick. Sprinkle with the oregano and another teaspoon of vegetable-broth seasoning. Layer a thin layer of lasagna noodles. Top with the remainder of the spaghetti sauce, the mushrooms, onions, the last teaspoon of vegetable-broth seasoning, and the 2 tablespoons of Parmesan, being careful to sprinkle it lightly so that it will cover the top. Cover with foil and bake at 350° for 45 minutes. Cut into squares; to serve, layer 2 squares so it will be thicker. The spinach flattens down during cooking.

Serves 4

LARGE GREEN SALAD W/ GARBANZO BEANS

4/4/9 CALORIES : 218
CAL FROM CARB. : 61%
CAL FROM PRO. : 17%
CAL FROM FAT : 22%

P/S RATIO   .61 : 1

DATE:

GRAM WT.	336.25	g	*RIBOFLN	.15	mg
CHOLSTRL.	0.00	mg	*NIACIN	1.40	mg
CALORIES	207.26	kcal	*VIT C	23.00	mg
*PROTEIN	9.68	g	*PANTO.	.55	mg
FAT	5.37	g	*B6	.08	mg
CARB.	33.12	g	*FOLACIN	111.81	mcg
CALCIUM	97.88	mg	*B12	0.00	mcg
PHOS.	186.17	mg	*MAGNES.	29.77	mg
IRON	5.06	mg	*ZINC	2.00	mg
SODIUM	215.03	mg	SAT. FAT	.60	g
*POTAS.	858.87	mg	MONO UNSAT.	3.30	g
*VIT A	1472.50	IU	POLYUNSAT.	.36	g
*THIAMIN	.19	mg	*FIBER	2.83	g

APPLE CORN MUFFINS

			4/4/9 CALORIES	: 226	
			CAL FROM CARB.	: 77%	
			CAL FROM PRO.	: 7%	
			CAL FROM FAT	: 16%	
P/S RATIO	.85 : 1				
DATE:					
GRAM WT.	125.75	g	RIBOFLN	.07	mg
CHOLSTRL.	0.00	mg	NIACIN	.33	mg
CALORIES	225.80	kcal	VIT C	1.53	mg
*PROTEIN	3.87	g	*PANTO.	.11	mg
*FAT	4.01	g	*B6	.03	mg
CARB.	43.96	g	*FOLACIN	4.30	mcg
CALCIUM	172.33	mg	*B12	.01	mcg
PHOS.	275.08	mg	*MAGNES.	8.42	mg
*IRON	.51	mg	*ZINC	.08	mg
SODIUM	26.95	mg	SAT. FAT	.50	g
*POTAS.	480.93	mg	MONO UNSAT.	2.56	g
*VIT A	61.08	IU	POLYUNSAT.	.42	g
THIAMIN	.04	mg	*FIBER	.40	g

SPINACH LASAGNA

			4/4/9 CALORIES	: 173	
			CAL FROM CARB.	: 72%	
			CAL FROM PRO.	: 17%	
			CAL FROM FAT	: 10%	
P/S RATIO	.11 : 1				
DATE:					
GRAM WT.	246.60	g	RIBOFLN	.30	mg
CHOLSTRL.	2.00	mg	NIACIN	3.06	mg
CALORIES	168.77	kcal	VIT C	40.59	mg
PROTEIN	7.65	g	*PANTO.	.83	mg
FAT	2.09	g	*B6	.21	mg
CARB.	31.45	g	*FOLACIN	36.33	mcg
CALCIUM	87.95	mg	*B12	.00	mcg
PHOS.	144.16	mg	MAGNES.	62.55	mg
IRON	3.00	mg	*ZINC	.51	mg
SODIUM	78.29	mg	SAT. FAT	.55	g
POTAS.	603.66	mg	MONO UNSAT.	.65	g
*VIT A	2948.05	IU	POLYUNSAT.	.06	g
THIAMIN	.24	mg	FIBER	1.32	g

DAY FOUR MENUS

_____Breakfast_____

Fruit 100
CORNMEAL WAFFLES 588
STRAWBERRY SYRUP 80
Herb Tea 25

_____Lunch_____

POTATO SOUP 258
Bread 56

_____Dinner_____

Green Salad 150
SPAGHETTI AND GREENS 159

                              Total   1416

                              Evening snack calories   384

Cornmeal Waffles

1¼	cups water	1	teaspoon baking powder
2	tablespoons olive oil		
1	cup whole-wheat flour	1	tablespoon honey
½	cup cornmeal or flour	2	egg whites, stiffly beaten

In the blender, blend together the water, oil, and honey. Add the flours a little at a time, along with the baking powder. Pour into a bowl and fold in the egg whites. Cook on a medium-hot waffle iron that has been sprayed with Pam. Serve with Butter Buds and/ or strawberry syrup.

Serves 2

Strawberry Syrup

½	cup mashed strawberries	2	teaspoons tapioca granules
½	cup apple juice	1	tablespoon honey

Cook the combined ingredients in a saucepan, bringing to a bubble and stirring constantly. Remove from the heat and let cool down to warm.

Serves 2

CORNMEAL WAFFLES
Per Single Serving

4/4/9 CALORIES : 588
CAL FROM CARB. : 53%
CAL FROM PRO. : 24%
CAL FROM FAT : 24%

P/S RATIO .76 : 1

DATE:

GRAM WT.	358.50	g	RIBOFLN	.78	mg
CHOLSTRL.	0.00	mg	NIACIN	3.26	mg
CALORIES	580.88	kcal	VIT C	.09	mg
*PROTEIN	34.96	g	*PANTO.	1.26	mg
*FAT	15.46	g	*B6	.21	mg
CARB.	77.64	g	*FOLACIN	61.11	mcg
CALCIUM	162.10	mg	*B12	.15	mcg
PHOS.	438.16	mg	*MAGNES.	89.11	mg
*IRON	2.69	mg	*ZINC	1.60	mg
SODIUM	372.92	mg	*SAT. FAT	1.87	g
*POTAS.	807.83	mg	*MONO UNSAT.	10.15	g
*VIT A	100.00	IU	*POLYUNSAT.	1.42	g
THIAMIN	.40	mg	*FIBER	1.58	g

STRAWBERRY SYRUP
Per Single Serving

4/4/9 CALORIES : 80
CAL FROM CARB. : 97%
CAL FROM PRO. : 1%
CAL FROM FAT : 1%

P/S RATIO 4.66 : 1

DATE:

GRAM WT.	111.15	g	RIBOFLN	.04	mg
CHOLSTRL.	0.00	mg	NIACIN	.19	mg
CALORIES	77.25	kcal	VIT C	21.79	mg
PROTEIN	.33	g	*PANTO.	.14	mg
FAT	.21	g	*B6	.04	mg
CARB.	19.72	g	FOLACIN	7.04	mcg
CALCIUM	9.91	mg	B12	0.00	mcg
PHOS.	12.33	mg	MAGNES.	6.35	mg
IRON	.42	mg	*ZINC	.16	mg
SODIUM	2.79	mg	SAT. FAT	.01	g
POTAS.	141.58	mg	MONO UNSAT.	.02	g
VIT A	10.75	IU	POLYUNSAT.	.08	g
THIAMIN	.02	mg	*FIBER	.32	g

Potato Soup

4	cups water	½	teaspoon extra-spicy "Mrs. Dash" or black pepper
5	large potatoes, peeled and quartered		
2	large carrots, scrubbed and chopped	1	clove garlic, minced
1	cup diced onions	3	tablespoons vegetable-broth seasoning
4	ounces fresh mushrooms, diced	3	tablespoons date "sugar"

Combine the water, potatoes, carrots, and onions in a large pot. Bring to a boil. Turn down the heat and simmer for 15 minutes. Blend the mixture in a blender until smooth. Return to the pot and add the mushrooms and seasonings. Simmer for 10 minutes more. Serve garnished with parsley or chopped chives.

Serves 4

Spaghetti and Greens

4	ounces spaghetti, preferably whole grain	1	tablespoon vegetable-broth seasoning
1	cup cooked dandelion greens (about 3.5 ounces raw)	1	clove fresh garlic, minced
1	tablespoon olive oil	⅛	teaspoon black pepper

Cook the spaghetti according to the package instructions but with just enough water to cover the dry pasta. When cooked, the pasta should have absorbed all of the water, leaving it just a little soupy, but not swimming in water. Do not drain, but toss with the remaining ingredients, using a fork to separate the greens, and mixing them throughout the pasta.

Serves 2

POTATO SOUP
Per Single Serving

4/4/9 CALORIES : 258
CAL FROM CARB. : 89%
CAL FROM PRO. : 10%
CAL FROM FAT : 1%

P/S RATIO   0 : 1

DATE:

GRAM WT.	415.79	g	*RIBOFLN	.17	mg
CHOLSTRL.	0.00	mg	*NIACIN	4.01	mg
CALORIES	251.75	kcal	*VIT C	52.50	mg
PROTEIN	6.71	g	*PANTO.	.34	mg
*FAT	.37	g	*B6	.68	mg
CARB.	57.48	g	*FOLACIN	32.01	mcg
CALCIUM	43.25	mg	*B12	0.00	mcg
PHOS.	158.62	mg	*MAGNES.	84.92	mg
*IRON	1.93	mg	*ZINC	.67	mg
SODIUM	29.21	mg	SAT. FAT	0.00	g
POTAS.	1031.52	mg	MONO UNSAT.	0.00	g
*VIT A	3982.50	IU	POLYUNSAT.	0.00	g
THIAMIN	.29	mg	FIBER	2.29	g

SPAGHETTI AND GREENS
Per Single Serving

4/4/9 CALORIES : 159
CAL FROM CARB. : 50%
CAL FROM PRO. : 9%
CAL FROM FAT : 42%

P/S RATIO   .61 : 1

DATE:

GRAM WT.	130.75	g	*RIBOFLN	.14	mg
CHOLSTRL.	0.00	mg	*NIACIN	.75	mg
CALORIES	156.65	kcal	*VIT C	9.50	mg
PROTEIN	3.55	g	*PANTO.	.00	mg
*FAT	7.35	g	*B6	.01	mg
CARB.	19.90	g	*FOLACIN	.09	mcg
CALCIUM	79.51	mg	*B12	.00	mcg
PHOS.	60.08	mg	MAGNES.	32.04	mg
*IRON	1.62	mg	*ZINC	.11	mg
SODIUM	24.00	mg	SAT. FAT	.90	g
*POTAS.	172.50	mg	MONO UNSAT.	4.95	g
*VIT A	6145.00	IU	POLYUNSAT.	.55	g
THIAMIN	.17	mg	FIBER	.77	g

CALORIES

_____ **Breakfast** _____

Fruit 100
COLD CEREAL* 170
DATE BRAN MUFFINS (2) with 1 tablespoon (unsweetened)
   Apple Butter 219
Herb Tea 25

_____ **Lunch** _____

SLOPPY MOES on 2 slices of Bread 464
Lettuce Leaf and Tomato Slices for garnish 15

_____ **Dinner** _____

GREEN SALAD ROMANA 84
YAMS, YES! 268
Mixed Vegetables** with Butter Buds (1 tablespoon Butter
   Buds for 1 cup vegetables) 157
   (**peas, carrots, corn, lima beans, green beans)
Fresh Fruit 100

                                        Total   1602

                              Evening snack calories   198

*COLD CEREAL—see examples on page 172.

Date Bran Muffins

1 ¼-ounce package active
   dry yeast
1 cup apple juice, warmed
1 tablespoon unsul-
   phured molasses

1 cup oat bran
¾ cup whole-wheat flour
½ cup chopped dates
2 egg whites
1 tablespoon olive oil

Dissolve the yeast in ¼ cup warm apple juice and add the molasses. Mix the oat bran, flour, and chopped dates and add to the yeast mixture. Stir in the egg whites, olive oil, and remaining apple juice. Let the mixture stand for 15 minutes while you preheat the oven to 350°. Spray muffin pan with Pam and pour in mixture until cups are two-thirds full. Bake 25 minutes or until muffins spring back when pressed lightly in the center.

Makes 12 muffins

Sloppy Moes

1 cup cooked barley
¾ cup unsalted spaghetti
   sauce

1 apple, peeled and cut
   into bite-size chunks
1 tablespoon vegetable-
   broth seasoning

Mix the cooked barley with the spaghetti sauce and raw apple. Mix in the vegetable-broth seasoning. Serve on toast. Garnish with a lettuce leaf and orange, pineapple, or tomato slices.

Serves 2

Green Salad Romana

6 outer leaves from head of romaine lettuce (save the inner leaves for a hearts of romaine salad)

¼ cup chopped green onions

1 small tomato, chopped

1 tablespoon olive oil

1 teaspoon vegetable-broth seasoning

1 tablespoon cider vinegar

1 tablespoon water

Tear the lettuce leaves into bite-size pieces. Toss with the remaining ingredients.

Serves 2

Yams, Yes!

2 small yams, peeled and cut into "carrot stick" pieces

1 tablespoon olive oil

1 tablespoon Parmesan cheese, grated

1 small onion, chopped

Toss all the ingredients together and put into a 1-quart casserole. Cover and bake at 350° for 1 hour. Serve hot. To brown better, remove the casserole lid the last 15 minutes.

Serves 2

DATE BRAN MUFFINS
Per Single Serving

4/4/9 CALORIES : 219
CAL FROM CARB. : 71%
CAL FROM PRO. : 14%
CAL FROM FAT : 16%

P/S RATIO   .63 : 1

DATE:

GRAM WT.	88.91	g	RIBOFLN	.16	mg
CHOLSTRL.	0.00	mg	NIACIN	1.63	mg
CALORIES	210.47	kcal	*VIT C	.38	mg
*PROTEIN	7.61	g	*PANTO.	.44	mg
*FAT	3.83	g	*B6	.12	mg
CARB.	38.88	g	*FOLACIN	44.60	mcg
CALCIUM	35.49	mg	*B12	.00	mcg
PHOS.	215.11	mg	MAGNES.	71.58	mg
IRON	1.41	mg	*ZINC	.42	mg
SODIUM	20.76	mg	*SAT. FAT	.30	g
*POTAS.	389.25	mg	*MONO UNSAT.	1.65	g
*VIT A	7.75	IU	*POLYUNSAT.	.19	g
THIAMIN	.38	mg	*FIBER	8.78	g

SLOPPY MOES
Per Single Serving

4/4/9 CALORIES : 464
CAL FROM CARB. : 86%
CAL FROM PRO. : 9%
CAL FROM FAT : 5%

P/S RATIO   .84 : 1

DATE:

GRAM WT.	277.21	g	RIBOFLN	.11	mg
CHOLSTRL.	0.00	mg	NIACIN	4.42	mg
CALORIES	447.80	kcal	VIT C	48.34	mg
PROTEIN	10.18	g	PANTO.	.59	mg
FAT	2.64	g	B6	.32	mg
CARB.	100.42	g	*FOLACIN	4.64	mcg
CALCIUM	37.41	mg	B12	.00	mcg
PHOS.	232.32	mg	MAGNES.	59.79	mg
IRON	3.70	mg	*ZINC	.14	mg
SODIUM	13.58	mg	SAT. FAT	.19	g
POTAS.	645.58	mg	MONO UNSAT.	.88	g
VIT A	1410.60	IU	POLYUNSAT.	.16	g
THIAMIN	.22	mg	FIBER	1.65	g

GREEN SALAD ROMANA

			4/4/9 CALORIES	: 84
			CAL FROM CARB.	: 21%
			CAL FROM PRO.	: 5%
			CAL FROM FAT	: 74%

P/S RATIO .61 : 1

DATE:

GRAM WT.	99.75	g	*RIBOFLN	.04	mg
CHOLSTRL.	0.00	mg	*NIACIN	.45	mg
CALORIES	80.15	kcal	*VIT C	19.50	mg
*PROTEIN	1.03	g	*PANTO.	.16	mg
FAT	6.97	g	*B6	.04	mg
CARB.	4.57	g	*FOLACIN	17.59	mcg
CALCIUM	31.38	mg	*B12	.00	mcg
PHOS.	24.95	mg	MAGNES.	11.44	mg
IRON	.85	mg	*ZINC	.27	mg
SODIUM	4.70	mg	SAT. FAT	.90	g
*POTAS.	219.87	mg	MONO UNSAT.	4.95	g
*VIT A	1185.00	IU	POLYUNSAT.	.55	g
*THIAMIN	.04	mg	*FIBER	.57	g

YAMS, YES!

			4/4/9 CALORIES	: 268
			CAL FROM CARB.	: 66%
			CAL FROM PRO.	: 7%
			CAL FROM FAT	: 27%

P/S RATIO .41 : 1

DATE:

GRAM WT.	208.13	g	RIBOFLN	.12	mg
CHOLSTRL.	2.00	mg	NIACIN	.95	mg
CALORIES	264.65	kcal	VIT C	33.50	mg
PROTEIN	4.74	g	*PANTO.	1.05	mg
FAT	8.20	g	*B6	.36	mg
CARB.	44.49	g	*FOLACIN	23.18	mcg
CALCIUM	103.51	mg	*B12	.00	mcg
PHOS.	116.58	mg	MAGNES.	47.00	mg
IRON	1.50	mg	ZINC	1.15	mg
SODIUM	69.00	mg	SAT. FAT	1.37	g
*POTAS.	478.00	mg	MONO UNSAT.	5.17	g
*VIT A	9282.50	IU	POLYUNSAT.	.56	g
THIAMIN	.12	mg	FIBER	1.53	g

Breakfast

Fruit	100
CINNAMON-RAISIN OATMEAL	159
Herb Tea	25

Lunch

MACARONI SALAD	319
Muffins (2)	200

Dinner

Green Salad	150
LENTIL STEW	162
Bread	56
Fresh Fruit	100
Total	1271

Evening snack calories 529

Cinnamon-Raisin Oatmeal

1¾	cups water	¾	teaspoon cinnamon
¾	cup oatmeal	¼	cup raisins

Bring the water to a boil. Stir in the oatmeal and cook for 5 minutes. Add the cinnamon and raisins and remove from heat. Serve with apple juice or ½ cup nonfat milk. Or serve with no liquid—it is delicious as is!

Serves 2

Macaroni Salad

1	cup uncooked salad macaroni (whole wheat)	1	cup cooked peas
1	tablespoon olive oil	4	tablespoons chopped pimientos
2	hard-cooked egg whites, chopped	2	tablespoons cider vinegar
1	tablespoon minced green onions	1	teaspoon prepared mustard
2	tablespoons minced sweet or dill pickle (whichever you prefer)	2	teaspoons vegetable-broth seasoning

Cook the macaroni according to the package directions. When the macaroni is cooked, drain and rinse, and immediately toss with the olive oil (to prevent sticking). Add the remaining ingredients in the order given, tossing with the vinegar, mustard, and vegetable-broth seasoning. Serve on a bed of lettuce, garnished with apple slices.

Serves 2

Lentil Stew

4 cups water
1 cup uncooked lentils
1 medium potato, scrubbed and cut into bite-size pieces
1 large carrot, scrubbed and cut into bite-size pieces
1 tablespoon tomato sauce
1 tablespoon vegetable-broth seasoning

Bring the water to a boil and add the lentils. Turn down the heat and simmer for 15 minutes. Add the potato and carrot and cook for 30 minutes more. Add the remaining ingredients and cook a final 10 to 15 minutes. Serve with bread or muffins and a salad.

Serves 4

Leftovers Suggestion: Toast a corn tortilla in a toaster and use warmed leftover lentil stew as a bean filling: Place 2 tablespoons in center of tortilla with 1 teaspoon or more of mild chile salsa. Roll and eat.

CINNAMON-RAISIN OATMEAL
Per Single Serving

			4/4/9 CALORIES	: 159	
			CAL FROM CARB.	: 80%	
			CAL FROM PRO.	: 10%	
			CAL FROM FAT	: 10%	

P/S RATIO 1.92 : 1

DATE:

GRAM WT.	198.12	g	RIBOFLN	.05	mg
CHOLSTRL.	0.00	mg	NIACIN	.29	mg
CALORIES	153.25	kcal	VIT C	.60	mg
PROTEIN	4.18	g	PANTO.	2.70	mg
FAT	1.88	g	B6	.41	mg
CARB.	31.81	g	FOLACIN	60.00	mcg
CALCIUM	25.37	mg	B12	0.00	mcg
PHOS.	120.25	mg	MAGNES.	43.80	mg
IRON	1.42	mg	ZINC	1.69	mg
SODIUM	394.37	mg	SAT. FAT	.40	g
POTAS.	245.62	mg	MONO UNSAT.	.60	g
VIT A	1.37	IU	POLYUNSAT.	.77	g
THIAMIN	.17	mg	FIBER	.59	g

MACARONI SALAD
Per Single Serving

			4/4/9 CALORIES	: 319	
			CAL FROM CARB.	: 62%	
			CAL FROM PRO.	: 16%	
			CAL FROM FAT	: 22%	

P/S RATIO .61 : 1

DATE:

GRAM WT.	321.00	g	*RIBOFLN	.29	mg
CHOLSTRL.	0.00	mg	*NIACIN	3.01	mg
CALORIES	316.90	kcal	*VIT C	38.25	mg
*PROTEIN	12.65	g	*PANTO.	.33	mg
FAT	7.85	g	*B6	.10	mg
CARB.	49.96	g	*FOLACIN	25.42	mcg
CALCIUM	37.51	mg	*B12	.02	mcg
PHOS.	151.83	mg	*MAGNES.	48.24	mg
IRON	3.51	mg	*ZINC	1.47	mg
*SODIUM	250.17	mg	SAT. FAT	.90	g
*POTAS.	260.00	mg	MONO UNSAT.	4.95	g
*VIT A	1190.00	IU	POLYUNSAT.	.55	g
*THIAMIN	.42	mg	*FIBER	1.98	g

LENTIL STEW
Per Single Serving

			4/4/9 CALORIES	: 162
			CAL FROM CARB.	: 77%
			CAL FROM PRO.	: 23%
			CAL FROM FAT	: 1%

P/S RATIO .59 : 1

DATE:

GRAM WT.	179.40	g	RIBOFLN	.09	mg
CHOLSTRL.	0.00	mg	NIACIN	1.60	mg
CALORIES	159.17	kcal	VIT C	12.35	mg
PROTEIN	9.27	g	*PANTO.	1.55	mg
*FAT	.13	g	B6	.61	mg
CARB.	31.23	g	FOLACIN	112.53	mcg
CALCIUM	36.43	mg	*B12	.00	mcg
PHOS.	157.34	mg	*MAGNES.	17.48	mg
IRON	2.64	mg	ZINC	1.22	mg
*SODIUM	10.67	mg	SAT. FAT	.00	g
POTAS.	558.92	mg	MONO UNSAT.	.03	g
*VIT A	2059.73	IU	POLYUNSAT.	.003	g
THIAMIN	.13	mg	FIBER	1.69	g

CALORIES

_____**Breakfast**_____

Fruit	100
FIBER FRENCH TOAST	74
Fruit Syrup (from Day Four, or store-bought;	
unsweetened, 2 tablespoons)	21
Herb Tea	25

_____**Lunch**_____

SPROUT SANDWICH	213
Lettuce Leaf and Pineapple Rings, unsweetened,	
as a garnish	50
Fresh Fruit	100

_____**Dinner**_____

ORIENTAL DINNER	480
Bread	56
Total	1119

Evening snack calories   681

Fiber French Toast

4	slices whole-grain bread	½	teaspoon cinnamon
1	cup apple juice	½	teaspoon vanilla
1	tablespoon tapioca granules	1	tablespoon date pieces
		1	ripe banana

Put all ingredients except bread into a blender in the order given. Blend for 3 minutes. In a bowl, dip bread into the mixture briefly and bake on a Pam-sprayed griddle. Let cook until browned; this takes a little bit longer than with egg batter. Serve with homemade or store-bought fruit syrup. Also can be served with just Butter Buds.

Serves 4

FIBER FRENCH TOAST
Per Single Serving

		4/4/9 CALORIES	: 74
		CAL FROM CARB.	: 96%
		CAL FROM PRO.	: 1%
		CAL FROM FAT	: 3%

P/S RATIO   .70 : 1

DATE:

GRAM WT.	95.38	g	RIBOFLN	.04	mg
CHOLSTRL.	0.00	mg	NIACIN	.27	mg
CALORIES	70.39	kcal	VIT C	3.15	mg
PROTEIN	.41	g	*PANTO.	.09	mg
FAT	.22	g	*B6	.18	mg
CARB.	17.78	g	FOLACIN	5.97	mcg
CALCIUM	6.90	mg	B12	0.00	mcg
PHOS.	11.59	mg	MAGNES.	11.29	mg
IRON	.35	mg	*ZINC	.07	mg
SODIUM	2.14	mg	*SAT. FAT	.06	g
POTAS.	205.39	mg	*MONO UNSAT.	.01	g
VIT A	24.89	IU	*POLYUNSAT.	.04	g
THIAMIN	.02	mg	FIBER	.33	g

Sprout Sandwich

4	slices whole-grain bread	1	teaspoon vegetable-broth seasoning
2	teaspoons prepared mustard	1	small tomato, sliced thin
¼	avocado	2	cups alfalfa sprouts

Spread 2 of the bread slices with ½ teaspoon mustard. On the remaining 2 slices of bread, layer the following: ⅛ of the avocado, ½ teaspoon vegetable-broth seasoning, ½ of the tomato, and a handful of sprouts. Top with the other slice of bread and cut in half. Serve each sandwich on a plate with lettuce leaf and unsweetened pineapple ring or orange or apple slices. You may garnish with a fresh or frozen strawberry for color.

Serves 2

Oriental Dinner

1	tablespoon olive oil	¼	cup water
½	large green pepper, sliced	1	tablespoon arrowroot flour
1	stalk of celery, chopped (about 1 cup)	1	cup water
¼	pound snow peas, deveined	1	tablespoon low-sodium soy sauce
½	small onion, chopped	1	tablespoon vegetable-broth seasoning
¼	pound mung sprouts	½	of an 8-ounce can of sliced water chestnuts
4	ounces fresh mushrooms, sliced	2	cups cooked rice
1	tablespoon sliced canned pimientos (optional, for color)		

In a skillet, sauté the green pepper, celery, snow peas, onion, sprouts, mushrooms, and pimiento in the olive oil. Place the vegetables in the skillet in the order given, so that the green pepper is cooked the longest, and so on. This will take approximately 15 minutes to complete. After the pimiento is added, mix the ¼ cup water with the arrowroot and stir into skillet. Allow the vegetables to cook more. Combine the 1 cup of water with the seasonings, mix in, and then add the chestnuts. Serve over 1 cup rice per person.

Serves 2

ORIENTAL DINNER
Per Single Serving

			4/4/9 CALORIES	: 480
			CAL FROM CARB.	: 72%
			CAL FROM PRO.	: 11%
			CAL FROM FAT	: 17%

P/S RATIO .61 : 1

DATE:

GRAM WT.	500.38	g	RIBOFLN	.36	mg
CHOLSTRL.	0.00	mg	NIACIN	5.39	mg
CALORIES	471.14	kcal	*VIT C	44.08	mg
PROTEIN	13.13	g	*PANTO.	5.40	mg
FAT	9.15	g	*B6	1.77	mg
CARB.	86.56	g	*FOLACIN	150.72	mcg
CALCIUM	95.85	mg	*B12	0.00	mcg
PHOS.	325.91	mg	*MAGNES.	124.71	mg
IRON	4.08	mg	*ZINC	1.43	mg
*SODIUM	1155.87	mg	*SAT. FAT	.90	g
*POTAS.	888.87	mg	*MONO UNSAT.	4.95	g
*VIT A	590.31	IU	*POLYUNSAT.	.55	g
THIAMIN	.46	mg	*FIBER	3.43	g

WEEK TWO SHOPPING LIST

( ) Is your pantry stocked with the baking and condiment staples?

( ) Is your pantry stocked with the food staples?
(Check for millet and split peas, barley, and cornmeal)

Fresh Foods

Oranges (recipe and
eat)
Carrots (half a dozen)
(Don't forget eggs)
Celery (1 stalk)
Cabbage (2 small heads)
Zucchini (half a dozen)
"Pink" Potatoes (2)
Fresh Mushrooms (16
ounces)
Green Pepper (1 large)
Fruit (2–3 servings per
day for 7 days)
Bananas (used in re-
cipes as well as eaten
plain)
Broccoli (1 head)
Purple Onion (1 large)
Parsley (1 bunch)
Yellow Summer Squash
(3 small)
Dried Apricots (⅓ cup)
(get a pound or more;
you'll use them)
Mustard Greens, fresh
young (1 bunch)
White Rose Potatoes (2
large)
Eggplant (1 large)
Cauliflower (1 head)
Leaf Lettuce for salads

Frozen Foods

Baby Lima beans
(10 ounce)
Green Beans (10 ounce)
Corn (10 ounce)
French-cut Green Beans
(10 ounce)
Black-eyed peas
(10 ounce)
Blueberries (1 small
package,
unsweetened)
Corn-on-the Cob (have
several packages on
hand)

Canned or Jar Foods

Kidney Beans (1 or more
cans)
Italian Tomatoes,
peeled and diced
(1 can)
Julienne beets (1 or
more cans, use in
salads)
Cannellini (1 15-ounce
can)
Pinto beans (if without
sugar) and if you
don't cook your own

Other

You'll use the following
pastas:
  "Orzo," a rice-like
  pasta
  "Spinach
  Spaghetti"
  "Soup Mix" (a
  mixture of rice,
  split peas, lentils,
  barley, pasta,
  etc., available
  where you buy
  rice and pasta)
  "Cavatelli"
  Spinach Pastina
  (tiny soup pasta)

Dessert ingredients
(check the recipes)

CALORIES

_____ **Breakfast** _____

Fruit 100
Cold Cereal 170
BLUEBERRY MUFFINS 249
Herb Tea 25

_____ **Lunch** _____

BLACK-EYED PEA SOUP 248
Bread w/ unsweetened Fruit Jam 77

_____ **Dinner** _____

ZUCCHINI CASSEROLE 97
STUFT MUSHROOMS 74
Bread 56
Fruit 100

                          Total   1196

                 Evening snack calories   604

Blueberry Muffins

1 cup apple juice	1 tablespoon baking powder
1 orange, peeled and sectioned	1 cup whole-wheat flour
1 small carrot, sliced	¾ cup oat bran
1 teaspoon vanilla	1 cup blueberries (fresh or frozen)
½ cup date sugar	2 egg whites, stiffly beaten
2 teaspoons cinnamon	
1 tablespoon olive oil	

In the blender, purée the apple juice, orange, and carrot together. Add the vanilla, date sugar, cinnamon, and olive oil while the blender is running. Pour mixture into a large bowl and, with a hand mixer, beat in the baking powder, flour, and bran. Fold in the berries, then the egg whites. Pour into Pam-sprayed, nonstick muffin pan, and bake in preheated 350° oven for 20 to 30 minutes, until center springs back when touched.

Makes 12 muffins

BLUEBERRY MUFFINS
Per Single Serving

			4/4/9 CALORIES	: 249	
			CAL FROM CARB.	: 76%	
			CAL FROM PRO.	: 11%	
			CAL FROM FAT	: 13%	

P/S RATIO   .65 : 1

DATE:

GRAM WT.	127.34	g	RIBOFLN	.10	mg
CHOLSTRL.	0.00	mg	NIACIN	1.17	mg
CALORIES	242.17	kcal	VIT C	13.00	mg
*PROTEIN	6.95	g	*PANTO.	.33	mg
*FAT	3.60	g	*B6	.11	mg
CARB.	47.72	g	*FOLACIN	16.87	mcg
CALCIUM	144.57	mg	*B12	.00	mcg
PHOS.	350.02	mg	*MAGNES.	63.48	mg
*IRON	1.14	mg	*ZINC	.59	mg
SODIUM	25.13	mg	*SAT. FAT	.31	g
*POTAS.	554.79	mg	*MONO UNSAT.	1.65	g
*VIT A	1366.83	IU	*POLYUNSAT.	.20	g
THIAMIN	.33	mg	*FIBER	6.77	g

Black-Eyed Pea Soup

4	cups water	¼	cup cooked kidney beans
1	cup chopped celery		
2	cups cut-up cabbage	½	cup cooked barley
4	rounded tablespoons orzo (ricelike pasta)	1	cup cooked black-eyed peas
1	medium zucchini, quartered and sliced	¼	cup unsalted spaghetti sauce
½	cup cooked baby lima beans	1	tablespoon vegetable-broth seasoning
		1	tablespoon olive oil

Put the water in a large pot and add the celery, cabbage, orzo, zucchini, lima beans, kidney beans, barley, and black-eyed peas. Cook for 20 minutes. Add the spaghetti sauce, seasoning, and olive oil and cook 10 more minutes.

Serves 4

Zucchini Casserole

1	large (approximately 8 x 2 inches) zucchini cut into ½-inch slices	1	stalk celery, chopped
½	onion, diced	1	(16 ounce) can Italian tomatoes, diced
2	small pink potatoes, un-peeled and diced	1	teaspoon olive oil
4	ounces fresh mush-rooms, sliced	1	tablespoon vegetable-broth seasoning
		1	teaspoon crushed basil leaves

Combine the fresh vegetables in a covered casserole. Add the remaining ingredients. Cover with the casserole lid and cook in the oven at 350° for 1 hour.

Serves 4

BLACK-EYED PEA SOUP
Per Single Serving

			4/4/9 CALORIES	: 248
			CAL FROM CARB.	: 69%
			CAL FROM PRO.	: 15%
			CAL FROM FAT	: 16%

P/S RATIO   .61 : 1

DATE:

GRAM WT.	240.47	g	RIBOFLN	.15	mg
CHOLSTRL.	0.00	mg	NIACIN	2.56	mg
CALORIES	240.10	kcal	*VIT C	40.40	mg
PROTEIN	9.74	g	*PANTO.	.62	mg
FAT	4.45	g	*B6	.21	mg
CARB.	42.72	g	*FOLACIN	59.12	mcg
CALCIUM	69.67	mg	*B12	.00	mcg
PHOS.	192.61	mg	*MAGNES.	65.96	mg
IRON	3.01	mg	*ZINC	.99	mg
SODIUM	77.61	mg	*SAT. FAT	.47	g
*POTAS.	644.43	mg	*MONO UNSAT.	2.62	g
*VIT A	684.55	IU	*POLYUNSAT.	.29	g
THIAMIN	.26	mg	FIBER	2.31	g

ZUCCHINI CASSEROLE
Per Single Serving

4/4/9 CALORIES : 97
CAL FROM CARB. : 73%
CAL FROM PRO. : 13%
CAL FROM FAT : 13%

P/S RATIO   .61 : 1

DATE:

GRAM WT.	265.51	g	RIBOFLN	.14	mg
CHOLSTRL.	0.00	mg	NIACIN	2.37	mg
CALORIES	91.31	kcal	VIT C	37.37	mg
PROTEIN	3.48	g	*PANTO.	.62	mg
FAT	1.55	g	*B6	.25	mg
CARB.	17.78	g	*FOLACIN	11.35	mcg
CALCIUM	39.75	mg	*B12	0.00	mcg
PHOS.	85.76	mg	MAGNES.	40.50	mg
IRON	1.34	mg	*ZINC	.46	mg
SODIUM	46.75	mg	SAT. FAT	.15	g
*POTAS.	692.37	mg	MONO UNSAT.	.82	g
*VIT A	1308.75	IU	POLYUNSAT.	.09	g
THIAMIN	.14	mg	FIBER	1.36	g

Stuft Mushrooms

4	tablespoons unsalted spaghetti sauce	1	slice whole-wheat bread
¼	green pepper	8	ounces fresh mushrooms, stems removed
1	tablespoon grated Parmesan cheese		

Blend all the ingredients except the mushrooms in a blender. Push the mixture down with a spoon when blender is off so it will blend smoothly. You may also use a food processer. Stuff the mushroom cavities with this mixture. Place the mushrooms on a Pam-sprayed, nonstick cookie sheet and bake at 450° for 15 minutes.

Serves 4

STUFT MUSHROOMS
Per Single Serving

			4/4/9 CALORIES	: 74
			CAL FROM CARB.	: 59%
			CAL FROM PRO.	: 20%
			CAL FROM FAT	: 20%

P/S RATIO   .25 : 1

DATE:

GRAM WT.	90.07	g	RIBOFLN	.20	mg
CHOLSTRL.	2.00	mg	NIACIN	2.23	mg
CALORIES	69.93	kcal	*VIT C	22.31	mg
PROTEIN	3.85	g	PANTO.	.89	mg
FAT	1.67	g	B6	.10	mg
CARB.	11.09	g	FOLACIN	13.27	mcg
CALCIUM	53.97	mg	*B12	.00	mcg
PHOS.	100.27	mg	MAGNES.	22.51	mg
IRON	1.25	mg	*ZINC	.44	mg
SODIUM	116.36	mg	SAT. FAT	.57	g
POTAS.	324.86	mg	MONO UNSAT.	.66	g
*VIT A	495.36	IU	POLYUNSAT.	.14	g
THIAMIN	.10	mg	FIBER	.74	g

DAY NINE MENUS

_____**Breakfast**_____

Fruit 100
CORNMEAL MUSH 182
Herb Tea 25

_____**Lunch**_____

SPINACH SPAGHETTI SOUP 272
Bread 56
Fresh Fruit 100

_____**Dinner**_____

BEET SALAD 48
Corn on the cob 81
1 large Baked Yam with Butter Buds (1 Tbsp.) 174
Fresh Fruit 100
                                    Total   1138

                        Evening snack calories   662

Cornmeal Mush

½ cup yellow cornmeal
1½ cups water

¼ cup raisins

Bring the water to a boil and stir in the cornmeal. Cook for 10 minutes, then stir in the raisins. (Add more water if you like it thinner; more cornmeal, a teaspoon at a time, if you like it thicker.) Serve with apple juice or nonfat milk, or leave plain.

Serves 2

Spinach Spaghetti Soup

7½ cups water
2 ounces spinach spaghetti
½ onion, chopped
½ medium green pepper, chopped fine
1 head broccoli (remove center stem and use only the flowerets and tender stems)

1 cup cooked barley
½ cup cooked garbanzo beans
3 tablespoons vegetable-broth seasoning
3 tablespoons unsalted spaghetti sauce

Bring the water to boiling in a large pot and add the spinach spaghetti, onion, green pepper, broccoli, barley, and beans. Let simmer for 20 minutes, then add the remaining ingredients and cook 10 minutes longer.

Serves 4

Beet Salad

2 cups julienne beets	1 tablespoon chopped parsley
2 teaspoons olive oil	1 tablespoon vegetable-broth seasoning
1 cup thinly sliced red onion	3 tablespoons vinegar

Toss all the ingredients together and let marinate 1 hour. If salad becomes too dry, add 1 teaspoon more olive oil.

Serves 4

CORNMEAL MUSH
Per Single Serving

4/4/9 CALORIES : 182
CAL FROM CARB. : 91%
CAL FROM PRO. : 7%
CAL FROM FAT : 2%

P/S RATIO .89 : 1

DATE:

GRAM WT.	52.62	g	RIBOFLN	.10	mg
CHOLSTRL.	0.00	mg	NIACIN	1.34	mg
CALORIES	179.75	kcal	VIT C	.60	mg
PROTEIN	3.30	g	*PANTO.	.00	mg
FAT	.50	g	*B6	.04	mg
CARB.	41.39	g	FOLACIN	3.01	mcg
CALCIUM	10.87	mg	B12	0.00	mcg
PHOS.	51:75	mg	MAGNES.	22.21	mg
IRON	1.37	mg	ZINC	.32	mg
SODIUM	2.37	mg	*SAT. FAT	.02	g
POTAS.	177.62	mg	*MONO UNSAT.	.00	g
VIT A	153.87	IU	*POLYUNSAT.	.02	g
THIAMIN	.18	mg	FIBER	.43	g

SPINACH SPAGHETTI SOUP
Per Single Serving

4/4/9 CALORIES : 272
CAL FROM CARB. : 82%
CAL FROM PRO. : 14%
CAL FROM FAT : 4%

P/S RATIO   .59 : 1

DATE:

GRAM WT.	221.65	g	RIBOFLN	.23	mg
CHOLSTRL.	0.00	mg	NIACIN	2.79	mg
CALORIES	260.66	kcal	*VIT C	101.68	mg
PROTEIN	9.68	g	*PANTO.	1.47	mg
FAT	1.17	g	*B6	.32	mg
CARB.	56.01	g	*FOLACIN	87.46	mcg
CALCIUM	95.67	mg	B12	.00	mcg
PHOS.	200.16	mg	*MAGNES.	48.64	mg
IRON	2.75	mg	*ZINC	.55	mg
SODIUM	16.26	mg	SAT. FAT	.01	g
POTAS.	500.38	mg	MONO UNSAT.	.10	g
VIT A	2200.45	IU	POLYUNSAT.	.01	g
THIAMIN	.21	mg	FIBER	2.24	g

BEET SALAD
Per Single Serving

4/4/9 CALORIES : 48
CAL FROM CARB. : 77%
CAL FROM PRO. : 10%
CAL FROM FAT : 12%

P/S RATIO   .61 : 1

DATE:

GRAM WT.	126.50	g	*RIBOFLN	.05	mg
CHOLSTRL.	0.00	mg	*NIACIN	.31	mg
CALORIES	45.59	kcal	*VIT C	9.50	mg
*PROTEIN	1.40	g	*PANTO.	.16	mg
FAT	.76	g	*B6	.08	mg
CARB.	9.35	g	*FOLACIN	15.39	mcg
CALCIUM	22.25	mg	*B12	.00	mcg
PHOS.	31.00	mg	MAGNES.	16.67	mg
IRON	.72	mg	*ZINC	.08	mg
SODIUM	40.11	mg	SAT. FAT	.08	g
*POTAS.	239.75	mg	MONO UNSAT.	.46	g
*VIT A	102.50	IU	POLYUNSAT.	.05	g
*THIAMIN	.03	mg	*FIBER	.86	g

BAKED YAM
Per Single Serving

4/4/9 CALORIES : 162
CAL FROM CARB. : 91%
CAL FROM PRO. : 6%
CAL FROM FAT : 3%

P/S RATIO   0 : 1

DATE:

GRAM WT.	113.88	g	RIBOFLN	.08	mg
CHOLSTRL.	0.00	mg	NIACIN	.80	mg
CALORIES	161.00	kcal	VIT C	25.00	mg
PROTEIN	2.40	g	PANTO.	.93	mg
FAT	.60	g	B6	.24	mg
CARB.	37.00	g	FOLACIN	13.66	mcg
CALCIUM	46.00	mg	B12	0.00	mcg
PHOS.	66.00	mg	MAGNES.	35.30	mg
IRON	1.00	mg	ZINC	.81	mg
SODIUM	14.00	mg	SAT. FAT	0.00	g
POTAS.	342.00	mg	MONO UNSAT.	0.00	g
VIT A	9230.00	IU	POLYUNSAT.	0.00	g
THIAMIN	.10	mg	FIBER	1.02	g

_____**Breakfast**_____

Fruit	100
ALL-FIBER WAFFLES/PANCAKES	383
Fruit Syrup (from Day Four, or store-bought; unsweetened, 2 tablespoons)	21
Herb Tea	25

_____**Lunch**_____

SOUP-MIX SOUP	176
Bread with unsweetened Jam (1 tablespoon)	66
Fresh Fruit	100

_____**Dinner**_____

Green Salad	150
MEXICAN BARLEY SUPPER	309
Fresh Fruit	100
Total	1430

Evening snack calories	370

All-Fiber Waffles/Pancakes

---

2 cups apple juice
2 teaspoons baking powder
1 tablespoon tapioca granules

1 teaspoon cinnamon
1 teaspoon vanilla
¾ cup oat bran
1 cup date pieces
1 cup whole-wheat flour

Blend all ingredients in the blender in the order given. Bake on a nonstick waffle iron, or a nonstick griddle that has been sprayed with Pam. Serve with Butter Buds or unsweetened fruit syrup or jam. These are quite sweet alone, so you will use less topping.

Serves 4

ALL FIBER WAFFLES/PANCAKES
Per Single Serving

			4/4/9 CALORIES	: 383	
			CAL FROM CARB.	: 85%	
			CAL FROM PRO.	: 9%	
			CAL FROM FAT	: 5%	
P/S RATIO	1.74 : 1				
DATE:					
GRAM WT.	201.72	g	RIBOFLN	.13	mg
CHOLSTRL.	0.00	mg	NIACIN	2.59	mg
CALORIES	361.10	kcal	VIT C	1.15	mg
*PROTEIN	9.19	g	*PANTO.	.67	mg
*FAT	2.23	g	*B6	.22	mg
CARB.	81.75	g	*FOLACIN	17.22	mcg
CALCIUM	105.51	mg	B12	0.00	mcg
PHOS.	370.00	mg	*MAGNES.	104.15	mg
*IRON	2.26	mg	*ZINC	.88	mg
SODIUM	6.85	mg	*SAT. FAT	.02	g
POTAS.	806.60	mg	*MONO UNSAT.	.00	g
VIT A	23.25	IU	*POLYUNSAT.	.04	g
THIAMIN	.51	mg	*FIBER	10.96	g

Soup-Mix Soup

1 cup "Soup Mix" (a mixture of rice, split peas, lentils, barley, pasta, etc., available where you buy rice)
6½ cups water
½ onion, chopped
1 wedge cabbage, cut up

1 cup cavatelli, dry (a kind of pasta, but any pasta will do)
6 heaping tablespoons unsalted spaghetti sauce
2 heaping tablespoons vegetable-broth seasoning
1 tablespoon olive oil

In a casserole dish with a cover, combine the soup mix with 2½ cups water. Cover and cook in the oven at 350° for 45 minutes. Place the remaining ingredients in a large pot, and cook in the 4 remaining cups of water. Add the casserole mixture to the vegetables in the pot and let cook for 5 minutes more.

Serves 4

Mexican Barley Supper

1 zucchini, sliced and quartered
4 ounces fresh mushrooms, sliced
1 tablespoon olive oil
4 tablespoons salsa (or however much you prefer)

½ cup water
1 cup cooked barley
1 tablespoon hulled sunflower seeds
1 tablespoon vegetable-broth seasoning
4 slices whole-wheat toast

Sauté the zucchini and mushrooms in the olive oil. Add the water and salsa and cook for 3 minutes. Add the barley, sunflower seeds, and seasoning. Serve over the toast.

Serves 4

SOUP MIX SOUP
Per Single Serving

4/4/9 CALORIES : 176
CAL FROM CARB. : 69%
CAL FROM PRO. : 10%
CAL FROM FAT : 21%

P/S RATIO .60 : 1

DATE:

GRAM WT.	136.99	g	RIBOFLN	.08	mg
CHOLSTRL.	0.00	mg	NIACIN	1.50	mg
CALORIES	174.52	kcal	*VIT C	15.29	mg
PROTEIN	4.67	g	*PANTO.	.57	mg
FAT	4.18	g	*B6	.19	mg
CARB.	30.48	g	*FOLACIN	13.22	mcg
CALCIUM	20.23	mg	*B12	.00	mcg
PHOS.	83.99	mg	*MAGNES.	24.10	mg
IRON	1.46	mg	*ZINC	.33	mg
SODIUM	42.20	mg	*SAT. FAT	.48	g
*POTAS.	237.20	mg	*MONO UNSAT.	2.69	g
*VIT A	362.77	IU	*POLYUNSAT.	.29	g
THIAMIN	.13	mg	FIBER	.51	g

MEXICAN BARLEY SUPPER
Per Single Serving

4/4/9 CALORIES : 309
CAL FROM CARB. : 73%
CAL FROM PRO. : 10%
CAL FROM FAT : 17%

P/S RATIO 1.69 : 1

DATE:

GRAM WT.	126.89	g	RIBOFLN	.12	mg
CHOLSTRL.	0.00	mg	NIACIN	3.10	mg
CALORIES	299.26	kcal	*VIT C	4.25	mg
PROTEIN	8.10	g	*PANTO.	.63	mg
FAT	5.84	g	*B6	.16	mg
CARB.	56.40	g	*FOLACIN	9.60	mcg
CALCIUM	44.84	mg	*B12	0.00	mcg
PHOS.	194.25	mg	*MAGNES.	43.59	mg
IRON	2.23	mg	*ZINC	.74	mg
SODIUM	336.81	mg	SAT. FAT	.67	g
*POTAS.	292.84	mg	MONO UNSAT.	2.98	g
*VIT A	278.59	IU	POLYUNSAT.	1.15	g
THIAMIN	.19	mg	FIBER	1.04	g

DAY ELEVEN MENUS

CALORIES

_____ **Breakfast**_____

Fruit 100
SPECIAL OATMEAL 250
Herb Tea 25

_____ **Lunch**_____

HEARTY SUMMER SOUP 122
Bread 56
Fresh Fruit 100

_____ **Dinner**_____

CHILI 451
CORNBREAD 311
Fresh Fruit 100

                              Total   1515

                    Evening snack calories   285

Special Oatmeal

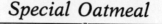

1 cup uncooked oatmeal	1 large ripe banana, mashed
2 cups boiling water	1 cup apple juice

Stir the oatmeal into the boiling water. Cook for 3 to 5 minutes, depending upon the texture you prefer. Remove from heat. Put half of mashed banana in each bowl. Pour oatmeal into bowls over banana. Use apple juice instead of milk.

Serves 2

Hearty Summer Soup

4½ cups water	1 15-ounce can (1½ cup) of cannellini, rinsed
¼ small head cabbage, cut up	4 tablespoons spinach pastina (tiny soup pasta)
1 cup frozen green beans	1 tablespoon tomato paste
3 yellow summer squash, sliced	2 tablespoons vegetable-broth seasoning

Combine all the ingredients in a large pot and simmer until the green beans are tender.

Serves 4

Chili

1	tablespoon olive oil	¾	cup unsalted spaghetti sauce
1	medium yellow onion, chopped	2	tablespoons vegetable-broth seasoning
3	cups cooked pinto beans with liquid	3 to 6	tablespoons mild chile salsa
1	cup cooked barley		

Sauté the onion in olive oil. Add with 1½ cups of the pinto beans and liquid to the blender. Blend coarsely. Pour the blended mixture into a pot with the remaining ingredients and simmer until flavors are thoroughly blended, about 10 minutes. 3 tablespoons mild salsa is about right for small children or those who prefer a very mild chili. Judge your preference accordingly.

Serves 4

Cornbread

1	cup apple juice	1	teaspoon vanilla
1	heaping cup cut-up cabbage	1	teaspoon olive oil
12	dates, pitted	1	cup corn flour
1	tablespoon baking powder	½	cup whole-wheat flour
		2	egg whites, stiffly beaten

Blend the apple juice with the cabbage, dates, baking powder, vanilla, and olive oil until thoroughly puréed. Pour into a mixing bowl and with a hand mixer add the corn flour and whole-wheat flour. Fold in the egg white and pour entire mixture into a Pam-sprayed, nonstick square or round pan and bake at 350° for 30 minutes.

Serves 4

SPECIAL OATMEAL
Per Single Serving

4/4/9 CALORIES : 250
CAL FROM CARB. : 82%
CAL FROM PRO. : 8%
CAL FROM FAT : 10%

P/S RATIO 1.73 : 1

DATE:

GRAM WT.	421.00	g	RIBOFLN	.12	mg
CHOLSTRL.	0.00	mg	NIACIN	.63	mg
CALORIES	242.50	kcal	VIT C	6.30	mg
PROTEIN	5.46	g	*PANTO.	3.74	mg
FAT	2.81	g	B6	.85	mg
CARB.	51.13	g	FOLACIN	90.20	mcg
CALCIUM	33.50	mg	B12	0.00	mcg
PHOS.	157.00	mg	MAGNES.	70.90	mg
IRON	2.03	mg	ZINC	2.33	mg
SODIUM	527.00	mg	SAT. FAT	.62	g
POTAS.	519.50	mg	MONO UNSAT.	.82	g
VIT A	47.00	IU	POLYUNSAT.	1.09	g
THIAMIN	.24	mg	FIBER	1.02	g

HEARTY SUMMER SOUP
Per Single Serving

4/4/9 CALORIES : 122
CAL FROM CARB. : 72%
CAL FROM PRO. : 23%
CAL FROM FAT : 5%

P/S RATIO 0 : 1

DATE:

GRAM WT.	210.96	g	RIBOFLN	.16	mg
CHOLSTRL.	0.00	mg	NIACIN	1.52	mg
CALORIES	116.67	kcal	VIT C	18.37	mg
PROTEIN	7.22	g	*PANTO.	.09	mg
FAT	.67	g	*B6	.04	mg
CARB.	22.23	g	*FOLACIN	15.30	mcg
CALCIUM	76.92	mg	B12	0.00	mcg
PHOS.	141.23	mg	*MAGNES.	22.08	mg
IRON	2.63	mg	*ZINC	1.50	mg
SODIUM	10.00	mg	SAT. FAT	0.00	g
POTAS.	512.89	mg	MONO UNSAT.	0.00	g
VIT A	698.90	IU	POLYUNSAT.	0.00	g
THIAMIN	.18	mg	FIBER	2.01	g

CHILI
Per Single Serving

4/4/9 CALORIES : 451
CAL FROM CARB. : 74%
CAL FROM PRO. : 15%
CAL FROM FAT : 11%

P/S RATIO   .60 : 1

DATE:

GRAM WT.	311.23	g	RIBOFLN	.17	mg
CHOLSTRL.	0.00	mg	NIACIN	3.53	mg
CALORIES	437.22	kcal	*VIT C	29.47	mg
PROTEIN	17.07	g	*PANTO.	1.23	mg
FAT	5.36	g	*B6	.19	mg
CARB.	83.89	g	*FOLACIN	255.77	mcg
CALCIUM	84.71	mg	*B12	.00	mcg
PHOS.	335.20	mg	*MAGNES.	33.49	mg
IRON	5.47	mg	*ZINC	1.74	mg
SODIUM	316.79	mg	SAT. FAT	.52	g
*POTAS.	905.54	mg	MONO UNSAT.	2.91	g
*VIT A	1026.80	IU	POLYUNSAT.	.32	g
THIAMIN	.28	mg	FIBER	3.05	g

CORNBREAD
Per Single Serving

4/4/9 CALORIES : 311
CAL FROM CARB. : 78%
CAL FROM PRO. : 8%
CAL FROM FAT : 13%

P/S RATIO   1.15 : 1

DATE:

GRAM WT.	171.90	g	RIBOFLN	.12	mg
CHOLSTRL.	0.00	mg	NIACIN	1.72	mg
CALORIES	302.97	kcal	VIT C	8.82	mg
*PROTEIN	6.70	g	*PANTO.	.43	mg
*FAT	4.63	g	*B6	.14	mg
CARB.	61.22	g	*FOLACIN	16.97	mcg
CALCIUM	192.98	mg	*B12	.01	mcg
PHOS.	346.94	mg	*MAGNES.	31.42	mg
*IRON	1.63	mg	*ZINC	.49	mg
SODIUM	31.85	mg	*SAT. FAT	.53	g
*POTAS.	724.55	mg	*MONO UNSAT.	2.72	g
*VIT A	135.60	IU	*POLYUNSAT.	.62	g
THIAMIN	.18	mg	*FIBER	1.36	g

_____**Breakfast**_____

Fruit	100
Cold Cereal	170
Bread with APRICOT BREAD SPREAD	127
Herb Tea	25

_____**Lunch**_____

OLD COUNTRY MUSTARD GREENS AND POTATOES ...	223
Bread	56
Fresh Fruit	100

_____**Dinner**_____

CABBAGE-MAC SOUP	196
Bread	56
Fresh Fruit	100
Total	1153

Evening snack calories 647

Apricot Bread Spread

⅓ cup dried apricots
⅓ cup pitted dates
¾ cup pineapple juice

1 teaspoon tapioca
   granules

Blend all ingredients in blender. Pour into a small saucepan and cook over medium heat for 5 minutes, stirring constantly. Cool and serve on whole-grain bread.

Serves 4

Old Country Mustard Greens and Potatoes

1 bunch young mustard greens (about 1 cup cooked)
2 large white-rose potatoes, cubed

1 rounded tablespoon tomato paste
1 teaspoon olive oil
1 teaspoon vegetable-broth seasoning

Simmer the greens in 3 inches of water until tender, about 30 minutes. Place the potatoes in a small saucepan with 1 inch of water. Cook 15 minutes. Drain most of the liquid off the potatoes and greens and mix them together. Toss with the tomato paste, oil, and seasoning.

Serves 2

Cabbage-Mac Soup

8	cups water	4 or 5	small end slices of egg-plant (no seeds)
½	Spanish onion		
1	small zucchini, sliced and quartered	1	cup canned garbanzo beans, rinsed
1	cup (whole-wheat) elbow macaroni	3	tablespoons unsalted spaghetti sauce
½	small head cabbage, chopped coarsely	2	tablespoons vegetable-broth seasoning
		1	tablespoon olive oil

Pour the water into a large pot, then add the remaining ingredients. Simmer until the macaroni is tender, about 20 minutes.

Serves 4

APRICOT BREAD SPREAD
Per Single Serving

			4/4/9 CALORIES	: 71
			CAL FROM CARB.	: 97%
			CAL FROM PRO.	: 3%
			CAL FROM FAT	: 0%

P/S RATIO   4.49 : 1

DATE:

GRAM WT.	62.32	g	RIBOFLN	.02	mg
CHOLSTRL.	0.00	mg	NIACIN	.47	mg
CALORIES	67.43	kcal	VIT C	5.10	mg
PROTEIN	.52	g	*PANTO.	.16	mg
FAT	.10	g	*B6	.07	mg
CARB.	17.39	g	FOLACIN	12.61	mcg
CALCIUM	13.33	mg	B12	0.00	mcg
PHOS.	13.16	mg	MAGNES.	12.02	mg
IRON	.45	mg	*ZINC	.11	mg
SODIUM	1.02	mg	*SAT. FAT	.00	g
POTAS.	190.66	mg	*MONO UNSAT.	.01	g
VIT A	324.25	IU	*POLYUNSAT.	.01	g
THIAMIN	.03	mg	FIBER	.40	g

OLD COUNTRY MUSTARD GREENS & POTATOES

			4/4/9 CALORIES	: 223
			CAL FROM CARB.	: 77%
			CAL FROM PRO.	: 12%
			CAL FROM FAT	: 11%

P/S RATIO   .61 : 1

DATE:

GRAM WT.	307.93	g	RIBOFLN	.19	mg
CHOLSTRL.	0.00	mg	NIACIN	4.05	mg
CALORIES	215.60	kcal	VIT C	73.50	mg
PROTEIN	6.62	g	*PANTO.	.11	mg
FAT	2.78	g	*B6	.48	mg
CARB.	43.22	g	*FOLACIN	57.92	mcg
CALCIUM	114.72	mg	*B12	.00	mcg
PHOS.	149.24	mg	MAGNES.	69.18	mg
IRON	2.94	mg	*ZINC	.59	mg
SODIUM	22.62	mg	SAT. FAT	.30	g
*POTAS.	1149.90	mg	MONO UNSAT.	1.65	g
*VIT A	4330.31	IU	POLYUNSAT.	.18	g
THIAMIN	.27	mg	FIBER	1.84	g

CABBAGE-MAC SOUP
Per Single Serving

			4/4/9 CALORIES	: 196
			CAL FROM CARB.	: 66%
			CAL FROM PRO.	: 15%
			CAL FROM FAT	: 19%

P/S RATIO   .61 : 1

DATE:

GRAM WT.	241.90	g	RIBOFLN	.15	mg
CHOLSTRL.	0.00	mg	NIACIN	1.79	mg
CALORIES	191.73	kcal	*VIT C	20.68	mg
PROTEIN	7.48	g	*PANTO.	.42	mg
FAT	4.22	g	*B6	.08	mg
CARB.	32.33	g	*FOLACIN	94.02	mcg
CALCIUM	53.30	mg	*B12	.00	mcg
PHOS.	133.70	mg	*MAGNES.	31.09	mg
IRON	2.47	mg	*ZINC	1.17	mg
SODIUM	9.63	mg	SAT. FAT	.46	g
*POTAS.	425.63	mg	MONO UNSAT.	2.58	g
*VIT A	342.95	IU	POLYUNSAT.	.28	g
THIAMIN	.21	mg	FIBER	1.60	g

DAY THIRTEEN MENUS

_____ **Breakfast** _____

Fruit 100
CREAM OF MILLET CEREAL 373
Herb Tea 25

_____ **Lunch** _____

CAULIFLOWER SOUP 383
Bread 56
Fresh Fruit 100

_____ **Dinner** _____

Baked Potato with 1 tablespoon Butter Buds 148
Brown Rice (1 cup) with low-sodium Soy Sauce 252
CRUMBED GREEN BEANS 56
Fresh Fruit 100

Total   1593

Evening snack calories   207

Cream of Millet Cereal

2½ cups water

1 cup millet, ground in blender to a flour (will yield a little less)

Boil the water and stir in the millet, stirring constantly for 1 minute. Lower the heat and cook for 5 more minutes. Serve with banana, raisins, and apple juice, or plain if you prefer.

Serves 2

Cauliflower Soup

5 cups water
1 small head of cauliflower, cut up
½ cup corn
1 cup lima beans
1 small zucchini, sliced and quartered

3 tablespoons spinach pastina
1½ cups cooked barley
4 rounded tablespoons unsalted spaghetti sauce
2 teaspoons olive oil
1½ tablespoons vegetable-broth seasoning

In a medium or large pot, bring the water to a boil with the remaining ingredients. Simmer for 20 minutes.

Serves 4

Crumbed Green Beans

---

1 package frozen French-style green beans

1 tablespoon olive oil

2 teaspoons vegetable-broth seasoning

½ cup whole-grain bread crumbs

Cook the beans and drain. Toss with the oil, vegetable-broth seasoning, and bread crumbs.

Serves 4

CAULIFLOWER SOUP
Per Single Serving

			4/4/9 CALORIES	: 383
			CAL FROM CARB.	: 80%
			CAL FROM PRO.	: 11%
			CAL FROM FAT	: 8%

P/S RATIO .60 : 1

DATE:

GRAM WT.	237.47	g	RIBOFLN	.15	mg
CHOLSTRL.	0.00	mg	NIACIN	3.54	mg
CALORIES	374.36	kcal	VIT C	51.78	mg
PROTEIN	11.24	g	*PANTO.	.98	mg
FAT	3.66	g	*B6	.36	mg
CARB.	76.85	g	*FOLACIN	18.62	mcg
CALCIUM	46.37	mg	*B12	.00	mcg
PHOS.	224.94	mg	MAGNES.	70.49	mg
IRON	3.59	mg	*ZINC	.21	mg
SODIUM	12.85	mg	SAT. FAT	.32	g
*POTAS.	485.16	mg	MONO UNSAT.	1.79	g
*VIT A	478.93	IU	POLYUNSAT.	.19	g
THIAMIN	.19	mg	FIBER	2.02	g

CRUMBED GREEN BEANS

4/4/9 CALORIES	:	59
CAL FROM CARB.	:	39%
CAL FROM PRO.	:	8%
CAL FROM FAT	:	53%

P/S RATIO   .65 : 1

DATE:

GRAM WT.	74.62	g	RIBOFLN	.06	mg
CHOLSTRL.	0.00	mg	NIACIN	.33	mg
CALORIES	56.95	kcal	*VIT C	3.50	mg
PROTEIN	1.42	g	*PANTO.	.10	mg
FAT	3.55	g	*B6	.04	mg
CARB.	5.75	g	*FOLACIN	19.46	mcg
CALCIUM	30.13	mg	*B12	.00	mcg
PHOS.	25.16	mg	MAGNES.	15.00	mg
IRON	.56	mg	ZINC	.25	mg
SODIUM	19.50	mg	SAT. FAT	.47	g
*POTAS.	106.50	mg	MONO UNSAT.	2.52	g
*VIT A	390.00	IU	POLYUNSAT.	.31	g
THIAMIN	.05	mg	FIBER	.68	g

BAKED POTATO
Per Single Serving

4/4/9 CALORIES	:	148
CAL FROM CARB.	:	89%
CAL FROM PRO.	:	11%
CAL FROM FAT	:	1%

P/S RATIO   0 : 1

DATE:

GRAM WT.	155.54	g	RIBOFLN	.07	mg
CHOLSTRL.	0.00	mg	NIACIN	2.70	mg
CALORIES	145.00	kcal	VIT C	31.00	mg
PROTEIN	4.00	g	*PANTO.	0.00	mg
FAT	.20	g	B6	.36	mg
CARB.	32.80	g	*FOLACIN	0.00	mcg
CALCIUM	14.00	mg	*B12	0.00	mcg
PHOS.	101.00	mg	MAGNES.	34.22	mg
IRON	1.10	mg	ZINC	.31	mg
SODIUM	6.00	mg	SAT. FAT	0.00	g
POTAS.	782.00	mg	MONO UNSAT.	0.00	g
*VIT A	0.00	IU	POLYUNSAT.	0.00	g
THIAMIN	.15	mg	FIBER	.93	g

BROWN RICE W/SOY SAUCE
Per Single Serving

			4/4/9 CALORIES	: 252
			CAL FROM CARB.	: 83%
			CAL FROM PRO.	: 13%
			CAL FROM FAT	: 4%

P/S RATIO   0 : 1

DATE:

GRAM WT.	231.00	g	RIBOFLN	.08	mg
CHOLSTRL.	0.00	mg	NIACIN	3.91	mg
CALORIES	254.00	kcal	VIT C	0.00	mg
PROTEIN	8.02	g	PANTO.	3.08	mg
FAT	1.20	g	B6	1.27	mg
CARB.	52.70	g	FOLACIN	42.80	mcg
CALCIUM	29.00	mg	B12	0.00	mcg
PHOS.	218.00	mg	MAGNES.	72.55	mg
IRON	1.98	mg	ZINC	.59	mg
SODIUM	2608.00	mg	SAT. FAT	0.00	g
POTAS.	265.00	mg	MONO UNSAT.	0.00	g
VIT A	0.00	IU	POLYUNSAT.	0.00	g
THIAMIN	.19	mg	*FIBER	.58	g

_____**Breakfast**_____

Fruit	100
CORN FLOUR WAFFLES	192
Butter Buds (2 tablespoons)	8
Herb Tea	25

_____**Lunch**_____

SPLIT PEA SOUP	296
Bread with unsweetened Fruit Jam	77

_____**Dinner**_____

Green Salad	150
BREADED EGGPLANT	168
Mixed Vegetables (1 cup) with Butter Buds	30
(1 tablespoon)	4
Fruit	100
Total	1150

Evening snack calories	650

Corn Flour Waffles

¾	cup water	2	teaspoons baking
1	cup pineapple juice		powder
1	small banana	1	cup oatmeal
¼	cup pitted dates	2	teaspoons olive oil
1	teaspoon vanilla	1	cup corn flour
1	tablespoon tapioca granules		

Blend all ingredients together in blender. Bake on a preheated, nonstick, Pam-sprayed griddle until done. These waffles will require about twice the cooking time as waffles with wheat flour and eggs, due to the nature of the ingredients.

Serves 4

Note: These are sweet enough without any syrup. Butter Buds are adequate, or applesauce.

Split Pea Soup

1½	cups uncooked split peas	¼	cup salsa
8	cups water	1	cup chopped yellow onion
1	cup apple juice	1	cup uncooked rice
1	cup chopped carrot (approximately 3 carrots)	3	tablespoons vegetable-broth seasoning
		1	tablespoon tomato paste

Soak the peas overnight. Cook all ingredients together in a pot, watching to make sure it does not boil over, until the peas are tender and the rice is done (at least 1 hour).

Serves 4

Breaded Eggplant

1	small green pepper	2	tablespoons sunflower seeds
1	small onion	4	pieces whole-wheat or whole-grain bread, crumbled
2	rounded tablespoons tomato paste		
2	egg whites	8	¼-inch-thick slices eggplant
2	teaspoons oregano		
1	teaspoon basil	2	small tomatoes, sliced thin
2	tablespoons vegetable-broth seasoning		
2	tablespoons grated Parmesan cheese		

In the blender, blend the green pepper, onion, tomato paste, egg whites, oregano, basil, vegetable-broth seasoning, cheese, and sunflower seeds. Pour this mixture over the bread crumbs in a large bowl. Mix thoroughly with a spoon. Arrange the eggplant slices on a nonstick, Pam-sprayed cookie sheet. Top with the blender mixture. Bake at 350° for 30 minutes. Top with fresh tomato slices before serving.

Serves 2

CORN FLOUR WAFFLES
Per Single Serving

4/4/9 CALORIES : 192
CAL FROM CARB. : 77%
CAL FROM PRO. : 6%
CAL FROM FAT : 17%

P/S RATIO   1.18 : 1

DATE:

GRAM WT.	228.72	g	RIBOFLN	.07	mg
CHOLSTRL.	0.00	mg	NIACIN	.62	mg
CALORIES	186.27	kcal	VIT C	10.07	mg
*PROTEIN	3.18	g	*PANTO.	2.03	mg
*FAT	3.66	g	*B6	.47	mg
CARB.	37.24	g	*FOLACIN	46.57	mcg
CALCIUM	131.96	mg	*B12	0.00	mcg
PHOS.	248.40	mg	*MAGNES.	43.20	mg
*IRON	1.11	mg	*ZINC	1.25	mg
SODIUM	263.04	mg	*SAT. FAT	.60	g
*POTAS.	590.14	mg	*MONO UNSAT.	2.06	g
*VIT A	34.81	IU	*POLYUNSAT.	.71	g
THIAMIN	.16	mg	*FIBER	.69	g

SPLIT PEA SOUP
Per Single Serving

4/4/9 CALORIES : 296
CAL FROM CARB. : 83%
CAL FROM PRO. : 14%
CAL FROM FAT : 3%

P/S RATIO   1.74 : 1

DATE:

GRAM WT.	352.22	g	RIBOFLN	.16	mg
CHOLSTRL.	0.00	mg	NIACIN	2.86	mg
CALORIES	291.10	kcal	*VIT C	14.07	mg
PROTEIN	10.30	g	*PANTO.	3.32	mg
FAT	1.08	g	*B6	1.00	mg
CARB.	61.63	g	*FOLACIN	66.80	mcg
CALCIUM	60.04	mg	*B12	0.00	mcg
PHOS.	188.73	mg	*MAGNES.	48.62	mg
IRON	2.88	mg	*ZINC	1.55	mg
SODIUM	546.12	mg	*SAT. FAT	.01	g
POTAS.	713.82	mg	*MONO UNSAT.	.00	g
VIT A	6369.40	IU	*POLYUNSAT.	.02	g
THIAMIN	.28	mg	FIBER	1.67	g

BREADED EGGPLANT
Per Single Serving

4/4/9 CALORIES : 168
CAL FROM CARB. : 58%
CAL FROM PRO. : 21%
CAL FROM FAT : 21%

P/S RATIO   1.88 : 1

DATE:

GRAM WT.	232.21	g	RIBOFLN	.19	mg
CHOLSTRL.	2.00	mg	NIACIN	2.04	mg
CALORIES	156.59	kcal	*VIT C	68.25	mg
PROTEIN	8.78	g	*PANTO.	.64	mg
FAT	4.05	g	*B6	.28	mg
CARB.	24.32	g	*FOLACIN	26.11	mcg
CALCIUM	95.65	mg	*B12	.01	mcg
PHOS.	169.15	mg	MAGNES.	52.07	mg
IRON	2.48	mg	*ZINC	1.13	mg
SODIUM	219.25	mg	SAT. FAT	.83	g
POTAS.	537.34	mg	MONO UNSAT.	.94	g
*VIT A	880.00	IU	POLYUNSAT.	1.56	g
THIAMIN	.25	mg	FIBER	2.10	g

MIXED VEGETABLES
Per Single Serving

4/4/9 CALORIES : 30
CAL FROM CARB. : 80%
CAL FROM PRO. : 17%
CAL FROM FAT : 3%

P/S RATIO   0 : 1

DATE:

GRAM WT.	45.50	g	RIBOFLN	.03	mg
CHOLSTRL.	0.00	mg	NIACIN	.50	mg
CALORIES	29.00	kcal	VIT C	3.75	mg
PROTEIN	1.45	g	PANTO.	.14	mg
FAT	.12	g	B6	.05	mg
CARB.	6.10	g	FOLACIN	7.28	mcg
CALCIUM	11.50	mg	B12	0.00	mcg
PHOS.	28.75	mg	*MAGNES.	0.00	mg
IRON	.60	mg	ZINC	.26	mg
SODIUM	24.00	mg	SAT. FAT	0.00	g
POTAS.	87.00	mg	MONO UNSAT.	0.00	g
VIT A	2252.50	IU	POLYUNSAT.	0.00	g
THIAMIN	.05	mg	FIBER	.54	g

WEEK THREE SHOPPING LIST

( ) Is your pantry stocked with the baking and condiment staples?

( ) Is your pantry stocked with the food staples?
(Check for rice, walnuts [raw], pinto beans, canned garbanzo and kidney beans, and barley)

Fresh Foods

Fruit (2–3 servings per day for 7 days)
Bananas (used in recipes as well as eaten plain)
"Pink" Potatoes (4 small)
Eggplant (1 small)
Zucchini (2 or 3)
Green Pepper (1 small)
(Don't forget eggs)
Spaghetti Squash (1 small)
Corn Tortillas (1 small package)
Leaf Lettuce for salads
Head Lettuce (recipe)
English Muffins, whole-grain (1 package)
Celery (is there some left over from last week?)
Apricots (fresh) (several small)
Tomatoes (fresh) (for recipes and salads)
Potatoes (you won't need but a few; do you have any left over from previous weeks?)

Frozen Foods

Peas (1 16-ounce package)
Italian Vegetables (1 20-ounce bag)
Corn (10-ounce package)
Apple Juice (get several to have on hand for recipes and drinking and cereal)

Canned or Jar Foods

Mushrooms (2 8-ounce cans)
Pitted, Moist Prunes (8-ounce can or bag)
Rosarita Vegetarian Refried Beans (1 16-ounce can)
Green Beans, unsalted (1 16-ounce can)
White Wine (1 small bottle for cooking)
Green and Wax Beans (1 16-ounce can)
Sesame Tahini (1 small jar or can)

Other

You'll use the following pastas:
    Alphabet Macaroni
    Macaroni

Dessert ingredients (check the recipes)

Breakfast

Fruit	100
Cold Cereal	170
Herb Tea	25

Lunch

Green Salad	150
PINK POTATOES AND PEAS	252
Yellow or Orange Vegetable (for example, 1 large ear of Corn)	81
Bread	56

Dinner

Carrot and Celery Sticks (1 small carrot; 1 stalk of celery)	34
RATATOUILLE ESPECIÀL	514
Bread	56
Fresh Fruit	100
Total	1538

Evening snack calories   262

Pink Potatoes and Peas

½ cup water
2 cups peas
½ cup chopped onion

4 small (approximately 3 inches long) red new potatoes
1 teaspoon olive oil
½ teaspoon sweet basil

Peel a small strip around the center of each potato. In a 1-quart casserole with a cover, place the water, peas and onion. Nestle the potatoes on top, drizzle with the olive oil, and sprinkle with basil. Cover and bake at 350° for 40 minutes.

Serves 4

PINK POTATOES AND PEAS
Per Single Serving

			4/4/9 CALORIES	: 252	
			CAL FROM CARB.	: 80%	
			CAL FROM PRO.	: 15%	
			CAL FROM FAT	: 6%	
P/S RATIO	.61	: 1			
DATE:					
GRAM WT.	329.87	g	RIBOFLN	.18	mg
CHOLSTRL.	0.00	mg	NIACIN	5.28	mg
CALORIES	248.06	kcal	VIT C	54.12	mg
PROTEIN	9.42	g	*PANTO.	.27	mg
FAT	1.65	g	*B6	.52	mg
CARB.	50.45	g	*FOLACIN	38.26	mcg
CALCIUM	40.25	mg	*B12	0.00	mcg
PHOS.	207.63	mg	MAGNES.	68.60	mg
IRON	2.96	mg	ZINC	1.27	mg
SODIUM	10.12	mg	SAT. FAT	.15	g
*POTAS.	1116.37	mg	MONO UNSAT.	.82	g
*VIT A	438.75	IU	POLYUNSAT.	.09	g
THIAMIN	.43	mg	FIBER	2.86	g

CARROT AND CELERY STICKS
Per Single Serving

			4/4/9 CALORIES	: 34
			CAL FROM CARB.	: 88%
			CAL FROM PRO.	: 9%
			CAL FROM FAT	: 3%

P/S RATIO   0 : 1

DATE:

GRAM WT.	88.75	g	RIBOFLN	.04	mg
CHOLSTRL.	0.00	mg	NIACIN	.46	mg
CALORIES	33.00	kcal	VIT C	7.66	mg
PROTEIN	.96	g	PANTO.	.27	mg
FAT	.13	g	B6	.11	mg
CARB.	7.66	g	FOLACIN	6.93	mcg
CALCIUM	33.66	mg	B12	0.00	mcg
PHOS.	30.66	mg	MAGNES.	20.24	mg
IRON	.56	mg	ZINC	.44	mg
SODIUM	55.00	mg	SAT. FAT	0.00	g
POTAS.	303.00	mg	MONO UNSAT.	0.00	g
VIT A	7976.66	IU	POLYUNSAT.	0.00	g
THIAMIN	.04	mg	FIBER	.82	g

CORN ON THE COB
Per Single Serving

			4/4/9 CALORIES	: 81
			CAL FROM CARB.	: 79%
			CAL FROM PRO.	: 12%
			CAL FROM FAT	: 9%

P/S RATIO   0 : 1

DATE:

GRAM WT.	77.00	g	RIBOFLN	.08	mg
CHOLSTRL.	0.00	mg	NIACIN	1.10	mg
CALORIES	70.00	kcal	VIT C	7.00	mg
PROTEIN	2.50	g	PANTO.	.41	mg
FAT	.80	g	B6	.12	mg
CARB.	16.20	g	FOLACIN	21.56	mcg
CALCIUM	2.00	mg	B12	0.00	mcg
PHOS.	69.00	mg	MAGNES.	36.96	mg
IRON	.50	mg	ZINC	.27	mg
*SODIUM	0.00	mg	SAT. FAT	0.00	g
POTAS.	151.00	mg	MONO UNSAT.	0.00	g
VIT A	310.00	IU	POLYUNSAT.	0.00	g
THIAMIN	.09	mg	FIBER	.53	g

Ratatouille Especiàl

2	cups water	½	cup onions, cut in chunks
2	cups eggplant, cut in chunks	1	cup cooked mushrooms
1	cup zucchini, cut in chunks	3	tablespoons unsalted spaghetti sauce
½	cup green pepper, cut in chunks	2	tablespoons vegetable-both seasoning
		4	cups cooked brown rice

In a large pot, combine the water with all the remaining ingredients except the rice. Cook 30 minutes over medium-low heat, until the green pepper is tender. Serve over hot cooked rice—1 cup per person.

Serves 4

RATATOUILLE ESPECIÀL
Per Single Serving

4/4/9 CALORIES : 514
CAL FROM CARB. : 85%
CAL FROM PRO. : 10%
CAL FROM FAT : 5%

P/S RATIO .59 : 1

DATE:

GRAM WT.	613.52	g	RIBOFLN	.27	mg
CHOLSTRL.	0.00	mg	NIACIN	7.34	mg
CALORIES	513.78	kcal	VIT C	39.93	mg
PROTEIN	12.58	g	*PANTO.	6.61	mg
FAT	2.93	g	*B6	2.60	mg
CARB.	109.73	g	*FOLACIN	96.18	mcg
CALCIUM	80.80	mg	B12	.00	mcg
PHOS.	355.04	mg	MAGNES.	148.17	mg
IRON	3.39	mg	*ZINC	1.40	mg
SODIUM	1110.13	mg	SAT. FAT	.01	g
POTAS.	694.63	mg	MONO UNSAT.	.10	g
*VIT A	426.70	IU	POLYUNSAT.	.01	g
THIAMIN	.48	mg	FIBER	2.99	g

CALORIES

_____Breakfast_____

Fruit	100
Cold Cereal	170
PRUNE MUFFINS	194
Herb Tea	25

_____Lunch_____

ALPHABET SOUP	222
Bread	56
Fresh Fruit	100

_____Dinner_____

Green Salad	150
SPAGHETTI SQUASH	326
Bread	56
Fresh Fruit	100
Total	1499

Evening snack calories 301

Prune Muffins

1	cup concentrated apple juice	8	ounces moist, pitted prunes (approximately 1 cup packed)
1	egg white		
1	teaspoon cinnamon	1	cup grated raw zucchini
1	tablespoon baking powder	1	cup oatmeal
		¾	cup oat bran
		¼	cup whole-wheat flour

In the blender, blend together the apple juice, egg white, cinnamon, baking powder, and prunes. In a bowl, combine the rest of the ingredients with the blender mixture, using a large spoon. Pour into Pam-sprayed, nonstick muffin pans and bake at 350° for 30 minutes.

Serves 12

PRUNE MUFFINS
Per Single Serving

			4/4/9 CALORIES	:	194
			CAL FROM CARB.	:	79%
			CAL FROM PRO.	:	12%
			CAL FROM FAT	:	8%
P/S RATIO	2.03 : 1				
DATE:					
GRAM WT.	190.91	g	RIBOFLN	.13	mg
CHOLSTRL.	0.00	mg	NIACIN	1.04	mg
CALORIES	185.79	kcal	VIT C	4.45	mg
*PROTEIN	6.04	g	*PANTO.	1.33	mg
*FAT	1.88	g	*B6	.24	mg
CARB.	38.62	g	*FOLACIN·	28.25	mcg
CALCIUM	152.40	mg	B12	.00	mcg
PHOS.	343.33	mg	*MAGNES.	70.02	mg
*IRON	1.60	mg	*ZINC	1.02	mg
SODIUM	185.96	mg	SAT. FAT	.18	g
POTAS.	690.29	mg	MONO UNSAT.	.35	g
VIT A	638.50	IU	POLYUNSAT.	.37	g
THIAMIN	.29	mg	*FIBER	7.02	g

Alphabet Soup

4 cups water
1 20-ounce package "Italian Vegetables" (zucchini, cauliflower, carrots, Italian green beans, lima beans), or an equivalent mixture

½ cup uncooked alphabet macaroni (2.6 ounces)
4 tablespoons unsalted spaghetti sauce
2 rounded tablespoons vegetable-broth seasoning

Combine all ingredients in a medium or large pot and simmer for 20 minutes.

Serves 2

Spaghetti Squash

1 small spaghetti squash (4 cups when cooked)
1½ cups unsalted spaghetti sauce
¼ cup water

1½ tablespoons vegetable-broth seasoning
2 teaspoons grated Parmesan cheese

Cut the squash in half, scoop out the seeds, and place cut side down in a pot with an inch of water. Cover the pot and steam the squash for 20 minutes. Remove from water and scoop out the strands with a fork. Combine spaghetti sauce with ¼ cup water and 1½ tablespoons vegetable-broth seasoning. Top squash strands with the sauce, and divide into 2 portions. Sprinkle each plateful with 1 teaspoon of the cheese.

Serves 2

ALPHABET SOUP
Per Single Serving

4/4/9 CALORIES : 222
CAL FROM CARB. : 79%
CAL FROM PRO. : 16%
CAL FROM FAT : 5%

P/S RATIO   .59 : 1

DATE:

GRAM WT.	288.07	g	RIBOFLN	.20	mg
CHOLSTRL.	0.00	mg	NIACIN	3.17	mg
CALORIES	212.93	kcal	VIT C	29.81	mg
PROTEIN	8.81	g	*PANTO.	.58	mg
FAT	1.26	g	*B6	.24	mg
CARB.	44.19	g	*FOLACIN	30.01	mcg
CALCIUM	56.97	mg	B12	.00	mcg
PHOS.	162.77	mg	*MAGNES.	19.19	mg
IRON	3.57	mg	ZINC	1.46	mg
SODIUM	99.86	mg	SAT. FAT	.05	g
POTAS.	525.86	mg	MONO UNSAT.	.29	g
VIT A	9467.86	IU	POLYUNSAT.	.03	g
THIAMIN	.35	mg	FIBER	2.46	g

SPAGHETTI SQUASH
Per Single Serving

4/4/9 CALORIES : 326
CAL FROM CARB. : 78%
CAL FROM PRO. : 12%
CAL FROM FAT : 10%

P/S RATIO   .31 : 1

DATE:

GRAM WT.	708.10	g	RIBOFLN	.62	mg
CHOLSTRL.	1.33	mg	NIACIN	4.54	mg
CALORIES	290.27	kcal	VIT C	128.88	mg
PROTEIN	10.19	g	*PANTO.	.11	mg
FAT	3.69	g	*B6	.12	mg
CARB.	63.45	g	*FOLACIN	5.51	mcg
CALCIUM	193.82	mg	*B12	.01	mcg
PHOS.	187.99	mg	MAGNES.	123.88	mg
IRON	7.17	mg	*ZINC	.30	mg
SODIUM	55.16	mg	SAT. FAT	.63	g
POTAS.	2131.82	mg	MONO UNSAT.	1.88	g
VIT A	8158.87	IU	POLYUNSAT.	.19	g
THIAMIN	.38	mg	FIBER	8.10	g

CALORIES

────────────── **Breakfast** ──────────────

Fruit 100
GRILLED APPLESAUCE SANDWICH 189
Herb Tea 25

────────────── **Lunch** ──────────────

TOSTADAS 208
Fresh Fruit 100

────────────── **Dinner** ──────────────

Green Salad 150
VEGELOAF 180
MUSHROOM GRAVY 158
Yellow Vegetable 81
Fresh Fruit 100

Total 1291

Evening snack calories 509

Grilled Applesauce Sandwich

4 teaspoons date sugar	8 tablespoons
1 teaspoon cinnamon	unsweetened
4 slices whole-grain bread	applesauce

Combine date sugar and cinnamon. Spread the bread with the applesauce and sprinkle with the date-cinnamon mixture. Place on a Pam-sprayed, nonstick cookie sheet. Grill under the broiler until bubbly. You may eat as is or as a sandwich.

Serves 2

Tostadas

4 corn tortillas	1 cup chopped tomatoes
1 16-ounce can Rosarita Vegetarian Refried Beans (or make your own)	4 tablespoons chopped sweet red onion
	2 cups chopped lettuce
3 tablespoons mild to hot salsa (according to preference)	4 teaspoons vegetable-broth seasoning
	Extra salsa for table service

Warm the tortillas on a Pam-sprayed, nonstick cookie sheet. Watch closely so that they do not burn. In a small saucepan, warm the beans with the salsa. Place ¼ of the mixture on one of the 4 tortillas, and top with ¼ cup of chopped tomatoes, 1 tablespoon of onion, ½ cup of lettuce, and sprinkle with 1 teaspoon of vegetable-broth seasoning. You may put the ingredients on the tortillas in any order you wish. Makes 4 tostadas.

Serves 2

Vegeloaf

2	cups canned green beans (no salt) (1 16-ounce can)	¼	cup raw walnut pieces (approximately ⅛ cup if chopped)
1	cup liquid from the green beans	2	tablespoons unsalted spaghetti sauce
1	egg white	2	cloves garlic
¾	cup cooked brown rice or barley	¼	cup cooked mushrooms
2	tablespoons vegetable-broth seasoning	2	cups whole-wheat bread crumbs, packed (4 slices of bread)

Blend the green beans with their liquid in the blender. Add the remaining ingredients except the bread crumbs and blend. Pour mixture into a bowl over the bread crumbs and combine. Pour into a nonstick, Pam-sprayed loaf pan and bake at 300° for 45 minutes.

Serves 4

GRILLED APPLESAUCE SANDWICH
Per Single Serving

4/4/9 CALORIES : 189
CAL FROM CARB. : 81%
CAL FROM PRO. : 11%
CAL FROM FAT : 7%

P/S RATIO 1.99 : 1

DATE:

GRAM WT.	119.00	g	RIBOFLN	.07	mg
CHOLSTRL.	0.00	mg	NIACIN	1.51	mg
CALORIES	179.16	kcal	*VIT C	.72	mg
PROTEIN	5.30	g	*PANTO.	.43	mg
FAT	1.63	g	*B6	.10	mg
CARB.	38.62	g	FOLACIN	15.35	mcg
CALCIUM	51.75	mg	B12	0.00	mcg
PHOS.	118.50	mg	*MAGNES.	40.75	mg
IRON	1.68	mg	ZINC	1.32	mg
SODIUM	265.33	mg	SAT. FAT	.20	g
POTAS.	181.99	mg	MONO UNSAT.	.60	g
*VIT A	17.50	IU	POLYUNSAT.	.40	g
THIAMIN	.12	mg	FIBER	1.12	g

TOSTADA
Per Single Serving

4/4/9 CALORIES : 208
CAL FROM CARB. : 75%
CAL FROM PRO. : 19%
CAL FROM FAT : 5%

P/S RATIO 4.28 : 1

DATE:

GRAM WT.	204.17	g	RIBOFLN	.11	mg
CHOLSTRL.	0.00	mg	NIACIN	1.55	mg
CALORIES	200.35	kcal	*VIT C	14.50	mg
PROTEIN	10.05	g	*PANTO.	.91	mg
FAT	1.32	g	*B6	.11	mg
CARB.	39.26	g	*FOLACIN	177.01	mcg
CALCIUM	55.17	mg	*B12	0.00	mcg
PHOS.	202.57	mg	*MAGNES.	29.06	mg
IRON	3.18	mg	*ZINC	1.72	mg
SODIUM	158.89	mg	SAT. FAT	.07	g
POTAS.	580.92	mg	MONO UNSAT.	.22	g
VIT A	755.41	IU	POLYUNSAT.	.30	g
THIAMIN	.21	mg	FIBER	2.16	g

VEGELOAF
Per Single Serving

				4/4/9 CALORIES	: 180
				CAL FROM CARB.	: 60%
				CAL FROM PRO.	: 14%
				CAL FROM FAT	: 26%

P/S RATIO 6.81 : 1

DATE:

GRAM WT.	158.45	g	*RIBOFLN	.12	mg
CHOLSTRL.	0.00	mg	*NIACIN	1.75	mg
CALORIES	172.29	kcal	*VIT C	6.45	mg
PROTEIN	6.65	g	*PANTO.	.97	mg
*FAT	5.20	g	B6	.36	mg
CARB.	27.12	g	*FOLACIN	25.53	mcg
CALCIUM	69.11	mg	B12	.00	mcg
PHOS.	136.63	mg	MAGNES.	51.24	mg
*IRON	2.35	mg	*ZINC	1.15	mg
SODIUM	251.27	mg	SAT. FAT	.39	g
POTAS.	257.02	mg	MONO UNSAT.	.97	g
*VIT A	431.34	IU	POLYUNSAT.	2.68	g
THIAMIN	.15	mg	FIBER	1.35	g

Mushroom Gravy

1 teaspoon safflower oil (or any flavorless type of oil)

¾ cup chopped onions

1 cup cooked mushroom pieces

1 tablespoon vegetable-broth seasoning

1 tablespoon arrowroot

1 cup water

1 tablespoon white wine

¼ teaspoon black pepper

1 tablespoon salsa

In a small (1 quart) saucepan, sauté the onions in the oil. Dissolve the vegetable-broth seasoning and arrowroot into 1 cup water. Add with the mushrooms to the onions. Cook gently until thickened (it will only take a minute or so), then add the white wine, pepper, and salsa. Serve over the vegeloaf. *Note:* You may want to double this recipe, it's so good!

Serves 4

CALORIES

_____Breakfast_____

Fruit	100
CAROB HOT CEREAL	181
Herb Tea	25

_____Lunch_____

Green Salad	150
ENGALIAN PIZZAS	598
Fresh Fruit	100

_____Dinner_____

Fruit Salad	145
ENCHILADAS	213
Total	1512

Evening snack calories   288

Carob Hot Cereal

2¼	cups water	½	teaspoon cinnamon
1	cup oatmeal	1	tablespoon raisins
1	tablespoon unsweetened carob powder	2	teaspoons honey

Bring the water to a boil. Stir in the oatmeal, carob, and cinnamon. Cook for 3 minutes. Remove from heat and stir in the raisins and honey. Let stand with lid on for 1 minute. No need to add any milk or juice—delicious as is!

Serves 2

Engalian Pizzas

4	whole-grain English muffins, halved	8	very thin slices green pepper
8	tablespoons unsalted spaghetti sauce (approximately ⅓ of a 15½-ounce jar)	8	tablespoons cooked, sliced mushrooms
16	teaspoons finely chopped onion (approximately ¼ of a small onion)	8	teaspoons grated Parmesan cheese

Place the halved muffins on a nonstick cookie sheet. Top each with 1 tablespoon spaghetti sauce, 2 teaspoons of onion, 1 slice of green pepper, and 1 tablespoon mushrooms. Sprinkle 1 teaspoon of the grated cheese evenly over the top. Bake at 350° for 15 minutes.

Serves 2

Fruit Salad

1 ripe banana, sliced thin
1 cup stone fruits, pitted and cut into chunks (peaches, apricots, nectarines, etc.)

1 cup seasonal fruits (strawberries, melon, kiwi, papaya, oranges, etc.)
½ cup pineapple chunks

Combine all ingredients together in a bowl.

Serves 2

Enchiladas

1 cup cooked pinto beans
⅔ cup unsalted spaghetti sauce
⅓ cup salsa (mild to hot according to taste preference)
1 cup cooked brown rice
1 tablespoon vegetable-broth seasoning
¼ cup chopped onions

½ cup salsa (mild to hot according to taste preference)
¼ cup unsalted spaghetti sauce
1 rounded tablespoon vegetable-broth seasoning
1 tablespoon grated Parmesan cheese
6 corn tortillas

Blend the pinto beans, ⅔ cup spaghetti sauce, and ⅓ cup salsa together coarsely in the blender. Transfer to a bowl and add the rice, 1 tablespoon vegetable-broth seasoning, and onions. Put 2 heaping tablespoons of the mixture into each corn tortilla and roll up. Place side by side in a 6 × 10-inch Pyrex baking dish which has been sprayed with Pam (or a nonstick dish of similar size). In a cup mix the ½ cup of salsa with the ¼ cup spaghetti sauce and 1 rounded tablespoon vegetable-broth seasoning and pour evenly over the rolled tortillas. Sprinkle the Parmesan cheese over all. Cover with foil and seal. Bake at 350° for 30 minutes. Makes 6.

Serves 2

CAROB HOT CEREAL
Per Single Serving

4/4/9 CALORIES : 181
CAL FROM CARB. : 78%
CAL FROM PRO. : 10%
CAL FROM FAT : 12%

P/S RATIO   1.98 : 1

DATE:

GRAM WT.	255.00	g	RIBOFLN	.06	mg
CHOLSTRL.	0.00	mg	NIACIN	.27	mg
CALORIES	177.00	kcal	VIT C	.12	mg
PROTEIN	4.95	g	PANTO.	3.62	mg
FAT	2.40	g	B6	.50	mg
CARB.	35.45	g	FOLACIN	79.66	mcg
CALCIUM	25.50	mg	B12	0.00	mcg
PHOS.	142.00	mg	MAGNES.	52.20	mg
IRON	1.60	mg	ZINC	2.31	mg
SODIUM	524.50	mg	SAT. FAT	.50	g
POTAS.	186.00	mg	MONO UNSAT.	.80	g
VIT A	.93	IU	POLYUNSAT.	1.00	g
THIAMIN	.19	mg	*FIBER	.53	g

ENGALIAN PIZZAS
Per Single Serving

4/4/9 CALORIES : 165
CAL FROM CARB. : 56%
CAL FROM PRO. : 14%
CAL FROM FAT : 30%

P/S RATIO   .50 : 1

DATE:

GRAM WT.	121.48	g	RIBOFLN	.18	mg
CHOLSTRL.	23.86	mg	NIACIN	1.61	mg
CALORIES	164.60	kcal	VIT C	42.56	mg
PROTEIN	5.80	g	*PANTO.	.29	mg
FAT	5.55	g	*B6	.10	mg
CARB.	23.31	g	*FOLACIN	6.10	mcg
CALCIUM	99.97	mg	*B12	.00	mcg
PHOS.	118.90	mg	*MAGNES.	14.93	mg
IRON	1.56	mg	*ZINC	.76	mg
SODIUM	246.06	mg	SAT. FAT	1.68	g
POTAS.	288.27	mg	MONO UNSAT.	2.58	g
*VIT A	606.99	IU	POLYUNSAT.	.85	g
THIAMIN	.13	mg	FIBER	.67	g

FRUIT SALAD
Per Single Serving

			4/4/9 CALORIES	:	145
			CAL FROM CARB.	:	90%
			CAL FROM PRO.	:	5%
			CAL FROM FAT	:	5%

P/S RATIO	2.00 : 1				
DATE:					
GRAM WT.	255.25	g	RIBOFLN	.15	mg
CHOLSTRL.	0.00	mg	NIACIN	1.48	mg
CALORIES	130.75	kcal	VIT C	58.97	mg
PROTEIN	1.79	g	PANTO.	.60	mg
FAT	.79	g	B6	.42	mg
CARB.	32.82	g	FOLACIN	31.10	mcg
CALCIUM	21.25	mg	B12	0.00	mcg
PHOS.	38.25	mg	MAGNES.	35.25	mg
IRON	.69	mg	ZINC	.33	mg
SODIUM	2.25	mg	SAT. FAT	.14	g
POTAS.	559.75	mg	MONO UNSAT.	.10	g
VIT A	530.25	IU	POLYUNSAT.	.28	g
THIAMIN	.09	mg	FIBER	1.43	g

ENCHILADAS
Per Single Serving

			4/4/9 CALORIES	:	213
			CAL FROM CARB.	:	79%
			CAL FROM PRO.	:	13%
			CAL FROM FAT	:	8%

P/S RATIO	1.17 : 1				
DATE:					
GRAM WT.	170.67	g	RIBOFLN	.09	mg
CHOLSTRL.	.66	mg	NIACIN	2.15	mg
CALORIES	206.59	kcal	*VIT C	24.92	mg
PROTEIN	6.97	g	*PANTO.	.82	mg
FAT	1.96	g	*B6	.27	mg
CARB.	42.29	g	*FOLACIN	63.93	mcg
CALCIUM	46.66	mg	*B12	.003	mcg
PHOS.	155.94	mg	*MAGNES.	37.30	mg
IRON	2.30	mg	*ZINC	.84	mg
SODIUM	620.48	mg	SAT. FAT	.29	g
POTAS.	494.76	mg	MONO UNSAT.	.64	g
VIT A	1189.15	IU	POLYUNSAT.	.34	g
THIAMIN	.19	mg	FIBER	1.39	g

DAY NINETEEN MENUS

CALORIES
_____ **Breakfast** _____

Fruit 100
BARLEY WITH FRUIT BREAKFAST PUDDING 517
Herb Tea 25

_____ **Lunch** _____

Green Salad 150
BAKED BEANS 155
Cornbread, Muffins, or Bread 56

_____ **Dinner** _____

4-BEAN SALAD 177
Corn on the Cob with Butter Buds (1 teaspoon) 106
Broccoli (1 cup) 51

Total 1337

Evening snack calories 463

Barley with Fruit Breakfast Pudding

1	cup cooked barley	¼	teaspoon cinnamon
2	tablespoons honey	½	teaspoon vanilla
¼	cup apple juice	2	tablespoons raisins
½	cup diced apples	1	tablespoon chopped
⅛	teaspoon nutmeg		walnuts

Mix all ingredients together and bake in a Pam-sprayed, nonstick casserole dish at 350° for 30 minutes.

Serves 2

BARLEY WITH FRUIT BREAKFAST PUDDING
Per Single Serving

			4/4/9 CALORIES	: 517	
			CAL FROM CARB.	: 86%	
			CAL FROM PRO.	: 7%	
			CAL FROM FAT	: 7%	

P/S RATIO   6.92 : 1

DATE:

GRAM WT.	196.25	g	RIBOFLN	.08	mg
CHOLSTRL.	0.00	mg	NIACIN	3.34	mg
CALORIES	497.75	kcal	VIT C	1.85	mg
PROTEIN	9.19	g	*PANTO.	.60	mg
FAT	3.80	g	B6	.30	mg
CARB.	111.89	g	*FOLACIN	1.83	mcg
CALCIUM	31.25	mg	B12	0.00	mcg
PHOS.	219.50	mg	MAGNES.	48.26	mg
IRON	2.71	mg	*ZINC	.34	mg
SODIUM	7.19	mg	SAT. FAT	.23	g
POTAS.	329.50	mg	MONO UNSAT.	.40	g
VIT A	30.94	IU	POLYUNSAT.	1.65	g
THIAMIN	.16	mg	*FIBER	1.00	g

Baked Beans

¾ cup celery, chopped small (pea size)
2 cups cooked pinto beans
⅓ cup unsalted spaghetti sauce
¼ cup water
¾ cup chopped onion

1 tablespoon natural catsup (made with honey)
1 tablespoon unsulphured blackstrap molasses
2 teaspoons vegetable-broth seasoning

Mix all the ingredients in a 2-quart casserole and cover. Bake at 350° for 45 minutes.

Serves 4

4-Bean Salad

1 16-ounce can green and wax beans
1 16-ounce can garbanzo beans, rinsed
1 16-ounce can kidney beans, rinsed
½ cup chopped green pepper

½ cup chopped onion (either yellow, red, or green)
4 tablespoons cider vinegar
1 tablespoon olive oil
1 tablespoon vegetable-broth seasoning
⅛ teaspoon black pepper

Combine all the ingredients in a bowl with a tight-sealing lid (such as Tupperware). Allow to marinate for at least an hour, gently shaking the bowl several times to mix the seasonings with the vegetables.

Serves 4

BAKED BEANS
Per Single Serving

4/4/9 CALORIES : 155
CAL FROM CARB. : 74%
CAL FROM PRO. : 21%
CAL FROM FAT : 5%

P/S RATIO .59 : 1

DATE:

GRAM WT.	177.17	g	RIBOFLN	.11	mg
CHOLSTRL.	0.00	mg	NIACIN	1.21	mg
CALORIES	149.64	kcal	*VIT C	15.62	mg
*PROTEIN	8.18	g	*PANTO.	.14	mg
*FAT	.94	g	*B6	.07	mg
CARB.	28.92	g	*FOLACIN	5.68	mcg
CALCIUM	101.08	mg	B12	.001	mcg
PHOS.	165.58	mg	*MAGNES.	26.86	mg
IRON	3.86	mg	*ZINC	1.53	mg
SODIUM	83.99	mg	SAT. FAT	.03	g
POTAS.	751.24	mg	MONO UNSAT.	.19	g
*VIT A	430.87	IU	POLYUNSAT.	.02	g
THIAMIN	.16	mg	*FIBER	1.83	g

4-BEAN SALAD
Per Single Serving

4/4/9 CALORIES : 177
CAL FROM CARB. : 60%
CAL FROM PRO. : 19%
CAL FROM FAT : 20%

P/S RATIO .61 : 1

DATE:

GRAM WT.	218.37	g	*RIBOFLN	.11	mg
CHOLSTRL.	0.00	mg	*NIACIN	.98	mg
CALORIES	169.07	kcal	*VIT C	29.62	mg
*PROTEIN	8.70	g	*PANTO.	.67	mg
FAT	4.08	g	*B6	.10	mg
CARB.	26.95	g	*FOLACIN	170.15	mcg
CALCIUM	74.00	mg	*B12	.00	mcg
PHOS.	159.29	mg	*MAGNES.	16.20	mg
IRON	3.56	mg	*ZINC	1.17	mg
SODIUM	167.28	mg	SAT. FAT	.45	g
*POTAS.	466.87	mg	MONO UNSAT.	2.47	g
*VIT A	162.50	IU	POLYUNSAT.	.27	g
*THIAMIN	.14	mg	*FIBER	2.38	g

————————**Breakfast**————————

Fruit	100
BREAKFAST BARS	208
Herb Tea	25

————————**Lunch**————————

HUMMUS SANDWICH	224
Fresh Fruit	100

————————**Dinner**————————

Green Salad	150
SPANISH RICE	156
Green Vegetable	51
Bread	56
Total	1070

Evening snack calories 730

Breakfast Bars

½	cup apple juice	1	tablespoon baking powder
1	small banana		
1	egg white	2½	ounces whole, pitted dates (approximately ½ cup)
½	teaspoon lemon extract		
½	teaspoon cinnamon		
1	tablespoon honey	3	fresh apricots, pitted (1½ inch in diameter)
½	cup oat bran		
		1	teaspoon vanilla

Combine the first eight ingredients in the blender. Pour into a Pam-sprayed, nonstick 10 × 1½-inch baking dish. Bake at 350° for 30 minutes. While mixture is baking, blend the dates, apricots, and vanilla in a small blender jar. You may need to stop the blender and press the mixture away from the blades a few times, as it is sticky. Top the bars with this after 30 minutes, and bake 10 minutes more at 400°.

Serves 4

BREAKFAST BARS
Per Single Serving

			4/4/9 CALORIES	: 208	
			CAL FROM CARB.	: 86%	
			CAL FROM PRO.	: 9%	
			CAL FROM FAT	: 5%	

P/S RATIO   .99 : 1

DATE:

GRAM WT.	151.42	g	RIBOFLN	.10	mg
CHOLSTRL.	0.00	mg	NIACIN	1.04	mg
CALORIES	196.50	kcal	VIT C	5.77	mg
*PROTEIN	4.77	g	*PANTO.	.32	mg
*FAT	1.18	g	*B6	.21	mg
CARB.	44.95	g	*FOLACIN	10.95	mcg
CALCIUM	191.65	mg	B12	.00	mcg
PHOS.	372.25	mg	*MAGNES.	53.10	mg
*IRON	1.02	mg	*ZINC	.24	mg
SODIUM	16.51	mg	*SAT. FAT	.06	g
POTAS.	858.00	mg	*MONO UNSAT.	.05	g
VIT A	748.87	IU	*POLYUNSAT.	.06	g
THIAMIN	.24	mg	*FIBER	6.91	g

Hummus Sandwich

¾	cup mashed garbanzo beans	1	tablespoon chopped fresh parsley
1	tablespoon sesame tahini	1	teaspoon vinegar
1	teaspoon minced garlic (2 cloves)	4	slices tomato
		4	slices whole-grain bread

In a blender, food processor, meat grinder, or with a potato masher, mix all the ingredients together, except the tomato and bread. Use ½ of the mixture for each sandwich, topping with the tomato slices.

Serves 2

Spanish Rice

2 cups cooked brown rice
¼ cup finely chopped green pepper
½ cup red onion (approximately ½ small onion)
1 tablespoon mild salsa
3 tablespoons unsalted spaghetti sauce
½ cup chopped fresh tomato (approximately 1 small tomato)
1 teaspoon vegetable-broth seasoning
½ cup apple juice
1 tablespoon grated Parmesan cheese

Combine all the ingredients except the Parmesan cheese. Sprinkle the cheese evenly over the top. Bake in a covered one-quart baking dish at 300° for 30 minutes.

Serves 4

HUMMUS SANDWICH
Per Single Serving

			4/4/9 CALORIES	: 224	
			CAL FROM CARB.	: 73%	
			CAL FROM PRO.	: 20%	
			CAL FROM FAT	: 8%	
P/S RATIO	2.00 : 1				
DATE:					
GRAM WT.	149.37	g	*RIBOFLN	.11	mg
CHOLSTRL.	0.00	mg	*NIACIN	2.05	mg
CALORIES	214.08	kcal	*VIT C	8.25	mg
*PROTEIN	11.10	g	*PANTO.	.91	mg
*FAT	1.99	g	*B6	.14	mg
CARB.	40.92	g	*FOLACIN	142.54	mcg
CALCIUM	83.91	mg	B12	0.00	mcg
PHOS.	224.54	mg	*MAGNES.	44.00	mg
*IRON	3.49	mg	*ZINC	2.16	mg
SODIUM	269.02	mg	SAT. FAT	.20	g
POTAS.	458.37	mg	MONO UNSAT.	.60	g
*VIT A	358.75	IU	POLYUNSAT.	.40	g
*THIAMIN	.21	mg	*FIBER	2.02	g

SPANISH RICE
Per Single Serving

			4/4/9 CALORIES	: 156
			CAL FROM CARB.	: 84%
			CAL FROM PRO.	: 10%
			CAL FROM FAT	: 6%

P/S RATIO   .07 : 1

DATE:

GRAM WT.	186.87	g	RIBOFLN	.05	mg
CHOLSTRL.	1.00	mg	NIACIN	1.67	mg
CALORIES	155.43	kcal	VIT C	20.16	mg
PROTEIN	3.77	g	*PANTO.	1.61	mg
FAT	1.11	g	*B6	.68	mg
CARB.	32.81	g	*FOLACIN	24.42	mcg
CALCIUM	41.12	mg	*B12	0.00	mcg
PHOS.	101.18	mg	*MAGNES.	37.44	mg
IRON	.95	mg	*ZINC	.47	mg
SODIUM	353.50	mg	SAT. FAT	.24	g
POTAS.	229.62	mg	MONO UNSAT.	.11	g
VIT A	314.62	IU	POLYUNSAT.	.01	g
THIAMIN	.12	mg	FIBER	.75	g

CALORIES

_____Breakfast_____

Fruit 100
POTATO PANCAKES 245
Butter Buds and Fruit Syrup (1 tablespoon each) 62
Herb Tea 25

_____Lunch_____

Fruit 100
GRILLED PINEAPPLE-BANANA SANDWICH 202
Applesauce (½ cup), unsweetened 55

_____Dinner_____

Green Salad 150
MACARONI AND CORN 436
Fresh Fruit 100

                          Total   1475

                  Evening snack calories   325

Potato Pancakes

1	cup water	½	cup corn flour
1	egg white	¼	cup oat bran
1	tablespoon honey	1	tablespoon baking
2	teaspoons safflower oil		powder
1	teaspoon vanilla	1½	cups oatmeal
1	cup chopped unpeeled potato (1 small potato)		

Blend the ingredients together in the blender in the order listed. Bake on a hot, Pam-sprayed, nonstick griddle or waffle iron. Serve with Butter Buds, unsweetened fruit syrup, and/or honey, and applesauce on the side.

Serves 4

POTATO PANCAKES
(2 Per Serving)

			4/4/9 CALORIES	: 245	
			CAL FROM CARB.	: 70%	
			CAL FROM PRO.	: 12%	
			CAL FROM FAT	: 18%	
P/S RATIO	1.53 : 1				
DATE:					
GRAM WT.	247.50	g	RIBOFLN	.09	mg
CHOLSTRL.	0.00	mg	NIACIN	.84	mg
CALORIES	244.32	kcal	VIT C	5.54	mg
*PROTEIN	7.65	g	*PANTO.	2.73	mg
*FAT	4.88	g	*B6	.42	mg
CARB.	43.09	g	*FOLACIN	63.17	mcg
CALCIUM	188.57	mg	*B12	.00	mcg
PHOS.	426.27	mg	*MAGNES.	62.94	mg
*IRON	1.61	mg	*ZINC	1.73	mg
SODIUM	406.44	mg	SAT. FAT	.71	g
*POTAS.	633.81	mg	MONO UNSAT.	2.37	g
*VIT A	50.00	IU	POLYUNSAT.	1.09	g
THIAMIN	.29	mg	*FIBER	3.64	g

Grilled Pineapple-Banana Sandwich

4	slices whole-grain bread	1	ripe banana, sliced
2	tablespoons crushed		lengthwise
	unsweetened pineapple	½	teaspoon cinnamon

Spread the pineapple on 2 slices of the bread. Cover with the strips of banana, then sprinkle each slice with ¼ teaspoon of cinnamon. Top with the other 2 slices of bread. Grill on a preheated, Pam-sprayed nonstick griddle until browned.

Serves 2

Macaroni and Corn

1	small onion, chopped	1	10-ounce package
½	green pepper, chopped		frozen corn
1	teaspoon olive oil	3	cups cooked macaroni
¾	cup unsalted spaghetti	1	tablespoon vegetable-
	sauce		broth seasoning

Sauté the onion and green pepper in the olive oil in a medium-sized saucepan. Add the spaghetti sauce, corn, seasoning, and macaroni. Cook until the corn is done, about 10 minutes. You may add water if you like it soupier.

Serves 2

GRILLED PINEAPPLE-BANANA SANDWICH
Per Single Serving

4/4/9 CALORIES : 202
CAL FROM CARB. : 80%
CAL FROM PRO. : 11%
CAL FROM FAT : 8%

P/S RATIO   1.48 : 1

DATE:

GRAM WT.	122.31	g	RIBOFLN	.12	mg
CHOLSTRL.	0.00	mg	NIACIN	1.75	mg
CALORIES	187.50	kcal	*VIT C	6.37	mg
PROTEIN	5.85	g	PANTO.	.54	mg
FAT	1.89	g	B6	.43	mg
CARB.	40.55	g	*FOLACIN	25.90	mcg
CALCIUM	54.87	mg	B12	0.00	mcg
PHOS.	125.62	mg	MAGNES.	57.06	mg
IRON	1.83	mg	ZINC	1.41	mg
SODIUM	264.81	mg	SAT. FAT	.30	g
POTAS.	376.81	mg	MONO UNSAT.	.62	g
*VIT A	50.62	IU	POLYUNSAT.	.45	g
THIAMIN	.16	mg	FIBER	1.13	g

MACARONI AND CORN
Per Single Serving

4/4/9 CALORIES : 436
CAL FROM CARB. : 77%
CAL FROM PRO. : 12%
CAL FROM FAT : 11%

P/S RATIO   .60 : 1

DATE:

GRAM WT.	503.59	g	RIBOFLN	.33	mg
CHOLSTRL.	0.00	mg	NIACIN	5.35	mg
CALORIES	416.43	kcal	VIT C	101.69	mg
PROTEIN	13.27	g	*PANTO.	1.11	mg
FAT	5.17	g	*B6	.44	mg
CARB.	84.27	g	*FOLACIN	38.87	mcg
CALCIUM	51.03	mg	*B12	.00	mcg
PHOS.	241.85	mg	MAGNES.	92.13	mg
IRON	4.84	mg	ZINC	1.81	mg
SODIUM	22.08	mg	SAT. FAT	.45	g
*POTAS.	870.33	mg	MONO UNSAT.	2.52	g
*VIT A	1911.10	IU	POLYUNSAT.	.27	g
THIAMIN	.52	mg	FIBER	2.12	g

WEEK FOUR SHOPPING LIST

( ) Is your pantry stocked with the baking and condiment staples?
(Some recipes call for thyme, bay leaf, paprika, sage)

( ) Is your pantry stocked with the food staples?
(Check for sesame seeds, sunflower seeds and cashews [a few], bulgur wheat, millet, spaghetti, fettucine [or other pastas], lentils)

Fresh Foods

Fruit (2–3 servings per day for 7 days)
Bananas (used in recipes as well as eaten plain)
(Don't forget eggs)
Tomatoes
Navel Oranges
Red Sweet Peppers
1 small Jicama
1 small Lime
A few dried Apricots
Fresh Mushrooms
Yellow Squash
Zucchini
Snow Peas, large handful
Fresh Bean Sprouts, large handful
Carrots
2 or 3 heads Leaf Lettuce
Green Onions
Baking Potatoes
Purple Onion, 1
Celery, small head
Dried Figs, 4-ounce bag
6 ounces Red Snapper (see Day Twenty-Six)
2 extra large Baking Apples
Parsley, 1 bunch
2 very large Fresh Green Peppers
1 tiny head of Cabbage
Some Fresh Green Cooking Vegetables

Frozen Foods

Frozen Peas, 1-pound bag
1 10-ounce package Corn and Lima Beans
Orange Juice, 1 can
1 package Frozen Mixed Vegetables
Corn-on-the-Cob

Canned or Jar Foods

Garbanzo Beans
Kidney Beans
Julienne Beets
Unsweetened Applesauce
Cooking Sherry
1 can Pineapple Chunks (get 2 if you'll use in fruit salad)
1 15-ounce can peeled Italian Tomatoes
1 small jar Sesame Tahini (may have to purchase at the health store)
Asparagus Spears

Other

Pita Pocket Bread
6 Whole Wheat Hamburger Buns
(Don't forget regular Whole-grain Bread)
1 quart Nonfat Milk (always optional)
Any dessert recipe ingredients

CALORIES

_____**Breakfast**_____

Fruit 100
HIGH-FIBER GRANOLA 564
1 cup Fruit Juice or Nonfat Milk 114
Herb Tea (with 1 teaspoon of honey) 48

_____**Lunch**_____

FALAFEL BURGERS 523
TAHINI SAUCE 56
Fresh Fruit 100

_____**Dinner**_____

Fresh Steamed Vegetable Platter 56
1 tablespoon Parmesan Cheese 21
JICAMA-ORANGE SALAD 63

Total   1645

Evening snack calories   155

High-Fiber Granola

1	cup oatmeal	¼	cup chopped dates or
½	cup oat bran		date pieces
2	tablespoons honey	⅛	cup unhulled sesame
2	teaspoons sesame, corn,		seeds
	or other oil	⅛	cup chopped cashews
1	tablespoon water	½	cup raisins (*add after*
			cooking; raisins are
			never cooked)

Toast the oatmeal and oat bran together on a large cookie sheet at 350° for 10 minutes. Mix together the honey, oil, and water. Toss the honey mixture with the dates, nuts, seeds, and then the oats mixture. Return to the oven on a Pam-sprayed cookie sheet and bake for 20 minutes more, stirring every few minutes. When the baking is done, add the raisins. Cool and serve.

Serves 2

HIGH FIBER GRANOLA
Per Single Serving

			4/4/9 CALORIES	: 564
			CAL FROM CARB.	: 66%
			CAL FROM PRO.	: 9%
			CAL FROM FAT	: 26%

P/S RATIO   2.46 : 1

DATE:

GRAM WT.	220.78	g	RIBOFLN	.17	mg
CHOLSTRL.	0.00	mg	NIACIN	1.79	mg
CALORIES	531.00	kcal	*VIT C	1.38	mg
PROTEIN	12.73	g	*PANTO.	2.17	mg
FAT	16.02	g	*B6	.38	mg
CARB.	92.57	g	*FOLACIN	44.23	mcg
CALCIUM	71.11	mg	*B12	0.00	mcg
PHOS.	391.87	mg	*MAGNES.	150.79	mg
IRON	2.71	mg	*ZINC	1.54	mg
*SODIUM	269.96	mg	*SAT. FAT	2.15	g
*POTAS.	720.25	mg	*MONO UNSAT.	5.90	g
*VIT A	22.62	IU	*POLYUNSAT.	5.29	g
THIAMIN	.59	mg	*FIBER	13.54	g

FRESH STEAMED VEGETABLE PLATTER
Per Single Serving

4/4/9 CALORIES : 122
CAL FROM CARB. : 71%
CAL FROM PRO. : 21%
CAL FROM FAT : 7%

P/S RATIO 0 : 1

DATE:

GRAM WT.	346.00	g	RIBOFLN	.35	mg
CHOLSTRL.	0.00	mg	NIACIN	2.65	mg
CALORIES	104.00	kcal	VIT C	120.50	mg
PROTEIN	6.70	g	*PANTO.	1.76	mg
FAT	1.05	g	*B6	.42	mg
CARB.	21.90	g	*FOLACIN	72.70	mcg
CALCIUM	130.00	mg	B12	0.00	mcg
PHOS.	155.50	mg	MAGNES.	69.68	mg
IRON	2.10	mg	*ZINC	.85	mg
*SODIUM	40.00	mg	SAT. FAT	0.00	g
POTAS.	710.50	mg	MONO UNSAT.	0.00	g
VIT A	10545.00	IU	POLYUNSAT.	0.00	g
THIAMIN	.25	mg	FIBER	3.37	g

FRESH STEAMED VEGETABLE PLATTER
Per Single Serving

4/4/9 CALORIES : 56
CAL FROM CARB. : 59%
CAL FROM PRO. : 34%
CAL FROM FAT : 7%

P/S RATIO   0 : 1

DATE:

GRAM WT.	230.00	g	RIBOFLN	.27	mg
CHOLSTRL.	0.00	mg	NIACIN	1.70	mg
CALORIES	45.00	kcal	VIT C	112.50	mg
PROTEIN	4.75	g	*PANTO.	1.33	mg
FAT	.50	g	*B6	.25	mg
CARB.	8.30	g	*FOLACIN	55.72	mcg
CALCIUM	103.50	mg	B12	0.00	mcg
PHOS.	97.00	mg	MAGNES.	41.12	mg
IRON	1.40	mg	*ZINC	.48	mg
SODIUM	14.50	mg	SAT. FAT	0.00	g
POTAS.	463.00	mg	MONO UNSAT.	0.00	g
VIT A	2250.00	IU	POLYUNSAT.	0.00	g
THIAMIN	.17	mg	FIBER	2.32	g

Falafel Burgers

1 cup boiling water
½ cup bulgur
2 cups canned garbanzo beans, drained
3 cloves garlic, minced
¼ cup lemon juice
1 teaspoon vegetable-broth seasoning
¼ teaspoon Tabasco

3 egg whites
1 teaspoon sesame, corn, or other oil
½ cup dry bread crumbs
12 fresh tomato slices
6 pita bread
6 tablespoons Tahini Sauce

Soak the bulgur in the boiling water for 20 minutes, then drain. In the blender (or food processor) combine the garbanzo beans, garlic, lemon juice, vegetable-broth seasoning, and Tabasco. In a large bowl beat the egg whites with the oil. Mix in the bread crumbs, puréed garbanzo mixture, and the drained bulgur. Shape mixture into 6 patties. On a Pam-sprayed, nonstick griddle, cook the patties about 5 minutes on each side. Serve immediately in pita pockets with tomato slices and 1 tablespoon tahini sauce for each pita.

Serves 3 (2 burgers each)

Tahini Sauce

3 tablespoons sesame tahini
2 tablespoons water (or more)
2 teaspoons lemon juice or vinegar

½ teaspoon sesame, corn, or other oil
1 or more cloves garlic, minced
Dash of cayenne pepper

In a small bowl, with a spoon stir the water, lemon juice, and oil with the tahini until thoroughly mixed. Stir in the garlic and cayenne pepper.

Makes 6 tablespoons

Jicama-Orange Salad

3 navel oranges   1 small jicama
2 sweet red peppers

Dressing

¼ cup vinegar   ⅛ teaspoon chile powder
1 tablespoon unrefined   or paprika
  corn oil   1 clove garlic, peeled and
2 teaspoons vegetable-   halved
  broth seasoning   1 teaspoon honey
⅛ teaspoon white pepper   Lime wedges for
                                    garnish

Remove the peel and the membrane from the oranges, separating
them into sections. Cut the peppers into long, thin strips. Cut the
jicama into matchstick strips, discarding any fibrous portions. (If
you've never used jicama before, note that the outer brown part is
discarded.) Combine the dressing ingredients in a jar with a tight-
fitting lid. Shake vigorously. Let stand as long as possible to
combine flavors. Toss the dressing together with the salad
ingredients just before serving. Garnish with lime wedges.
Variation: Add other tropical fruits, or cut-up apple.

Serves 4

FALAFEL BURGERS
Per Single Serving (2 Burgers)

			4/4/9 CALORIES	: 523
			CAL FROM CARB.	: 70%
			CAL FROM PRO.	: 18%
			CAL FROM FAT	: 12%

P/S RATIO   1.58 : 1

DATE:

GRAM WT.	346.84	g	*RIBOFLN	.36	mg
CHOLSTRL.	0.00	mg	*NIACIN	4.09	mg
CALORIES	515.18	kcal	*VIT C	23.35	mg
PROTEIN	23.59	g	*PANTO.	1.59	mg
*FAT	7.21	g	*B6	.19	mg
CARB.	91.46	g	*FOLACIN	243.01	mcg
CALCIUM	133.50	mg	*B12	.02	mcg
PHOS.	347.66	mg	*MAGNES.	56.00	mg
*IRON	5.68	mg	ZINC	2.62	mg
SODIUM	487.16	mg	*SAT. FAT	1.22	g
POTAS.	808.91	mg	*MONO UNSAT.	2.63	g
*VIT A	557.41	IU	*POLYUNSAT.	1.93	g
THIAMIN	.52	mg	*FIBER	2.82	g

TAHINI SAUCE
Per Single Serving (1 tablespoon)

			4/4/9 CALORIES	: 56
			CAL FROM CARB.	: 2%
			CAL FROM PRO.	: 0%
			CAL FROM FAT	: 98%

P/S RATIO   .12 : 1

DATE:

GRAM WT.	9.65	g	*RIBOFLN	.002	mg
CHOLSTRL.	15.50	mg	*NIACIN	.004	mg
CALORIES	55.26	kcal	*VIT C	.77	mg
PROTEIN	.09	g	*PANTO.	.001	mg
*FAT	6.12	g	*B6	.005	mg
CARB.	.29	g	*FOLACIN	.44	mcg
CALCIUM	1.96	mg	*B12	0.00	mcg
PHOS.	2.73	mg	*MAGNES.	.41	mg
*IRON	.01	mg	ZINC	.01	mg
SODIUM	58.74	mg	*SAT. FAT	3.62	g
POTAS.	6.59	mg	*MONO UNSAT.	1.75	g
*VIT A	217.08	IU	*POLYUNSAT.	.43	g
THIAMIN	.002	mg	*FIBER	.00	g

JICAMA-ORANGE SALAD
Per Single Serving

4/4/9 CALORIES : 63
CAL FROM CARB. : 90%
CAL FROM PRO. : 8%
CAL FROM FAT : 2%

P/S RATIO 1.65 : 1

DATE:

GRAM WT.	138.25	g	RIBOFLN	.06	mg
CHOLSTRL.	0.00	mg	NIACIN	.47	mg
CALORIES	59.00	kcal	VIT C	133.77	mg
PROTEIN	1.47	g	*PANTO.	.24	mg
FAT	.22	g	*B6	.05	mg
CARB.	14.39	g	*FOLACIN	29.77	mcg
CALCIUM	44.00	mg	B12	0.00	mcg
PHOS.	25.50	mg	*MAGNES.	9.75	mg
IRON	.34	mg	*ZINC	.06	mg
*SODIUM	0.00	mg	SAT. FAT	.01	g
*POTAS.	177.75	mg	MONO UNSAT.	.02	g
VIT A	1981.75	IU	POLYUNSAT.	.02	g
THIAMIN	.11	mg	FIBER	1.10	g

JICAMA-ORANGE SALAD DRESSING
Per Single Serving (½ cup)

4/4/9 CALORIES : 39
CAL FROM CARB. : 23%
CAL FROM PRO. : 0%
CAL FROM FAT : 77%

P/S RATIO 4.70 : 1

DATE:

GRAM WT.	20.96	g	*RIBOFLN	.001	mg
CHOLSTRL.	0.00	mg	*NIACIN	.01	mg
CALORIES	38.41	kcal	*VIT C	.05	mg
*PROTEIN	.06	g	*PANTO.	.00	mg
*FAT	3.40	g	*B6	.007	mg
CARB.	2.45	g	*FOLACIN	.09	mcg
*CALCIUM	.48	mg	*B12	0.00	mcg
*PHOS.	1.70	mg	*MAGNES.	.57	mg
*IRON	.01	mg	*ZINC	.04	mg
SODIUM	1.42	mg	SAT. FAT	.42	g
POTAS.	7.79	mg	MONO UNSAT.	.82	g
*VIT A	40.62	IU	POLYUNSAT.	2.00	g
*THIAMIN	.002	mg	*FIBER	.02	g

CALORIES

_____ **Breakfast** _____

Fruit 100
CROCKPOT OATMEAL WITH APRICOT 119
Herb Tea 25

_____ **Lunch** _____

REFRIGERATOR SOUP 300
Bread with 1 tablespoon Apple Butter 89
Fresh Fruit 100

_____ **Dinner** _____

PASTA ORIENTAL 330
Muffins with 2 teaspoons Butter Buds 249
Fresh Fruit 100
                                                                          ─────
                                        Total   1412

                                Evening snack calories   388

Crockpot Oatmeal With Apricot

1¼ cups water
½ cup oatmeal
½ cup apple juice

¼ cup chopped dried apricots
⅛ cup millet

Put all the ingredients into a crockpot and turn on low overnight (approximately 8 hours). This may also be cooked the normal way, using a small saucepan, according to package directions. Watch it carefully, adding water if needed.

Serves 2

Refrigerator Soup

When the refrigerator is bulging with various fresh vegetables that have been partially used, it's time to make refrigerator soup! Fill your large pot half full of water, then add the following categories of ingredients, chopped, diced, chunked, etc., according to your personal preference (this is a partial list, typical of what you may have on hand):

For Thickness:	For Flavor:	Mostly for Bulk:	For Heartiness:
Potato, peeled and chunked	Spaghetti sauce, unsalted	Zucchini	Barley
Macaroni	Salsa	Yellow squash	Rice
Spaghetti, broken	Tomatoes	Summer squash	Lentils
Any pasta	Oregano	Eggplant	Split peas
	Garlic	Carrots	Beans, cooked (kidney, garbanzo, etc.)
	Onions		Peas
	Vegetable-broth seasoning		
	Parsley		
	Cabbage		
	Green Pepper		
	Celery		

Pasta Oriental

4 ounces fettucine or tagliarini (before cooking
1 small onion, chopped
8 ounces fresh mushrooms, sliced
2 cloves garlic, minced
1 cup thinly sliced yellow squash
1 cup thinly sliced zucchini
1 cup snow peas, strings removed

1 cup fresh bean sprouts (optional)
1 cup chopped tomatoes
1 tablespoon olive oil
3 tablespoons Butter Buds
¾ cup water
1 tablespoon arrowroot
½ teaspoon cayenne pepper
3 tablespoons vegetable-broth seasoning

Following package instructions, cook fettucine. Sauté the onion, mushrooms, garlic, squash, zucchini, snow peas, sprouts, and tomatoes in the olive oil. Cover and let steam on low while the fettucine is cooking in a separate pot. Heat Butter Buds, water, and arrowroot powder together in a small saucepan to make a sauce. Drain the cooked pasta and toss with the cooked vegetables, sauce, pepper, and vegetable-broth seasoning. Serve hot.

Serves 2

CROCKPOT OATMEAL WITH APRICOT
Per Single Serving

4/4/9 CALORIES : 119
CAL FROM CARB. : 82%
CAL FROM PRO. : 9%
CAL FROM FAT : 9%

P/S RATIO   1.99 : 1

DATE:

GRAM WT.	190.75	g	RIBOFLN	.04	mg
CHOLSTRL.	0.00	mg	NIACIN	.42	mg
CALORIES	115.75	kcal	VIT C	.77	mg
PROTEIN	2.75	g	*PANTO.	1.86	mg
FAT	1.31	g	B6	.27	mg
CARB.	24.29	g	FOLACIN	40.55	mcg
CALCIUM	19.00	mg	B12	0.00	mcg
PHOS.	83.25	mg	MAGNES.	31.20	mg
IRON	1.34	mg	ZINC	1.18	mg
SODIUM	264.00	mg	SAT. FAT	.26	g
POTAS.	267.50	mg	MONO UNSAT.	.42	g
VIT A	634.00	IU	POLYUNSAT.	.52	g
THIAMIN	.10	mg	FIBER	.62	g

PASTA ORIENTAL
Per Single Serving

4/4/9 CALORIES : 330
CAL FROM CARB. : 62%
CAL FROM PRO. : 16%
CAL FROM FAT : 22%

P/S RATIO   .61 : 1

DATE:

GRAM WT.	549.50	g	*RIBOFLN	.53	mg
CHOLSTRL.	0.00	mg	*NIACIN	6.51	mg
CALORIES	316.15	kcal	*VIT C	64.50	mg
PROTEIN	13.30	g	*PANTO.	1.47	mg
*FAT	8.17	g	*B6	.39	mg
CARB.	51.11	g	*FOLACIN	46.64	mcg
CALCIUM	110.04	mg	*B12	0.00	mcg
PHOS.	282.51	mg	MAGNES.	90.60	mg
*IRON	4.25	mg	*ZINC	2.18	mg
SODIUM	21.62	mg	*SAT. FAT	.90	g
*POTAS.	992.87	mg	*MONO UNSAT.	4.95	g
*VIT A	1950.00	IU	*POLYUNSAT.	.55	g
THIAMIN	.57	mg	FIBER	4.12	g

_____ **Breakfast** _____

Fruit	100
CARROT WAFFLES	289
Applesauce	55
Herb Tea	25

_____ **Lunch** _____

CHEF SALAD	301
HONEY-LEMON DRESSING	224
Bread or Muffins	56
Fresh Fruit	100

_____ **Dinner** _____

TWICE-BAKED POTATOES	129
ZUCCATASH	73
Fresh Fruit	100
Total	1452

Evening snack calories   348

Carrot Waffles

½	cup apple juice	1	teaspoon baking
¼	cup chopped carrots		powder
2	teaspoons corn or	¾	cup whole-wheat flour
	sesame oil	2	egg whites, stiffly beaten
1	tablespoon honey		

Blend together the juice and chopped carrots. While the blender is running, add the oil, honey, and baking powder. Pour into a bowl and mix in the flour. Fold in the egg whites. Bake on Pam-sprayed, nonstick waffle iron. Serve with Butter Buds and applesauce.

Serves 2

CARROT WAFFLES
Per Single Serving

4/4/9 CALORIES	:	289
CAL FROM CARB.	:	70%
CAL FROM PRO.	:	13%
CAL FROM FAT	:	17%

P/S RATIO   4.64 : 1

DATE:

GRAM WT.	171.03	g	RIBOFLN	.16	mg
CHOLSTRL.	0.00	mg	NIACIN	2.17	mg
CALORIES	276.65	kcal	VIT C	1.79	mg
*PROTEIN	9.58	g	*PANTO.	.63	mg
*FAT	5.52	g	*B6	.19	mg
CARB.	50.52	g	*FOLACIN	23.56	mcg
CALCIUM	140.33	mg	*B12	.02	mcg
PHOS.	345.75	mg	*MAGNES.	59.32	mg
*IRON	1.89	mg	*ZINC	1.32	mg
SODIUM	60.41	mg	*SAT. FAT	.57	g
POTAS.	584.20	mg	*MONO UNSAT.	1.10	g
*VIT A	1513.00	IU	*POLYUNSAT.	2.68	g
THIAMIN	.27	mg	*FIBER	1.30	g

APPLESAUCE
Per Single Serving

4/4/9 CALORIES : 55
CAL FROM CARB. : 100%
CAL FROM PRO. : 0%
CAL FROM FAT : 0%

P/S RATIO   1.70 : 1

DATE:

GRAM WT.	122.00	g	RIBOFLN	.03	mg
CHOLSTRL.	0.00	mg	NIACIN	.22	mg
CALORIES	53.00	kcal	VIT C	1.45	mg
PROTEIN	.20	g	PANTO.	.11	mg
FAT	.06	g	B6	.03	mg
CARB.	13.77	g	FOLACIN	.70	mcg
CALCIUM	3.50	mg	B12	0.00	mcg
PHOS.	9.00	mg	MAGNES.	3.50	mg
IRON	.14	mg	ZINC	.03	mg
SODIUM	2.50	mg	SAT. FAT	.01	g
POTAS.	91.50	mg	MONO UNSAT.	.00	g
VIT A	35.00	IU	POLYUNSAT.	.01	g
THIAMIN	.01	mg	FIBER	.65	g

Chef Salad

1	small head leafy green lettuce	2	tablespoons chopped green onion
1	cup canned garbanzo beans, rinsed	1	tablespoon hulled sun-flower seeds
½	cup canned kidney beans, rinsed	1	cup unsweetened julienne beets
½	cup frozen peas, rinsed to thaw	1	large tomato, in chunks
		6	asparagus spears Honey-Lemon Dressing

Wash lettuce, let drain, and tear into bite-size pieces. Combine all the ingredients. Reserve the asparagus spears for a garnish. Toss with the Honey-Lemon Dressing. Divide into two portions, heaping each onto a large, chilled plate. (Keep plates in freezer during preparation of the vegetables.) Lay the asparagus spears over the top.

Serves 2

Honey-Lemon Dressing

3 tablespoons lemon juice
1 tablespoon honey
1 tablespoon vegetable-broth seasoning

2 tablespoons water
3 tablespoons oil

Blend or shake together.

Serves 2-4

Twice-Baked Potatoes

4 baking potatoes
2 egg whites
2 tablespoons Butter Buds
1 tablespoon Parmesan cheese
1 teaspoon olive oil

1 tablespoon finely chopped onion
1 teaspoon crushed, dried thyme
⅛ teaspoon pepper
Paprika (approximately ⅛ teaspoon for each potato)

Bake the potatoes for 50 minutes at 400°. Slice ¼ inch lengthwise off each potato. Scoop out the pulp and place in a mixing bowl. Reserve the shells. Beat the potato pulp with all the remaining ingredients except the paprika. Return the mixture to the shells, sprinkle with the paprika, and bake at 350° for 15 minutes.

Serves 4

CHEF SALAD
Per Single Serving

4/4/9 CALORIES : 301
CAL FROM CARB. : 67%
CAL FROM PRO. : 24%
CAL FROM FAT : 10%

P/S RATIO   5.26 : 1

DATE:

GRAM WT.	477.28	g	RIBOFLN	.31	mg
CHOLSTRL.	0.00	mg	NIACIN	3.14	mg
CALORIES	285.12	kcal	*VIT C	39.75	mg
PROTEIN	17.76	g	*PANTO.	1.68	mg
FAT	3.29	g	*B6	.27	mg
CARB.	50.40	g	*FOLACIN	339.45	mcg
CALCIUM	122.68	mg	*B12	.00	mcg
PHOS.	352.18	mg	*MAGNES.	56.99	mg
IRON	6.44	mg	*ZINC	3.58	mg
SODIUM	103.65	mg	SAT. FAT	.25	g
POTAS.	1138.18	mg	MONO UNSAT.	.42	g
VIT A	1522.18	IU	POLYUNSAT.	1.35	g
THIAMIN	.53	mg	FIBER	4.91	g

HONEY-LEMON DRESSING
Per Single Serving

4/4/9 CALORIES : 224
CAL FROM CARB. : 19%
CAL FROM PRO. : 0%
CAL FROM FAT : 81%

P/S RATIO   .61 : 1

DATE:

GRAM WT.	53.55	g	RIBOFLN	.007	mg
CHOLSTRL.	0.00	mg	NIACIN	.07	mg
CALORIES	216.95	kcal	VIT C	10.59	mg
PROTEIN	.14	g	*PANTO.	.04	mg
FAT	20.25	g	*B6	.01	mg
CARB.	10.61	g	*FOLACIN	3.31	mcg
CALCIUM	2.03	mg	*B12	.00	mcg
PHOS.	2.24	mg	MAGNES.	1.81	mg
IRON	.13	mg	ZINC	.13	mg
SODIUM	.69	mg	*SAT. FAT	2.70	g
*POTAS.	34.00	mg	*MONO UNSAT.	14.85	g
*VIT A	4.50	IU	*POLYUNSAT.	1.65	g
THIAMIN	.007	mg	*FIBER	.00	g

TWICE-BAKED POTATOES
Per Single Serving

			4/4/9 CALORIES	: 129
			CAL FROM CARB.	: 74%
			CAL FROM PRO.	: 16%
			CAL FROM FAT	: 11%

P/S RATIO   .25 : 1

DATE:

GRAM WT.	157.87	g	RIBOFLN	.10	mg
CHOLSTRL.	1.00	mg	NIACIN	2.02	mg
CALORIES	128.69	kcal	VIT C	22.25	mg
PROTEIN	5.14	g	*PANTO.	.04	mg
FAT	1.60	g	*B6	.24	mg
CARB.	23.77	g	*FOLACIN	12.41	mcg
CALCIUM	30.00	mg	*B12	.01	mcg
PHOS.	85.01	mg	MAGNES.	32.58	mg
IRON	.84	mg	ZINC	.32	mg
SODIUM	52.50	mg	SAT. FAT	.38	g
*POTAS.	583.75	mg	MONO UNSAT.	.93	g
*VIT A	9.83	IU	POLYUNSAT.	.09	g
THIAMIN	.12	mg	FIBER	.69	g

Zuccatash

1 medium zucchini (approximately 1½ cups cut up), sliced and quartered

1 10-ounce package frozen corn and lima beans

1 cup water

1 teaspoon olive oil

1 rounded teaspoon tomato paste

2 teaspoons vegetable-broth seasoning

Cook all ingredients together in a small pot until the zucchini is tender, about 12 minutes.

Serves 4

ZUCCATASH
Per Single Serving

4/4/9 CALORIES : 73
CAL FROM CARB. : 63%
CAL FROM PRO. : 21%
CAL FROM FAT : 16%

P/S RATIO   .61 : 1

DATE:

GRAM WT.	134.36	g	RIBOFLN	.09	mg
CHOLSTRL.	0.00	mg	NIACIN	.96	mg
CALORIES	71.06	kcal	VIT C	10.91	mg
PROTEIN	3.92	g	*PANTO.	.06	mg
FAT	1.36	g	*B6	.04	mg
CARB.	11.64	g	*FOLACIN	6.90	mcg
CALCIUM	35.24	mg	*B12	0.00	mcg
PHOS.	58.02	mg	MAGNES.	38.37	mg
IRON	1.63	mg	*ZINC	.31	mg
SODIUM	3.45	mg	SAT. FAT	.15	g
*POTAS.	240.46	mg	MONO UNSAT.	.82	g
*VIT A	381.30	IU	POLYUNSAT.	.09	g
THIAMIN	.05	mg	FIBER	1.44	g

CALORIES
———————————— **Breakfast** ————————————

Fruit	100
Cold Cereal	170
APPLESAUCE MUFFINS	223
Herb Tea	25

———————————— **Lunch** ————————————

MINEGHETTI SOUP	169
Bread with Apple Butter	89
Fresh Fruit	100

———————————— **Dinner** ————————————

WHEAT PILAF	219
Corn on the Cob	81
Green Vegetable	51
Fresh Fruit	100
Total	1327

Evening snack calories   473

Applesauce Muffins

1 egg white	2 teaspoons oil
1 teaspoon vanilla	¾ cup oat bran
2 tablespoons honey	¾ cup raisins
1 teaspoon cinnamon	½ cup water
2 teaspoons baking soda	1 cup whole-wheat flour
1½ cups unsweetened applesauce	

Combine the ingredients with a hand mixer, in the order given. Pour into Pam-sprayed, nonstick muffin pans. Bake at 350° for 40 minutes.

Makes 12 muffins

APPLESAUCE MUFFINS
Per Single Serving

4/4/9 CALORIES : 223
CAL FROM CARB. : 74%
CAL FROM PRO. : 12%
CAL FROM FAT : 13%

P/S RATIO .66 : 1

DATE:

GRAM WT.	93.12	g	RIBOFLN	.10	mg
CHOLSTRL.	0.00	mg	NIACIN	.55	mg
CALORIES	213.26	kcal	VIT C	1.38	mg
PROTEIN	6.90	g	*PANTO.	.09	mg
FAT	3.33	g	*B6	.06	mg
CARB.	41.68	g	*FOLACIN	1.99	mcg
CALCIUM	33.42	mg	*B12	.00	mcg
PHOS.	222.01	mg	MAGNES.	75.71	mg
IRON	.86	mg	ZINC	.13	mg
SODIUM	13.31	mg	SAT. FAT	.23	g
*POTAS.	371.29	mg	MONO UNSAT.	1.10	g
*VIT A	18.87	IU	POLYUNSAT.	.15	g
THIAMIN	.41	mg	*FIBER	12.59	g

Mineghetti Soup

6 cups water
1 cup zucchini chunks (1 small zucchini)
½ cup diced red onion (¼ medium onion
1½ cups eggplant chunks (¼ small eggplant)
2 ounces spaghetti, broken
1½ cups diced yellow squash (2 small squash)

½ cup chopped celery (1 stalk)
½ cup cooked mushrooms
1 cup cooked kidney beans
1 cup frozen peas
5 heaping tablespoons unsalted spaghetti sauce
2 tablespoons vegetable-broth seasoning

Combine all of the ingredients in a large pot in the order listed. Begin cooking while you prepare the ingredients, adding them as they are ready. Simmer until the vegetables are tender (20 minutes minimum once the spaghetti is added).

Serves 4

Wheat Pilaf

½ cup finely chopped onion

2 tablespoons Butter Buds

2 teaspoons unrefined sesame or corn oil

1 cup bulgur

2 tablespoons vegetable-broth seasoning

2 cups water

Juice of 1 orange (about ¼ cup)

1 tablespoon cooking sherry

½ cup finely chopped dried figs

2 tablespoons sesame seeds

1 teaspoon finely grated orange peel

Sauté the onion in the oil until soft. Stir in the bulgur to coat with the oil, then add the Butter Buds and the vegetable-broth seasoning mixed with 2 cups water. Add the orange juice and sherry. Cover and simmer over low heat for ½ hour. Stir in the figs, sesame seeds, and orange peel. Cover again and continue to cook for 10 minutes. Serve hot.

Serves 4

MINEGHETTI SOUP
Per Single Serving

4/4/9 CALORIES : 169
CAL FROM CARB. : 72%
CAL FROM PRO. : 22%
CAL FROM FAT : 6%

P/S RATIO   .59 : 1

DATE:

GRAM WT.	377.54	g	RIBOFLN	.27	mg
CHOLSTRL.	0.00	mg	NIACIN	3.33	mg
CALORIES	158.89	kcal	*VIT C	33.88	mg
PROTEIN	9.39	g	*PANTO.	.88	mg
FAT	1.12	g	*B6	.17	mg
CARB.	30.62	g	*FOLACIN	106.79	mcg
CALCIUM	83.29	mg	B12	.00	mcg
PHOS.	186.86	mg	*MAGNES.	56.86	mg
IRON	3.52	mg	*ZINC	1.54	mg
SODIUM	74.10	mg	SAT. FAT	.03	g
POTAS.	724.72	mg	MONO UNSAT.	.18	g
*VIT A	1087.41	IU	POLYUNSAT.	.01	g
THIAMIN	.32	mg	FIBER	3.35	g

WHEAT PILAF
Per Single Serving

4/4/9 CALORIES : 219
CAL FROM CARB. : 68%
CAL FROM PRO. : 10%
CAL FROM FAT : 21%

P/S RATIO   3.72 : 1

DATE:

GRAM WT.	136.01	g	RIBOFLN	.08	mg
CHOLSTRL.	0.00	mg	NIACIN	1.85	mg
*CALORIES	204.84	kcal	VIT C	11.80	mg
PROTEIN	5.66	g	*PANTO.	.59	mg
FAT	5.26	g	*B6	.20	mg
CARB.	37.57	g	*FOLACIN	13.73	mcg
CALCIUM	47.52	mg	*B12	0.00	mcg
PHOS.	154.08	mg	*MAGNES.	55.46	mg
IRON	1.47	mg	*ZINC	.89	mg
*SODIUM	4.50	mg	*SAT. FAT	.62	g
*POTAS.	321.45	mg	*MONO UNSAT.	1.39	g
*VIT A	130.58	IU	*POLYUNSAT.	2.32	g
THIAMIN	.22	mg	*FIBER	1.67	g

CALORIES

_____ **Breakfast** _____

Fruit 100
ORANGE PANCAKES 256
ORANGE SAUCE 121
Herb Tea 25

_____ **Lunch** _____

LENTIL-POTATO BURGERS 340
Fresh Fruit Salad (banana, pineapple, apple, orange,
   peach, berries) 224

_____ **Dinner** _____

Green Salad 150
COMPANY SKILLET FISH 398
Fresh Fruit 100

                       Total   1714

        Evening snack calories   86

Orange Pancakes

½ cup orange juice
¼ cup liquid Butter Buds
1 egg white
1 tablespoon orange-juice concentrate
½ cup whole-wheat flour
1½ teaspoons baking powder
2 tablespoons ground nuts or seeds (sunflower seeds, sesame, almond, walnut, or pecan)
2 teaspoons oil

Blend all ingredients in a blender, adding the dry ingredients slowly until mixture has the consistency of pancake batter. Bake on a hot Pam-sprayed, nonstick griddle. Serve with Orange Sauce or your favorite fruit syrup.

Serves 2

Orange Sauce

¼ cup orange juice
1 thin slice orange
1 tablespoon arrowroot
2 tablespoons honey

Combine the orange juice, orange slice, and arrowroot in a double boiler and cook, stirring, until thick. Remove from heat and stir in the honey.

Serves 2

ORANGE PANCAKES
Per Single Serving

4/4/9 CALORIES : 256
CAL FROM CARB. : 54%
CAL FROM PRO. : 13%
CAL FROM FAT : 33%

P/S RATIO 2.75 : 1

DATE:

GRAM WT.	134.58	g	RIBOFLN	.11	mg
CHOLSTRL.	0.00	mg	NIACIN	1.99	mg
CALORIES	246.45	kcal	*VIT C	36.48	mg
*PROTEIN	8.48	g	*PANTO.	.51	mg
*FAT	9.44	g	*B6	.14	mg
CARB.	34.81	g	*FOLACIN	54.98	mcg
CALCIUM	195.94	mg	*B12	.01	mcg
PHOS.	451.26	mg	*MAGNES.	47.90	mg
*IRON	1.75	mg	*ZINC	.77	mg
SODIUM	29.81	mg	*SAT. FAT	1.11	g
*POTAS.	764.81	mg	*MONO UNSAT.	4.16	g
*VIT A	77.45	IU	*POLYUNSAT.	3.07	g
THIAMIN	.41	mg	*FIBER	1.08	g

FRESH FRUIT SALAD
Per Single Serving

4/4/9 CALORIES : 224
CAL FROM CARB. : 91%
CAL FROM PRO. : 4%
CAL FROM FAT : 5%

P/S RATIO 2.05 : 1

DATE:

GRAM WT.	387.00	g	RIBOFLN	.18	mg
CHOLSTRL.	0.00	mg	NIACIN	1.47	mg
CALORIES	203.50	kcal	VIT C	100.95	mg
PROTEIN	2.40	g	PANTO.	.80	mg
FAT	1.24	g	B6	.52	mg
CARB.	51.24	g	FOLACIN	55.60	mcg
CALCIUM	53.00	mg	B12	0.00	mcg
PHOS.	50.00	mg	MAGNES.	47.50	mg
IRON	.98	mg	ZINC	.38	mg
SODIUM	2.75	mg	SAT. FAT	.20	g
POTAS.	720.00	mg	MONO UNSAT.	.13	g
VIT A	488.00	IU	POLYUNSAT.	.41	g
THIAMIN	.18	mg	FIBER	2.19	g

Lentil-Potato Burgers

2 cups mashed potatoes (4 medium potatoes)	½ cup chopped pecans
1 onion, chopped	6 whole-wheat buns
1 tablespoon unrefined oil	Natural mustard
	Catsup
½ teaspoon sage	Onion slices
2 cups cooked lentils	Tomato slices
	Lettuce

Peel potatoes, cook until done, and blend with some cooking liquid in blender until smooth. Combine the onion, oil, and sage in pan and simmer to partially cook the onion. Add the lentils and pecans and mix well. Form into small burgers and place on a Pam-sprayed, nonstick cookie sheet. Cover with foil and bake at 400° for 20 minutes. Serve on whole-wheat burger buns with natural mustard, catsup, onion slices, tomato slices, and lettuce.

Makes 6 burgers

Company Skillet Fish

2 teaspoons unrefined oil (sesame, corn, or olive)	2 cups zucchini, cut into chunks
1 tablespoon minced green pepper	3 tablespoons mild salsa
1 tablespoon minced tomato	6 ounces red snapper (or other similar low-fat fish), cut into chunks
½ cup minced onion	1½ cup cooked brown rice
1 clove garlic, minced	¼ cup water

Sauté the green pepper, tomato, onion, garlic, and zucchini chunks in the oil until the green pepper is partially soft. Add the salsa, fish chunks, brown rice, and water. Simmer over low heat for 15 to 20 minutes until the fish is thoroughly cooked.

Serves 2

ORANGE SAUCE
Per Single Serving

4/4/9 CALORIES : 121
CAL FROM CARB. : 76%
CAL FROM PRO. : 16%
CAL FROM FAT : 8%

P/S RATIO .07 : 1

DATE:

GRAM WT.	69.91	g	RIBOFLN	.06	mg
CHOLSTRL.	14.16	mg	NIACIN	1.26	mg
CALORIES	116.70	kcal	*VIT C	15.68	mg
PROTEIN	4.88	g	PANTO.	.21	mg
FAT	1.13	g	B6	.06	mg
CARB.	23.18	g	*FOLACIN	2.48	mcg
CALCIUM	7.73	mg	B12	.30	mcg
PHOS.	53.85	mg	MAGNES.	10.79	mg
IRON	.60	mg	ZINC	1.07	mg
SODIUM	11.37	mg	*SAT. FAT	.57	g
POTAS.	132.37	mg	*MONO UNSAT.	.37	g
*VIT A	62.00	IU	*POLYUNSAT.	.04	g
THIAMIN	.07	mg	*FIBER	.11	g

LENTIL-POTATO BURGERS
Per Single Serving

4/4/9 CALORIES : 340
CAL FROM CARB. : 55%
CAL FROM PRO. : 13%
CAL FROM FAT : 31%

P/S RATIO 1.61 : 1

DATE:

GRAM WT.	217.08	g	RIBOFLN	.17	mg
*CHOLSTRL.	0.00	mg	NIACIN	2.14	mg
CALORIES	333.63	kcal	*VIT C	10.00	mg
PROTEIN	11.30	g	*PANTO.	1.32	mg
*FAT	11.98	g	*B6	.39	mg
CARB.	47.06	g	*FOLACIN	77.10	mcg
CALCIUM	78.17	mg	*B12	0.00	mcg
PHOS.	186.27	mg	*MAGNES.	34.96	mg
IRON	2.85	mg	*ZINC	1.39	mg
*SODIUM	415.50	mg	*SAT. FAT	1.29	g
*POTAS.	490.50	mg	*MONO UNSAT.	7.15	g
*VIT A	50.83	IU	*POLYUNSAT.	2.08	g
THIAMIN	.30	mg	FIBER	1.55	g

COMPANY SKILLET FISH
Per Single Serving

			4/4/9 CALORIES	: 398	
			CAL FROM CARB.	: 52%	
			CAL FROM PRO.	: 26%	
			CAL FROM FAT	: 22%	
P/S RATIO	4.70 : 1				
DATE:					
GRAM WT.	467.62	g	*RIBOFLN	.23	mg
*CHOLSTRL.	0.00	mg	*NIACIN	11.26	mg
CALORIES	397.59	kcal	*VIT C	29.00	mg
PROTEIN	26.13	g	*PANTO.	2.28	mg
*FAT	9.84	g	*B6	.98	mg
CARB.	51.60	g	*FOLACIN	34.07	mcg
CALCIUM	98.18	mg	*B12	0.00	mcg
PHOS.	371.03	mg	*MAGNES.	77.39	mg
*IRON	2.93	mg	*ZINC	1.29	mg
*SODIUM	721.12	mg	*SAT. FAT	.56	g
*POTAS.	522.75	mg	*MONO UNSAT.	1.10	g
*VIT A	2287.08	IU	*POLYUNSAT.	2.66	g
THIAMIN	.28	mg	FIBER	2.00	g

CALORIES

Breakfast

Fruit	100
BAKED APPLE	190
Muffins or Toast with Apple Butter	148
Herb Tea	25

Lunch

Baked Potato with Mushroom Gravy (see recipe for Gravy on Day Seventeen)	306
GREEN PEPPER AND PINEAPPLE SKEWERS	165
Fresh Fruit	100

Dinner

Green Salad	150
SPAGHETTI WITH MARINARA SAUCE	221
Fresh Fruit	100
Total	1505

Evening snack calories 295

Baked Apple

2	extra-large baking apples (Pippin or some other tart apple)	1	tablespoon raisins
		2	tablespoons honey
1	tablespoon finely chopped dates	1	teaspoon cinnamon
		2	teaspoons lemon juice

Wash the outside of the apples. Don't peel them. Cut out the center core from the top down, leaving about ¼ inch uncut on the very bottom to hold the sweeteners. Mix the dates, raisins, honey, cinnamon, and lemon juice together. Pour half of the mixture into each apple center. Place the apples in a nonstick baking dish. Bake at 300° for 1 hour.

Serves 2

BAKED APPLE
Per Single Serving

			4/4/9 CALORIES	: 190
			CAL FROM CARB.	: 97%
			CAL FROM PRO.	: 1%
			CAL FROM FAT	: 2%
P/S RATIO	1.75 : 1			

DATE:					
GRAM WT.	171.59	g	RIBOFLN	.03	mg
CHOLSTRL.	0.00	mg	NIACIN	.35	mg
CALORIES	173.78	kcal	VIT C	8.65	mg
PROTEIN	.58	g	PANTO.	.17	mg
FAT	.53	g	B6	.09	mg
CARB.	46.10	g	FOLACIN	5.62	mcg
CALCIUM	16.14	mg	B12	0.00	mcg
PHOS.	17.85	mg	MAGNES.	10.25	mg
IRON	.56	mg	ZINC	.27	mg
SODIUM	3.65	mg	*SAT. FAT	.08	g
POTAS.	243.28	mg	*MONO UNSAT.	.02	g
VIT A	78.04	IU	*POLYUNSAT.	.15	g
THIAMIN	.03	mg	*FIBER	1.24	g

Green Pepper and Pineapple Skewers

1 can unsweetened pineapple chunks

3 large green peppers, cut into 2-inch-square chunks

3 tablespoons tomato paste

3 tablespoons honey

2 tablespoons cider vinegar

⅛ teaspoon cinnamon

*⅛ teaspoon cloves

*⅛ teaspoon allspice

*Note: Alternatively, use ½ teaspoon cinnamon, no cloves or allspice.

Combine tomato paste, honey, vinegar, and spice(s). Marinate the green pepper chunks and pineapple in this mixture for 30 to 60 minutes. Thread the pineapple and pepper chunks alternately on skewers. On an outdoor barbecue or under a broiler, barbecue, turning often. Since skewers vary in length, the number used varies. The recipe will usually serve 3.

Spaghetti with Marinara Sauce

1	tablespoon olive oil	1	tablespoon honey
¼	cup chopped onions	½	teaspoon grated lemon rind
¼	cup minced carrot	1	tablespoon minced fresh parsley
1	large clove garlic, minced	4	ounces uncooked pasta, cooked
⅛	teaspoon black pepper		Optional: Add vegetable-broth seasoning, to taste, just before serving.
1	15-ounce can peeled Italian tomatoes, diced		
1	small bay leaf, crushed		
⅛	teaspoon dried thyme Optional: 4 ounces low-fat fish (red snapper, halibut, etc.), broiled or steamed		

Cook the pasta according to label directions while making the sauce. Drain pasta just before adding the sauce to prevent sticking together. Sauté the onions, carrot, and garlic for about 5 minutes in the olive oil. Add the pepper, tomatoes, bay leaf, and thyme. Cook 5 minutes more. Add the fish if you are using it. Lower the heat and cook gently for fifteen minutes, stirring often. Add the honey and lemon rind and heat through for two minutes. Spoon over pasta and garnish with parsley.

Serves 2

GREEN PEPPER AND PINEAPPLE SKEWERS
Per Single Serving

			4/4/9 CALORIES	:	165
			CAL FROM CARB.	:	94%
			CAL FROM PRO.	:	5%
			CAL FROM FAT	:	1%

P/S RATIO   4.86 : 1

DATE:

GRAM WT.	230.70	g	*RIBOFLN	.12	mg
CHOLSTRL.	0.00	mg	*NIACIN	1.37	mg
CALORIES	150.77	kcal	*VIT C	144.11	mg
*PROTEIN	2.20	g	*PANTO.	.27	mg
FAT	.33	g	*B6	.26	mg
CARB.	38.82	g	*FOLACIN	7.63	mcg
CALCIUM	26.77	mg	B12	0.00	mcg
PHOS.	40.43	mg	MAGNES.	33.67	mg
IRON	1.70	mg	*ZINC	.68	mg
SODIUM	22.02	mg	SAT. FAT	.00	g
POTAS.	475.47	mg	MONO UNSAT.	.008	g
*VIT A	992.29	IU	POLYUNSAT.	.02	g
*THIAMIN	.19	mg	*FIBER	1.83	g

SPAGHETTI WITH MARINARA SAUCE
Per Single Serving

			4/4/9 CALORIES	:	221
			CAL FROM CARB.	:	61%
			CAL FROM PRO.	:	9%
			CAL FROM FAT	:	30%

P/S RATIO   .61 : 1

DATE:

GRAM WT.	331.50	g	*RIBOFLN	.17	mg
CHOLSTRL.	0.00	mg	*NIACIN	2.47	mg
CALORIES	210.27	kcal	*VIT C	64.34	mg
PROTEIN	4.97	g	*PANTO.	.09	mg
*FAT	7.46	g	*B6	.06	mg
CARB.	33.78	g	*FOLACIN	4.51	mcg
CALCIUM	54.13	mg	*B12	0.00	mcg
PHOS.	111.70	mg	MAGNES.	42.50	mg
*IRON	2.11	mg	*ZINC	.55	mg
SODIUM	20.87	mg	SAT. FAT	.90	g
*POTAS.	819.50	mg	MONO UNSAT.	4.95	g
*VIT A	4081.25	IU	POLYUNSAT.	.55	g
THIAMIN	.24	mg	*FIBER	1.79	g

CALORIES

Breakfast

Fruit	100
OVEN-BAKED FRENCH TOAST	280
Butter Buds and/or Syrup	4
Herb Tea	25

Lunch

CREAM OF VEGETABLE SOUP	219
Corn Bread (see Day Eleven menus)	311
Fresh Fruit	100

Dinner

Green Salad	150
STUFFED GREEN PEPPERS	219
Corn on the Cob	81
Fresh Fruit	100
Total	**1589**

Evening snack calories   211

Oven-Baked French Toast

2	ripe bananas	1	teaspoon sesame or
2	egg whites		corn oil
¼	teaspoon cinnamon	4	slices whole-wheat
1	teaspoon vanilla		bread

In the blender, blend together the bananas, egg whites, cinnamon, vanilla, and oil. Pour into a large bowl, and dip the bread into the mixture. Arrange the bread on a Pam-sprayed, nonstick cookie sheet. Bake in a preheated 350° oven for 15 to 20 minutes or until done. Turn bread toasted side up when serving. Serve with Butter Buds, fruit syrup, and/or apple sauce.

Serves 2

OVEN-BAKED FRENCH TOAST
Per Single Serving

			4/4/9 CALORIES	: 280
			CAL FROM CARB.	: 72%
			CAL FROM PRO.	: 14%
			CAL FROM FAT	: 14%
P/S RATIO	2.64 : 1			

DATE:					
GRAM WT.	199.26	g	RIBOFLN	.26	mg
CHOLSTRL.	0.00	mg	NIACIN	2.04	mg
CALORIES	263.03	kcal	*VIT C	10.30	mg
PROTEIN	9.73	g	*PANTO.	.75	mg
FAT	4.41	g	*B6	.75	mg
CARB.	50.92	g	*FOLACIN	41.80	mcg
CALCIUM	61.00	mg	*B12	.02	mcg
PHOS.	140.00	mg	MAGNES.	75.00	mg
IRON	1.96	mg	ZINC	1.51	mg
SODIUM	315.00	mg	SAT. FAT	.69	g
POTAS.	632.00	mg	MONO UNSAT.	1.19	g
*VIT A	92.00	IU	POLYUNSAT.	1.83	g
THIAMIN	.17	mg	FIBER	1.37	g

Cream of Vegetable Soup

4 cups water	4 tablespoons whole-wheat flour or arrow-root powder
2 cups frozen mixed vegetables (peas, carrots, corn, limas, green beans)	2 teaspoons unrefined oil or olive oil
	1 tablespoon vegetable-broth seasoning

Partially thaw the frozen vegetables. Blend them in the blender with the water, add the remaining ingredients, and blend until smooth. Cook in saucepan on low heat until bubbly, about 12 to 15 minutes. Stir often.

Serves 2

Stuffed Green Peppers

2 very large fresh green peppers	1 tablespoon hulled sun-flower seeds
1 cup cooked brown rice	2 teaspoons vegetable-broth seasoning
¼ cup unsalted spaghetti sauce	⅓ cup shredded cabbage

Cut peppers in half, remove white cores, and steam in 1 inch of water, cut side down, for 10 minutes. Mix the remaining ingredients and use to stuff the peppers. Place in a nonstick casserole, cover, and bake at 350° for 30 minutes. Serve with extra sauce if desired.

Serves 2

CREAM OF VEGETABLE SOUP
Per Single Serving

4/4/9 CALORIES : 219
CAL FROM CARB. : 64%
CAL FROM PRO. : 14%
CAL FROM FAT : 22%

P/S RATIO   4.70 : 1

DATE:

GRAM WT.	201.53	g	RIBOFLN	.14	mg
CHOLSTRL.	0.00	mg	NIACIN	2.65	mg
CALORIES	206.06	kcal	VIT C	15.00	mg
PROTEIN	7.80	g	*PANTO.	.72	mg
FAT	5.33	g	*B6	.27	mg
CARB.	35.05	g	*FOLACIN	34.82	mcg
CALCIUM	52.12	mg	*B12	0.00	mcg
PHOS.	170.75	mg	*MAGNES.	16.95	mg
IRON	2.90	mg	ZINC	1.46	mg
SODIUM	96.50	mg	*SAT. FAT	.56	g
POTAS.	403.50	mg	*MONO UNSAT.	1.10	g
*VIT A	9010.00	IU	*POLYUNSAT.	2.66	g
THIAMIN	.30	mg	FIBER	2.52	g

STUFFED GREEN PEPPERS
Per Single Serving

4/4/9 CALORIES : 194
CAL FROM CARB. : 73%
CAL FROM PRO. : 11%
CAL FROM FAT : 16%

P/S RATIO   4.47 : 1

DATE:

GRAM WT.	262.27	g	RIBOFLN	.14	mg
CHOLSTRL.	0.00	mg	NIACIN	2.65	mg
CALORIES	188.39	kcal	*VIT C	164.31	mg
PROTEIN	5.65	g	*PANTO.	1.78	mg
FAT	3.45	g	*B6	.93	mg
CARB.	35.48	g	*FOLACIN	32.00	mcg
CALCIUM	38.57	mg	*B12	.00	mcg
PHOS.	149.79	mg	MAGNES.	58.36	mg
IRON	2.22	mg	*ZINC	.77	mg
SODIUM	297.06	mg	SAT. FAT	.30	g
POTAS.	512.71	mg	MONO UNSAT.	.71	g
VIT A	947.55	IU	POLYUNSAT.	1.38	g
THIAMIN	.30	mg	FIBER	2.34	g

High-Fiber Desserts

Yummy Birthday Cake

A truly moist, delicious cake with lots of fiber and *no* added fats!
Of course, it isn't just for birthdays.

3 egg whites	1 teaspoon cinnamon
½ cup raw honey	1 cup water
1 tablespoon baking soda	1 cup oat bran
½ cup grated carrot	1 cup whole-wheat flour
(1 small carrot)	1 cup date pieces
1 cup grated zucchini	
(1 small zucchini)	

Cream together the egg whites, honey, and baking soda. Stir in
the carrot and zucchini. Add the cinnamon and water and mix
with a hand mixer. While the mixer is running, add the bran and
flour, then the date pieces. Pour into two 8 × 1½-inch nonstick
round cake pans that have been sprayed with Pam. Bake in
preheated 350° oven for 30 minutes. Fill and top with Filling and
Frosting below.

Filling and Frosting

1 cup apple juice	3 tablespoons tapioca
½ cup date pieces	granules
1 teaspoon vanilla	

Put ingredients into blender and blend for 2 minutes or until
dates are dispersed throughout. Pour into saucepan and cook for
5 minutes, stirring continuously. Remove from heat and cool
down to warm before filling and frosting the cake. Cake can be
served warm.

Serves 8

Strawberry-topped "Little Cakes"

½ cup whole-wheat flour
½ cup oat bran
1 teaspoon baking powder
1 teaspoon baking soda
½ cup date "sugar"

½ cup finely ground walnuts
2 tablespoons Butter Buds liquid
¼ cup plus 1 tablespoon water

Blend all the ingredients with a fork until doughy. Shape into little cakes. Place on a Pam-sprayed, nonstick baking sheet. Bake at 350° for 25 to 30 minutes or until done.

Strawberry Topping

1 cup strawberries
1 cup apple juice

3 tablespoons tapioca granules

In a saucepan, cook all ingredients, mashing the strawberries with a fork. Cook until bubbly and thickened, about 5 minutes. Remove from heat and cool until just warm. Serve over the little cakes. Top with fresh strawberries and a sprinkle of date sugar.

Makes 2 cups

Company Apple-Blueberry Cobbler

1 quart jar of water-packed blueberries (or equivalent amount of frozen blueberries, thawed)

2 large apples, peeled and cut into chunks

¼ cup almonds

¼ cup uncooked oatmeal

½ teaspoon cinnamon

1 cup apple juice

1 teaspoon vanilla

2 teaspoons tapioca granules

1 cup chopped dates

Pour the blueberries and chunks of apple into a 9 × 14-inch Pyrex baking dish. In the blender, chop the almonds, oatmeal, and cinnamon fine. Remove mixture and purée the remaining ingredients with the apple juice. Stir the liquid mixture into the berries and apples until well mixed. Sprinkle with the dry mixture. Bake in a preheated 350° oven for 30 minutes. Let cool. Serve either warm or cold.

Serves 8

YUMMY BIRTHDAY CAKE
Per Single Serving

```
                                    4/4/9 CALORIES    : 250
                                    CAL FROM CARB.  : 85%
                                    CAL FROM PRO.   : 11%
                                    CAL FROM FAT    :  4%
```

P/S RATIO   1.00 : 1

DATE:

GRAM WT.	103.93	g	RIBOFLN	.13	mg
CHOLSTRL.	0.00	mg	NIACIN	1.59	mg
CALORIES	235.19	kcal	VIT C	3.12	mg
PROTEIN	6.90	g	*PANTO.	.43	mg
FAT	1.30	g	*B6	.10	mg
CARB.	53.24	g	*FOLACIN	11.56	mcg
CALCIUM	36.02	mg	B12	.00	mcg
PHOS.	175.87	mg	MAGNES.	65.99	mg
IRON	1.20	mg	ZINC	.77	mg
SODIUM	25.07	mg	*SAT. FAT	.00	g
POTAS.	377.87	mg	*MONO UNSAT.	.00	g
VIT A	846.12	IU	*POLYUNSAT.	.00	g
THIAMIN	.31	mg	*FIBER	7.08	g

FILLING AND FROSTING
Per Single Serving

```
                                    4/4/9 CALORIES    : 59
                                    CAL FROM CARB.  : 98%
                                    CAL FROM PRO.   :  2%
                                    CAL FROM FAT    :  0%
```

P/S RATIO   1.74 : 1

DATE:

GRAM WT.	45.27	g	RIBOFLN	.01	mg
CHOLSTRL.	0.00	mg	NIACIN	.27	mg
CALORIES	56.31	kcal	VIT C	.28	mg
PROTEIN	.27	g	*PANTO.	.08	mg
FAT	.09	g	*B6	.03	mg
CARB.	14.53	g	FOLACIN	1.61	mcg
CALCIUM	6.00	mg	B12	0.00	mcg
PHOS.	7.37	mg	MAGNES.	5.03	mg
IRON	.25	mg	*ZINC	.04	mg
SODIUM	1.29	mg	*SAT. FAT	.00	g
POTAS.	110.31	mg	*MONO UNSAT.	.00	g
VIT A	5.81	IU	*POLYUNSAT.	.01	g
THIAMIN	.01	mg	FIBER	.31	g

STRAWBERRY-TOPPED "LITTLE CAKES"
Per Single Serving

4/4/9 CALORIES : 306
CAL FROM CARB. : 59%
CAL FROM PRO. : 9%
CAL FROM FAT : 31%

P/S RATIO   8.81 : 1

DATE:

GRAM WT.	56.12	g	RIBOFLN	.06	mg
CHOLSTRL.	0.00	mg	NIACIN	.91	mg
CALORIES	293.41	kcal	VIT C	.25	mg
*PROTEIN	7.03	g	*PANTO.	.30	mg
*FAT	10.76	g	*B6	.16	mg
CARB.	45.67	g	*FOLACIN	5.70	mcg
CALCIUM	86.06	mg	B12	0.00	mcg
PHOS.	294.50	mg	*MAGNES.	70.22	mg
*IRON	1.17	mg	*ZINC	.77	mg
SODIUM	1.71	mg	*SAT. FAT	.67	g
POTAS.	336.04	mg	*MONO UNSAT.	1.43	g
VIT A	5.00	IU	*POLYUNSAT.	5.95	g
THIAMIN	.32	mg	*FIBER	6.67	g

STRAWBERRY TOPPING
Per Single Serving

4/4/9 CALORIES : 63
CAL FROM CARB. : 97%
CAL FROM PRO. : 2%
CAL FROM FAT : 2%

P/S RATIO   4.66 : 1

DATE:

GRAM WT.	105.55	g	RIBOFLN	.03	mg
CHOLSTRL.	0.00	mg	NIACIN	.14	mg
CALORIES	62.75	kcal	VIT C	21.70	mg
PROTEIN	.34	g	*PANTO.	.12	mg
FAT	.22	g	*B6	.04	mg
CARB.	15.33	g	FOLACIN	7.02	mcg
CALCIUM	10.00	mg	B12	0.00	mcg
PHOS.	13.00	mg	MAGNES.	6.18	mg
IRON	.39	mg	*ZINC	.06	mg
SODIUM	2.45	mg	SAT. FAT	.01	g
POTAS.	137.25	mg	MONO UNSAT.	.02	g
VIT A	10.75	IU	POLYUNSAT.	.08	g
THIAMIN	.02	mg	FIBER	.33	g

COMPANY APPLE-BLUEBERRY COBBLER
Per Single Serving

4/4/9 CALORIES : 178
CAL FROM CARB. : 81%
CAL FROM PRO. : 4%
CAL FROM FAT : 15%

P/S RATIO   2.37 : 1

DATE:

GRAM WT.	174.26	g	RIBOFLN	.10	mg
CHOLSTRL.	0.00	mg	NIACIN	1.09	mg
CALORIES	163.78	kcal	*VIT C	3.43	mg
PROTEIN	1.77	g	*PANTO.	.42	mg
FAT	3.10	g	*B6	.13	mg
CARB.	36.06	g	FOLACIN	13.25	mcg
CALCIUM	27.77	mg	B12	0.00	mcg
PHOS.	48.16	mg	MAGNES.	26.86	mg
IRON	.84	mg	*ZINC	.26	mg
SODIUM	18.77	mg	*SAT. FAT	.21	g
POTAS.	294.26	mg	*MONO UNSAT.	1.50	g
VIT A	101.87	IU	*POLYUNSAT.	.51	g
THIAMIN	.07	mg	FIBER	2.07	g

Frozen Banana Pie

20	almonds	1	tablespoon unsweetened carob powder
¼	cup oatmeal		
4	large, soft dates		
3	medium-size ripe bananas	1	teaspoon vanilla (optional)
		1	tablespoon honey (optional)

Grind together the almonds, oatmeal, and dates in the smallest blender glass; have the dry ingredients nearest the blades to prevent sticking. You may have to remove the jar and clean the blades once or twice. When blended to a moist powder, pour into a pie pan. In a clean blender glass, purée the bananas with the carob powder. If desired, add vanilla and honey. Pour this on top of the dry mixture. Top with slices of extra banana as a decorative touch. Freeze overnight or until firm. Before serving, thaw for a few minutes, but no more.

Serves 4 to 6

Punkin' Pie

½	cup date pieces	1	teaspoon pumpkin pie spice
¼	cup oat bran		
1	cup pineapple juice	1	tablespoon molasses
2	cups canned pumpkin	2	tablespoons honey
		3	egg whites, stiffly beaten

Grind the date pieces and oat bran together in a 1-cup blender glass until the dates are in tiny bits. Pour this mixture into the bottom of a round glass or nonstick pie pan. Toast for 10 minutes at 350°. Remove from oven. Blend the remaining ingredients together except the egg whites. Use a spoon or spatula to push the ingredients down if they don't mix easily. Pour this mixture into a large bowl and fold in the egg whites. Pour into the pie pan and bake at 350° for 30 minutes.

Serves 8

FROZEN BANANA PIE
Per Single Serving

			4/4/9 CALORIES	: 234	
			CAL FROM CARB.	: 53%	
			CAL FROM PRO.	: 8%	
			CAL FROM FAT	: 39%	

P/S RATIO   2.13 : 1

DATE:

GRAM WT.	126.55	g	RIBOFLN	.26	mg
CHOLSTRL.	0.00	mg	NIACIN	1.28	mg
CALORIES	215.92	kcal	*VIT C	7.72	mg
PROTEIN	4.64	g	PANTO.	.59	mg
FAT	10.22	g	B6	.55	mg
CARB.	31.05	g	FOLACIN	30.32	mcg
CALCIUM	50.82	mg	B12	0.00	mcg
PHOS.	117.86	mg	MAGNES.	78.72	mg
IRON	1.28	mg	ZINC	.54	mg
SODIUM	34.38	mg	*SAT. FAT	.96	g
POTAS.	538.72	mg	*MONO UNSAT.	6.53	g
VIT A	73.20	IU	*POLYUNSAT.	2.06	g
THIAMIN	.10	mg	FIBER	1.10	g

PUNKIN' PIE
Per Single Serving

			4/4/9 CALORIES	: 114	
			CAL FROM CARB.	: 87%	
			CAL FROM PRO.	: 10%	
			CAL FROM FAT	: 4%	

P/S RATIO   5.00 : 1

DATE:

GRAM WT.	123.75	g	RIBOFLN	.09	mg
CHOLSTRL.	0.00	mg	NIACIN	.75	mg
CALORIES	107.09	kcal	*VIT C	6.79	mg
*PROTEIN	2.95	g	PANTO.	.42	mg
*FAT	.45	g	B6	.08	mg
CARB.	24.95	g	*FOLACIN	8.58	mcg
CALCIUM	30.97	mg	B12	.00	mcg
PHOS.	50.62	mg	MAGNES.	25.00	mg
IRON	.66	mg	*ZINC	.23	mg
SODIUM	21.47	mg	*SAT. FAT	.00	g
POTAS.	326.84	mg	*MONO UNSAT.	.00	g
*VIT A	3928.68	IU	*POLYUNSAT.	.00	g
THIAMIN	.09	mg	*FIBER	2.57	g

Popcorn

Good news! You don't have to give up a favorite munchie!

½	cup popcorn kernels	2	teaspoons dry Butter Buds

Pop the popcorn without oil in the hot air popper, or for a toastier taste, in the campfire popper. Sprinkle on the Butter Buds or dip the popcorn into the Buds since they have a tendency to fall to the bottom of the bowl.

Makes 9 cups

Easy Cookies

Full of fiber and flavor!

1	cup banana purée (2 medium bananas)	⅓	cup chopped almonds
½	cup date pieces	1	teaspoon vanilla
		1½	cups uncooked oatmeal

Pour the banana purée into a bowl and add the remaining ingredients. Mix well with a spoon. Drop by the tablespoonful onto a Pam-sprayed, nonstick cookie sheet. Bake at 375° for 18 to 20 minutes.

Makes 24 cookies

Carob-Date Brownies

2	egg whites	3	rounded tablespoons carob powder
1	tablespoon molasses		
1	tablespoon honey	½	cup oat bran
1½	teaspoons vanilla	½	cup apple juice
1	cup grated zucchini	1	cup flour
		¾	cup chopped dates

Beat together the egg whites, molasses, honey, and vanilla for 1 minute. Slowly, while beating, add the remaining ingredients. Bake in a Pam-sprayed, nonstick brownie pan (9" square cake pan 1½ inches deep) at 350° for 30 minutes.

Serves 9

POPCORN
Per Single Serving

			4/4/9 CALORIES	: 23
			CAL FROM CARB.	: 78%
			CAL FROM PRO.	: 13%
			CAL FROM FAT	: 9%
P/S RATIO	0 : 1			

DATE:

GRAM WT.	6.00	g	RIBOFLN	.01	mg
CHOLSTRL.	0.00	mg	NIACIN	.10	mg
CALORIES	23.00	kcal	VIT C	0.00	mg
PROTEIN	.80	g	*PANTO.	0.00	mg
FAT	.30	g	B6	.01	mg
CARB.	4.60	g	*FOLACIN	0.00	mcg
CALCIUM	1.00	mg	B12	0.00	mcg
PHOS.	17.00	mg	*MAGNES.	0.00	mg
IRON	.20	mg	ZINC	.24	mg
*SODIUM	0.00	mg	*SAT. FAT	0.00	g
*POTAS.	0.00	mg	MONO UNSAT.	.10	g
*VIT A	0.00	IU	POLYUNSAT.	.20	g
*THIAMIN	0.00	mg	FIBER	.13	g

EASY COOKIES
Per Single Serving

			4/4/9 CALORIES	: 97
			CAL FROM CARB.	: 67%
			CAL FROM PRO.	: 8%
			CAL FROM FAT	: 25%

P/S RATIO   2.08 : 1

DATE:

GRAM WT.	90.02	g	RIBOFLN	.07	mg
CHOLSTRL.	0.00	mg	NIACIN	.44	mg
CALORIES	92.45	kcal	*VIT C	1.71	mg
PROTEIN	2.21	g	PANTO.	1.02	mg
FAT	2.68	g	B6	.25	mg
CARB.	16.43	g	FOLACIN	25.99	mcg
CALCIUM	17.52	mg	B12	0.00	mcg
PHOS.	59.02	mg	MAGNES.	30.47	mg
IRON	.66	mg	ZINC	.65	mg
SODIUM	131.26	mg	*SAT. FAT	.31	g
POTAS.	187.95	mg	*MONO UNSAT.	1.51	g
VIT A	19.04	IU	*POLYUNSAT.	.65	g
THIAMIN	.07	mg	FIBER	.47	g

CAROB-DATE BROWNIES
Per Single Serving

			4/4/9 CALORIES	: 140
			CAL FROM CARB.	: 84%
			CAL FROM PRO.	: 12%
			CAL FROM FAT	: 4%

P/S RATIO   1.74 : 1

DATE:

GRAM WT.	77.16	g	RIBOFLN	.08	mg
CHOLSTRL.	0.00	mg	NIACIN	1.18	mg
CALORIES	131.80	kcal	*VIT C	2.25	mg
*PROTEIN	4.31	g	*PANTO.	.29	mg
*FAT	.75	g	*B6	.08	mg
CARB.	29.27	g	*FOLACIN	8.34	mcg
CALCIUM	26.56	mg	B12	.004	mcg
PHOS.	108.50	mg	MAGNES.	41.19	mg
IRON	.95	mg	*ZINC	.48	mg
SODIUM	13.31	mg	*SAT. FAT	.002	g
POTAS.	266.58	mg	*MONO UNSAT.	.0006	g
*VIT A	77.52	IU	*POLYUNSAT.	.004	g
THIAMIN	.18	mg	*FIBER	3.47	g

Raisin Oatmeal Bars

½	cup water	¾	cup oatmeal
2	teaspoons tapioca granules	¼	cup chopped walnuts
		½	cup pitted dates
1	cup raisins	½	cup whole-wheat flour
2	tablespoons date sugar	½	teaspoon baking soda
		½	cup apple juice

Add ½ cup water slowly to the tapioca granules, stirring well. Pour over the raisins and the date sugar in a small saucepan and heat over medium heat, stirring constantly until thickened. Remove from heat. Grind the oatmeal with the walnuts. Pour into a bowl. Grind the dates with the flour. Pour into bowl with the oatmeal mixture. Add the baking soda. Moisten with apple juice. Spread batter on a Pam-sprayed, 10 × 6-inch Pyrex or nonstick baking dish. Spread raisin mixture on top and bake at 350° for 25 minutes.

Serves 8

Non-Fat Carob Ice Cream

4	ounces nonfat milk	1	heaping teaspoon carob powder
1½	ripe bananas (approximately ¾ cup)	1	teaspoon lecithin
1	teaspoon honey	½	teaspoon vanilla

Put all ingredients into ice-cream maker and prepare according to the machine you are using. Or you can freeze the bananas and milk and blend with the other ingredients in a blender or purée through a Champion juicer, for a "soft-serve" type of ice cream.

Serves 1 or 2

RAISIN OATMEAL BARS
Per Single Serving

			4/4/9 CALORIES	: 181
			CAL FROM CARB.	: 80%
			CAL FROM PRO.	: 6%
			CAL FROM FAT	: 14%

P/S RATIO   6.55 : 1

DATE:

GRAM WT.	82.20	g	RIBOFLN	.04	mg
CHOLSTRL.	0.00	mg	NIACIN	.78	mg
CALORIES	167.84	kcal	VIT C	.80	mg
PROTEIN	2.82	g	*PANTO.	.54	mg
FAT	2.92	g	*B6	.17	mg
CARB.	36.01	g	*FOLACIN	12.32	mcg
CALCIUM	22.42	mg	B12	0.00	mcg
PHOS.	78.13	mg	*MAGNES.	28.57	mg
IRON	1.06	mg	*ZINC	.57	mg
SODIUM	52.27	mg	*SAT. FAT	.24	g
POTAS.	285.75	mg	*MONO UNSAT.	.43	g
VIT A	8.31	IU	*POLYUNSAT.	1.61	g
THIAMIN	.11	mg	FIBER	.80	g

NON-FAT CAROB ICE CREAM
Per Single Serving

			4/4/9 CALORIES	: 203
			CAL FROM CARB.	: 75%
			CAL FROM PRO.	: 23%
			CAL FROM FAT	: 2%

P/S RATIO   .27 : 1

DATE:

GRAM WT.	117.87	g	RIBOFLN	.55	mg
CHOLSTRL.	6.00	mg	NIACIN	.75	mg
CALORIES	197.04	kcal	VIT C	9.70	mg
PROTEIN	11.73	g	PANTO.	1.29	mg
FAT	.63	g	B6	.59	mg
CARB.	38.24	g	FOLACIN	31.23	mcg
CALCIUM	382.04	mg	B12	1.21	mcg
PHOS.	307.16	mg	MAGNES.	57.10	mg
IRON	.37	mg	ZINC	1.39	mg
SODIUM	161.41	mg	SAT. FAT	.30	g
POTAS.	873.83	mg	MONO UNSAT.	.09	g
VIT A	79.00	IU	POLYUNSAT.	.08	g
THIAMIN	.16	mg	*FIBER	.42	g

June Apricot Cobbler

If you have an apricot tree, this recipe is especially for you!

2¾	cups mashed fresh apricots (remove pit, but leave unpeeled; this is about 25 small [1½-inch diameter] apricots)	1	cup pitted dates
		1	teaspoon cinnamon
		2	tablespoon tapioca granules
		⅓	cup oatmeal
		⅓	cup dates
1	cup apple juice	½	teaspoon cinnamon

Spread the apricots evenly in the bottom of a 6 × 10-inch baking dish. Pour apple juice in a graduated blender and measure the 1 cup dates by displacement: When the liquid reaches the 2-cup mark, you've added 1 cup of dates. Purée juice and dates. Add the cinnamon and tapioca while blender is running. Make the cobbler topping by grinding together in a clean, dry blender jar the oatmeal, ⅓ cup dates, and cinnamon. Sprinkle over the apricot mixture. Bake at 350° for 35 to 40 minutes or until bubbly and top is browned.

Serves 8

Peach Cobbler

1	cup pineapple juice	1	20-ounce bag Freestone Peaches, unsweetened, or equivalent fresh
¾	cup pitted dates		
1	teaspoon vanilla		
1	teaspoon cinnamon	1	tablespoon whole almonds
1	tablespoon tapioca		
		¼	cup pitted dates
		⅓	cup oatmeal

Blend the juice, dates, vanilla, cinnamon, and tapioca. In a Pyrex baking dish or nonstick dish, layer the peaches; pour the juice mixture over all. Grind the remaining ingredients as a topping and sprinkle evenly over the top. Bake at 350° for 45 minutes.

Serves 8

JUNE APRICOT COBBLER
Per Single Serving

			4/4/9 CALORIES	: 144
			CAL FROM CARB.	: 93%
			CAL FROM PRO.	: 4%
			CAL FROM FAT	: 3%

P/S RATIO   2.25 : 1

DATE:

GRAM WT.	125.30	g	RIBOFLN	.05	mg
CHOLSTRL.	0.00	mg	NIACIN	.99	mg
CALORIES	132.40	kcal	VIT C	5.61	mg
PROTEIN	1.55	g	*PANTO.	.50	mg
FAT	.47	g	*B6	.11	mg
CARB.	33.60	g	FOLACIN	11.66	mcg
CALCIUM	20.15	mg	B12	0.00	mcg
PHOS.	30.14	mg	MAGNES.	17.52	mg
IRON	.80	mg	*ZINC	.32	mg
SODIUM	23.89	mg	*SAT. FAT	.04	g
POTAS.	389.68	mg	*MONO UNSAT.	.12	g
VIT A	1406.21	IU	*POLYUNSAT.	.09	g
THIAMIN	.05	mg	FIBER	1.04	g

PEACH COBBLER
Per Single Serving

			4/4/9 CALORIES	: 122
			CAL FROM CARB.	: 88%
			CAL FROM PRO.	: 5%
			CAL FROM FAT	: 7%

P/S RATIO   2.40 : 1

DATE:

GRAM WT.	121.90	g	RIBOFLN	.08	mg
CHOLSTRL.	0.00	mg	NIACIN	.91	mg
CALORIES	112.00	kcal	*VIT C	118.08	mg
PROTEIN	1.74	g	*PANTO.	.35	mg
FAT	1.01	g	*B6	.09	mg
CARB.	26.77	g	*FOLACIN	13.87	mcg
CALCIUM	23.63	mg	B12	0.00	mcg
PHOS.	39.67	mg	*MAGNES.	17.25	mg
IRON	.78	mg	*ZINC	.20	mg
*SODIUM	22.74	mg	*SAT. FAT	.07	g
*POTAS.	201.78	mg	*MONO UNSAT.	.43	g
VIT A	2517.62	IU	*POLYUNSAT.	.17	g
THIAMIN	.09	mg	FIBER	1.52	g

Pineapple-Banana or Strawberry-Coconut Popsicles

1	32-ounce bottle of juice (the best are juices with banana or coconut juice [not the fat] added)	16	2-ounce juice molds

Pour 2 ounces of juice into each mold, seal, and freeze until hard. If the bottle of juice is $1.69, each popsicle is only 10¢. A great quick treat . . . especially in summer!

Strawberry-Topped Cake #2

1	pint fresh strawberries, washed and sliced	⅔	cup whole-wheat flour
2	tablespoons raw honey	⅓	cup date "sugar"
3	egg whites	1	teaspoon vanilla
½	cup water	3	teaspoons baking powder

Drizzle the strawberries with the honey. Set aside. With a hand mixer beat the egg whites while adding water, flour, date sugar, and vanilla slowly. Add the baking powder last. Pour into a Pam-sprayed, nonstick round cake pan and bake at 350° for 30 minutes. Cool. Cut into individual servings and top each with fresh, sliced strawberries.

Serves 6

STRAWBERRY-TOPPED CAKE #2
Per Single Serving

			4/4/9 CALORIES	: 142
			CAL FROM CARB.	: 87%
			CAL FROM PRO.	: 11%
			CAL FROM FAT	: 3%

P/S RATIO   9.23 : 1

DATE:

GRAM WT.	99.86	g	RIBOFLN	.09	mg
CHOLSTRL.	0.00	mg	NIACIN	.73	mg
CALORIES	135.38	kcal	VIT C	28.22	mg
*PROTEIN	3.78	g	*PANTO.	.36	mg
*FAT	.45	g	*B6	.07	mg
CARB.	30.91	g	*FOLACIN	16.57	mcg
CALCIUM	123.11	mg	B12	.01	mcg
PHOS.	225.72	mg	*MAGNES.	22.11	mg
*IRON	.68	mg	*ZINC	.46	mg
SODIUM	26.72	mg	*SAT. FAT	.01	g
POTAS.	404.50	mg	*MONO UNSAT.	.02	g
VIT A	13.66	IU	*POLYUNSAT.	.09	g
THIAMIN	.08	mg	*FIBER	.57	g

PART V
Patient Testimonials

Case History

Glenora Barker arrived at the Institute on May 12, 1986, taking 64 units of insulin per day. She had been on insulin for 13 years and during that time had been chronically and constantly overweight. When she started insulin, she weighed 180 pounds. Over those 8 years she gained an additional 21 pounds and entered the Institute at 201.

All along the way, physicians had told her that she could get off insulin with a diet and exercise program, but this had never been successfully implemented.

Here at the Institute, we initiated her program with a modified fast and discontinued insulin completely. This can be done under direct control, and in her case, her blood sugar did not go up. It was somewhat high upon arrival while on insulin, 299, and after one week on the program without insulin it had dropped to 255.

She and her husband left the Institute, returned to Florida, and stayed on the regimen without insulin and her blood sugar staying within the 220–280 range. Over this time she lost 50 pounds, down to 151, and her husband lost 30 pounds, from 200 to 170, both of them enthusiastically adapting to the program like ducks to water.

Eight months after they left the Institute I received the following letter from her husband, six months after they had adjusted on the program.

Dear Dr. Whitaker:

People ask—what do we eat? My reply: we eat anything we want to. However, if you think for one minute we would eat red meat, fats, sugar, salt or dairy products, except for skim milk and a few other things, you are out of your mind. The benefits my loving wife and myself have received by deleting these foods from our diet is so great that we will continue it for the rest of our lives. In addition, we will also stay on the vitamin program, designed by Dr. Whitaker, that complements this diet and continue to exercise on a regular basis as well.

We feel so great, we have excess energy and our mental

outlook has been reversed completely. We look forward to another glorious day which always seems too short for all the things we want to do. We are truly alive.

Between us, we have lost 80 pounds in six months. Glenora has lost 50 and I have lost 30. In addition, my wife has not had an insulin shot in six months, and she had been on insulin daily for eight years and was taking 65 units when we arrived at the Institute in California.

Of interest to me, is that we require so much less sleep now than we did. I used to get up about 8:00 A.M., go to work, and be so tired that I would need a nap every afternoon before going back to work until 6:00 P.M. After work I would go home, sit in a lounge chair and watch a little TV before going to bed around 9:00 P.M. I then would get up at 8:00 A.M. to repeat the cycle.

NOW, I do not need an afternoon nap and if I go to bed before 11:00, I am up by 5:00 A.M., ready to do anything and everything. Our children and employees now say, "Stay out of the way, here comes dad, he will run you over." We get things done and love it. Our attitude continues to spiral upward. Many people who knew us, have seen this remarkable change in our mental attitude. We were at times quite depressed. Now we truly glory at being alive.

We also love to share our experience with others in our shop and personal lives. Actually, Glenora's doctors have been telling both of us that diet and exercise were powerful and could get Glenora off of insulin, but the program was simply not implemented. I guess they expected us just to figure out how to do it ourselves. We share with our friends and family how valuable the experience at the Institute has been. We never would have believed such good things could happen to us without the two weeks we spent there, following through completely on the program designed for us. I guess it all seems so simple now. If you want a program of vigorous diet and exercise, go to where they teach diet and exercise, not to places that simply say it might work.

Dr. Whitaker, we truly thank you.

Don Barker
Miami, Florida

Dear Dr. Whitaker:

Your program has been of great benefit in bringing about a new feeling of well being. I feel well and sleep well, I felt no ill effects from the new life-style. I'm particularly pleased that I have been able to stay off the oral diabetic medication (Orinase) since attending your Institute in September of 1985. My weekly blood sugar measurements are averaging about 130 and I expect these will reduce even more with the added exercise and reduced weight.

My doctor now considers me a miracle. He never believed that your diet program would work and said that I would always need medicine. He now tells me to "keep doing whatever you are doing."

Thank you very much for your help.

Sincerely yours,
Leland P. Robinson

Dear Dr. Whitaker:

Your program has changed my life—all for the better. My weight is under control having lost 15 pounds, and I no longer have blood pressure problems, or require blood pressure medication. My attitude and stamina have greatly improved. My blood sugar levels have been in line, perhaps a bit on the high side, but much better than before the program.

My "quality of life" is at a much higher level than prior to this program.

Thank you very much.

Sigmund Czarnecki
Woodstock, Connecticut

Dear Dr. Whitaker:

Since I got straightened out at your clinic, the quality of my life has greatly improved. I don't sleep as much as I used to, but my sleep is more satisfying and I am not reluctant to get up early in the morning if I awaken at that time. I feel that my work is done better and faster. My concentration has improved, but I am hoping for more improvement. My moods are mostly good and I can say without reservation that the past few years have been the best of my life, despite the diabetes. I can't thank you enough. As you know, I am still on insulin, 42 units, and my blood sugars fluctuate still quite widely, 60–300, generally in the 150 to 220 range. As you know, my blood sugar upon entering the Institute had reached 387, and when I left, it had dropped to 134.

I feel I'm doing quite well.

> *John Gilbert*
> *Nassau, Bahamas*

Dear Dr. Whitaker:

I do believe that my participation in Dr. Whitaker's program has saved my sight. On May 13, 1985, I arrived at his clinic, I was 56 years old and had been a diabetic for 18 years. I had been treated for the first 4 years with the oral drug, DBI, and I have been on insulin ever since. Like most diabetics, my insulin requirement gradually and slowly increased until I was taking 55 units when I entered.

I did not get off of insulin completely, but reduced my insulin from 55 units to 20 units a day.

Before I entered Dr. Whitaker's Wellness Institute, I had been having bleeding episodes in my eyes and had had laser treatments. When I arrived at the Institute, my cholesterol level was 240, triglycerides were 852 and my blood sugar was 187.

When I left the Institute my cholesterol had dropped to 236, my triglycerides were down to 203, and on much less insulin, my fasting glucose was 126.

For a year and a half after that, and up to the present I have not had any more bleeding in my eyes. In addition, my cholesterol level has stayed low and my very high triglycerides have also stayed low. My opthalmologist is baffled as to what happened.

Prior to going to Dr. Whitaker's Institute, he had mentioned that the Institute was a good idea, but it was likely too late for me as the eye problems would probably continue. After a year and a half of no further damage, he was pleasantly surprised and told me to "keep doing whatever you are doing."

Since that time I am now able to drive, and I'm back in business as a real estate agent doing better than ever. I couldn't be happier or more satisfied with the result.

> *Majorie Atwood*
> *Sacramento, California*

Dr. Whitaker's Comment:

I was indeed pleased with Majorie Atwood's progress, particularly because the damage to the eyes seems to have been slowed considerably.

I think one of the major reasons for this success was the use of MaxEPA fish oil. When she arrived both her cholesterol and triglyceride levels were elevated, and were successfully brought down with our overall program plus the MaxEPA.

Dr. Margaret J. Albreck, professor of medicine at West Virginia University school of Medicine in Morgan Town, used substantial doses of fish oil and found it beneficial in 8 obese diabetic patients. Their triglyceride level fell from 530 to 333, the HDL cholesterol leveled, the platelet aggregation decreased, meaning abnormal clotting was reduced. It is these changes which may have had a significantly beneficial effect upon stopping the progression of eye damage in Majorie.

Dear Dr. Whitaker:

I had been an insulin dependent diabetic for about 9 years before I went to see Dr. Whitaker. Upon entering the Institute, my major concern was painful tingling in both of my feet and ankles. Dr. Whitaker explained that this was a very common condition among insulin diabetics called peripheral neuropathy, a condition where the nerves degenerate and symptoms of pain and numbness follow. The pain had been getting worse for several months.

Upon arrival I was taking 40 units of insulin, but following Dr. Whitaker's diet regimen, my insulin requirement dropped to 24 units. Dr. Whitaker started me on Yohimbine, a drug that is commonly used to improve male sexual function. In some cases the drug has been shown to reduce the pains of diabetic peripheral neuropathy.

In my case, it was like a miracle drug. Almost immediately after taking the drug all the pains in my feet and ankles disappeared. I had no discomfort for over a year, except on those occasions in which I did not take the Yohimbine for a few days. However, immediately after restarting Yohimbine, the pains would disappear.

The overall experience of the Institute was extremely beneficial, and I put the principles to work in my life and stayed with them. I am still taking insulin, 28 units, but feel better now, a year and a half after leaving the Institute, than I had for four years before going.

John Mauzy
Golden, Colorado

Dr. Whitaker's Comment:

Yohimbine has received quite a reputation as an enhancer of male sexual function. Studies in men and in animals indicate that it seems to enhance male sexual desire and function. In addition, a few uncontrolled studies have shown that Yohimbine does relieve the painful nervous tingling of diabetic peripheral neuropathy. Certainly more studies need to be done with this potential use of the drug, but in John's case, and in several others, it has seemed to relieve the symptoms of this condition.

Testimonial

Dear Dr. Whitaker:

When I arrived at your office in June of 1986, I had been on insulin for approximately six months. As you know, my blood sugar in January of 1986 was found to be 287 and it went to 300 plus. My glycohemoglobin was approximately 16 and my fasting blood glucose levels were way above 200. After starting on insulin, shortly after that, I began having significant hypoglycemic reactions. My glycohemoglobin fell rapidly, but I was continued on insulin.

When I came to you, you and I were both concerned about the hypoglycemic reactions, so we decided to go without insulin under close control.

It has been nine months now and I have not gone back on insulin. I am very happy that my glycohemoglobin and blood sugar levels stay within normal limits and that I have measurements of C-Peptide that document my body is producing insulin.

I truly love the dietary regimen and exercise. I feel so much healthier, vibrant and alive. You have no idea how happy I am to be off of daily injection.

I know, as you have told me, that I will most likely have to have insulin down the road. However, I am happy for the past nine months, and frankly, I see no end in sight to my improved health.

Somehow, and I know there is no proof of this, I think the vitamins and minerals are contributing to my improved status.

I will always be grateful for your attention, concern and help.

Sincerely,
Vasken Imasdounian

Case History

D A V I D   C O E

David, a 33-year-old moderately obese man was now in big trouble. He had been bothered with obesity for most of his life and the tendency to gain or lose 75 pounds over a several month period. Following one of his rapid weight loss regimens, he developed exceedingly high blood fat levels and an elevated blood glucose level. On December 2, 1986, his triglyceride level measured 1047, his cholesterol level a whopping 346, and his blood sugar level had risen to 267.

His general practitioner started him on Micronase, a new generation medication for diabetes. He had told David that he probably would have to have insulin within the year. Unfortunately, no dietary intervention or the use of MaxEPA supplementation had been advocated.

David came to the Institute for a second opinion. We immediately stopped the Micronase and put him on a trial of high carbohydrates, high fiber, low-fat diet outlined in this book. We also used substantial amounts of MaxEPA fish oil which has been shown to be very effective at lowering elevated triglyceride levels. David responded quite well, very rapidly, and even predictably. On Feburary 2, 1987, his triglyceride level had fallen to 182, his cholesterol level had fallen to 172, and blood sugar level was a healthy normal 102.

David's case represents how intimately the blood sugar level is associated with the blood fat level. When triglyceride levels are elevated, one can expect the blood sugar level to go up as well. With marked elevation in triglycerides, full blown diabetes can be expected. Therefore, the first priority in any patient with elevated blood fat levels is to lower the fat levels and the blood sugar level will generally follow.

PAUL ZIMMERMAN

My husband was deteriorating right before my eyes. We'd been married over 40 years, built a successful business together, enjoyed "the good life." But for years, I'd been helplessly watching him go downhill: He'd had a heart attack at the age of 45, surgery to replace arteries in his legs at 51, four bypass operations before 57, and his diabetes had worsened to the point where now, at age 65, he was taking 55 units of insulin by injection every day.

The surgery improved the circulation in his legs for several years, but the pain had returned and now Paul could walk no farther than 50 yards. Another catheterization and special X-rays were done. They showed that his arteries and even the plastic grafts were rapidly closing up with fat and cholesterol. Another operation would not help, his doctor said, and he had no choice but to send us home.

We expected gangrene to set in, and then the surgeon would have to amputate Paul's legs. Diabetes and its terrible complications had a stranglehold on my husband, and we had both lost hope.

Then I read an article by Julian Whitaker, M.D., about how a diet, exercise, vitamin and mineral program can be used to treat the very problems that were killing my husband. We were skeptical—Paul had been under medical supervision for 10 years, and he was getting worse—but we had nothing to lose. We went to California to see Dr. Whitaker and enter his clinic.

We spent two weeks there, experiencing the specialized diet and the vitamin and exercise program, learning how to do them at home. In four weeks, Paul was completely off insulin with normal blood sugars. In six weeks, he had lost 22 pounds and was able to walk three to four miles a day, nonstop, without pain. Even the pins and needles sensations in his feet, so common with diabetics, had improved.

His blood cholesterol—we now understand how important this test is—had dropped from 196 to 148. After eight weeks on this program, his doctor at home repeated the studies of circulation in his legs and found a 66 percent improvement in the right leg and a 42 percent improvement in the left leg. He told us he'd never seen such rapid improvement, and that Paul would probably not lose his legs.

What more can be said? During our stay, Dr. Whitaker and his staff made sure we understood exactly how to follow the program once we were home. Now, eight months later, Paul is closely following the program that saved his life, and he's improving every day. He recently passed a new milestone: Now he's completely off all heart medication!

Six months after Paul Zimmerman left the institute, I received the following letter from his vascular surgeon.

Dear Dr. Whitaker:

Enclosed please find the copies of the last two peripheral vascular studies done with exercise on Paul Zimmerman. You will note that the first one is dated 8/24/81 and the recent one 2/23/82. If you will turn to the second page, in the lower left hand corner, you will note the arm to ankle index was increased from .55 to .71; on the left from .66 to .75. Also, you will note that the wave forms have obviously improved. I am sure that you will agree with me that this is not only a very pleasant surprise, but solid proof that improvement can be made in these patients with diet and exercise. You may feel free to use our studies for any use that you may wish to put them to.

Parenthetically, I should add that Paul continues to feel well and continues his diet and exercise program. I told him that if he continues, in the next 3 to 6 months, he should be able to go up to the mountains and do the trout fishing that he enjoys so much. He sends along his best regards as do I.

Sincerely yours,
Dr. D.C.

Dear Dr. Whitaker:

Even though I was taking 130 units of insulin and seventeen prescription pills every day of my life, I was surprised to be at the Whitaker Clinic. After reading about Dr. Whitaker and the Institute in *Prevention* magazine, my wife had recommended we go. For the past two years she had literally begged me to go.

But I was not easily persuaded. As a "workaholic" who can't remember missing a day's work in the last thirty-five years, except for a one-night stay in the hospital after the removal of a "melanoma" mole, I wanted to try everything else first. And I did!

When I was diagnosed as "early onset diabetes," my personal reaction was perhaps typical. Trying to forestall the thought of the traditional insulin, I ran the gamut on Orinase and Diabenese. I even cheated by taking more than the doctor prescribed, hoping to avoid the needle. But the blood sugar levels kept rising, so I finally gave in and started on a modest level of insulin injections.

For nine months I had dutifully gone to the hospital twice a week for two blood tests. These automatically resulted in an increase of insulin intake until I reached the 130-units-per-day mark. In answer to my question, "Will this situation ever be better?" the doctor just flatly told me, "No."

At this time I was also taking medication for high blood pressure and atrial fibrillation, resulting in the daily intake of the seventeen prescription pills daily.

While I'm grateful for the limited number of doctors who have literally saved my life in specific situations—Dr. Whitaker tops that list—I've surely had my share of medical kiss-offs of the "keep taking your present medications and call me if you need help" type!

When I finally arrived at the Whitaker Clinic I was taking 130 units of insulin per day (44 of humulin R and 86 of humulin NPH) for diabetes, 2 hydrochlorothiazide, 8 "micro K" potassium pills, and 2 Midamor (another diuretic) for high blood pressure, plus 1 digoxin and 4 verapamil tablets for atrial fibrillation controll.

Diet had hardly been mentioned all during this build-up of my "pathological museum." We had been told to use salt sparingly, and we cut out all sugar, thinking it was the culprit.

What a shocker we received at the Whitaker Institute. Dr. Whitaker placed me on a nonfat diet, and increased my exercise schedule. In two days I was totally "off insulin," and within a week I had discontinued all prescription pills. My blood sugar levels were, for the very first time in years, safely within the desired range of 80–120, my blood pressure remained at the same, or lower, levels I had achieved under medication, and my pulse was normal. At the end of the first week I had dropped six pounds. I really was a new person!

The clinic's nonfat diet, prepared personally by a registered nurse/professional nutritionist, was simple, adequate, and, best of all, understandable. Taking time to exercise was a scheduled luxury, and a totally new life-style was formulated—health, attitude, and commitment being the keys.

We will be forever grateful for the Whitaker Institute and the wonderful people associated with it.

Ray and Ad Kimball
Littleton, Colorado
June 6, 1984

BIBLIOGRAPHY

"Adult-Onset Diabetes Show Atherogenic Lipid Patterns." *Medical World News*. January 8, 1979, p. 56.

Anderson, James W., et al. "Beneficial Effects of a High Carbohydrate, High Fiber Diet on Hyperglycemic Diabetic Men." *American Journal of Clinical Nutrition 29*: 895–899, 1976.

Biometric Society. "Report of the Committee for Assessment of Biometric Aspects of Controlled Trials of the Hypoglycemic Agents." *Journal of the American Medical Association 231*: 583–608, 1975.

Bosco, Dominic. *The People's Guide to Vitamins and Minerals*. Chicago: Contemporary Books, 1980.

Calvert, G. D. *Medical World News*, Jan. 8, 1979, p. 56.

Campbell, Peter, et al. "Pathogenesis of the Dawn Phenomenon in Patients with Insulin-Dependent Diabetes Mellitus." *New England Journal of Medicine 312*: 1473–1479, 1985.

Chalmers, Thomas C., ed. "Settling the UGDE Controversy." *Journal of the American Medical Association 231*: 624–625 1975.

Colata, Gina. "How Important Is Dietary Calcium in Preventing Osteoporosis." *Science 233*: 519–520, 1986.

Cooper, W. D. "Cardiac Arrhythmias Following Acute Myocardial Infarction: Associations with the Serum Potassium Level and Prior Diuretic Therapy." *European Heart Journal 5*: 464, 1984.

Cornfield, Jerome. "The University Group Diabetes Program: A Further Study of the Mortality Finding." *Journal of the American Medical Association 217*: 1676–1687, 1971.

Coustan, Donald R. "A Randomized Clinical Trial of the Insulin Pump vs. Intensive Conventional Therapy in Diabetic Pregnancies. *Journal of the American Medical Association 255*: 631–636, 1986.

Cryer, Philip E. "Glucose Counterregulation, Hypoglycemia, and Intensive Insulin Therapy in Diabetes Mellitus. *New England Journal of Medicine 313*: 232–241, 1985.

Davidson, John. *Clinical Diabetes Mellitus, A Problem Oriented Approach.* New York: Thieme, Inc., 1986.

Davidson, John K. "The FDA and Hypoglycemic Drugs." *Journal of the American Medical Association 232*: 854, 1975.

"Diabetes Diagnoses Grounded on GTT Are Wrong Most of Time." *Family Practice News*: 1, October 15, 1979.

Dupree, John. "Near Normal Glycemic Control Does Not Slow Progression of Mild Diabetic Retinopathy." Paper presented to American Diabetes Association meeting, 1983.

"Fish Oil May Ease Arthritis Pain." *Medical World News.* July 14, 1986, p. 9.

General Practitioner Research Group, "Calcium Pantothenate in Arthritic Conditions." *Practitioner 224*: 208, 1980.

Gonzalez, Elizabeth Rashe. "Exercise Therapy Rediscovered for Diabetes, But What Does It Do?" *Journal of the American Medical Association 242*: 1591, 1979.

Greene, Eva-lynne. "Well-Being Up With Captopril, Down With Two Other Agents." *Medical Tribune.* September 17, 1986, page 8.

Hadden, D. R. "Myocardial Infarction in Maturity-Onset Diabetes, A Retrospective Study." *Lancet 1*: 335–338, 1972.

Hendler, Sheldon Saul. *The Complete Guide of Anti-Aging Nutrients.* New York: Simon & Schuster, 1985.

Himsworth, H. P. "The Dietetic Factor Determining the Glucose Tolerance and Sensitivity to Insulin of Healthy Men. *Clinical Science 2*: 67–94, 1935.

Johnson, Nancy E. "Effect of Level of Protein Intake of Urinary and Fecal Calcium and Calcium Retention of Young Adult Males." *Journal of Nutrition 100*: 1425–1430, 1970.

Kempner, Walter. "Treatment of Hypertension Vascular Disease with Rice Diet." *American Journal of Medicine 4*: 545–577, 1948.

Klachko, D. M., et al. "Blood Glucose Levels During Walking in Normal and Diabetic Subjects." *Diabetes 21*: 89–100, 1972.

Knatterud, Genell L., et al. "Hypoglycemic Agents on Vascular Complications in Patients with Adult-Onset Diabetes." *Journal of the American Medical Association 240*: 37–42, 1978.

The Kroc Collaboratine Study Group. "Blood Glucose and the Evolution of Diabetic Retinopathy and the Albuminuria." *New England Journal of Medicine 311*: 1365–1372, 1984.

The Kroc Collaborative Study Group. "Hopes for Whole Pancreas, Islet Cell Transplant Falter." *Internal Medicine News.* September 1–14, 1986.

Kuller, Lewis H. "Unexpected Effects of Treating Hypertension in Men with Electrocardiographic Abnormalities: A Critical Analysis." *Circulation 73*: 114–123, 1986.

Lauritzen, Torsten. "Two-Year Experience with Continuous Subcutaneous Insulin Infusion in Relation to Retinopathy and Neuropathy." *Diabetes 34 [Suppl. 3]*: 74–79, 1985.

Lernmark, Ake. "Islet Cell Surface Antibodies in Juvenile Diabetes Mellitus." *New England Journal of Medicine 299*: 375–380, 1978.

Levey, Gerald S., and Roger F. Palmer. "Effect of Tolbutamide on Adenyl Cyclase in Rabbit and Human Heart and Contractility of Isolated Rabbit Atria." *Journal of Clinical Endocrinology 33*: 317–334, 1971.

Lorenzi, Mara, and Michael Goldman. "Improved Diabetic Control and Retinopathy." *New England Journal of Medicine 308*: 1600, 1983.

McDougall, John. *McDougall's Medicine, A Challenging Second Opinion.* Piscataway, New Jersey: New Century Press, 1985.

Mather, H. M. "Hypomagnesaemis in Diabetes." *Acta Clinica Chemica 95*: 235–242, 1979.

Mazess, Richard B. "Bone Mineral Content of North Alaskan Eskimos." *American Journal of Clinical Nutrition 27*: 916–925, 1974.

Medical World News, July 14, 1986, p. 9.

Merrimee, Thomas, et al. "Insulin Like Growth Factors, Studies in Diabetes With and Without Retinopathy." *New England Journal of Medicine 309*: 527–530, 1983.

Mertz, Walter. "Effects and Metabolism of Glucose Tolerance Factor." *Nutrition Review 33*: 1929, 1975.

Miranda, Perla M., and David L. Horwitz. "High-Fiber Diets in the Treatment of Diabetes Mellitus." *Annals of Internal Medicine 88*: 482–486, 1978.

Mitch, William E., et al. "The Effect of a Keto Acid–Amino Acid Supplement to a Restricted Diet on the Progression of Chronic Renal Failure." *New England Journal of Medicine 311*: 623–629, 1984.

Morgan, T. O. "Failure of Therapy to Improve Prognosis in Elderly Males with Hypertension." *Australia Medical Journal 2*: 27, 1980.

Nutrition Search, Inc. *Nutrition Almanac.* New York: McGraw-Hill Paperbacks, 1979.

Parham, Barbara. "What's Wrong With Eating Meat?" Denver: Ananda Marga Publications, 1981.

Peterson, Lyle. *Cardiovascular Rehabilitation: A Comprehensive Approach.* New York: Macmillan, 1983.

Phillipson, B. E., et al. "Reduction of Plasma Lipids, Lipoproteins, and Apoproteins by Dietary Fish Oils in Patients with Hypertriglyceridemia." *New England Journal of Medicine 312*: 1210–1216, 1985.

Rabinowitch, I. M. "Effects of the High Carbohydrate–Low Calorie Diet Upon Carbohydrate Tolerance in Diabetes Mellitus." *Canadian Medical Association Journal 33*: 136–144, 1935.

Rabinowitch, I. M. "Experiences with a High Carbohydrate–Low Calorie Diet for the Treatment of Diabetes Mellitus." *Canadian Medical Association Journal 23*: 489–498, 1930.

Rabinowitch, I. M. "The Present Status of the High Carbohydrate–Low Calorie Diet for the Treatment of Diabetes." *Canadian Medical Association Journal 26*: 141–148, 1932.

Roberts, Hyman J. "Perspective on Vitamin E as Therapy." *Journal of the American Medical Association 256*: 129, 1981.

Rose, W. C. "Amino Acid Requirements of Man." *Journal of Biological Chemistry 217*: 997–1004, 1955.

Rudman, Daniel. "Megadose Vitamins. Use and Misuse (editorial)." *New England Journal of Medicine 309*: 488, 1983.

Sackler, Arthur M. "On the Nonsense of Official Recommended Daily Allowances (RDAs)." *Medical Tribune*, Sept. 18, 1985, p. 46.

Samsum, W. D. "The Use of High Carbohydrate Diets in the Treatment of Diabetes Mellitus." *Journal of the American Medical Association: 86:* 178–181, January 16, 1926.

Schaumburg, Herbert. "Sensory Neuropathy from Pyridoxine Abuse." *New England Journal of Medicine 309*: 1445–1448, 1983.

Schor, Stanley. "The University Group Diabetes Program, A Statistician Looks at the Mortality Results." *Journal of the American Medical Association 217*: 1671–1675, 1971.

Seifter, Eli, Ph.D., et al. "Impaired Wound Healing in Streptozotic Diabetes: Prevention by Supplementary Vitamin A." *Annals of Surgery 194*: 42–50, 1982.

Somogyi, Michael. *Bulletin of the St. Louis Jewish Hospital Medical Staff*, May 1951.

Somogyi, Michael. "Dietary and Insulin Therapy of Diabetes." *Bulletin of the Saint Louis Jewish Hospital Medical Staff:* 1–16, October 1949.

Srikanta, S. "Islet-Cell Antibodies and BETA-Cell Function in Monozygotic Triplets and Twins Initially Discordant for Type 1 Diabetes Mellitus." *New England Journal of Medicine 308*: 322–325, 1983.

Struthers, A. D. "Prior Thiazide Diuretic Treatment Increases Adrenaline-Induced Hypokalemia." *Lancet 1*: 1358, 1985.

Sweeney, J. Shirley. "Dietary Factors That Influence the Dextrose Tolerance Test." *Archives of Internal Medicine 40*: 818–830, 1927.

"Tight Control Trial Needs More Diabetics." *Medical World News*, Feb. 23, 1987, p. 6.

"University Group Diabetes Program: A Study of the Effects of Hypoglycemic Agents on Vascular Complications in Patients with Adult-Onset Diabetes. 11. Mortality Results." *Diabetes 19 [Suppl]*: 814, 1970.

"University Group Diabetes Program." *Journal of the American Medical Association 218*: 1400–1410, 1971.

Walker, Ruth. "Calcium Retention in the Adult Human Male As Affected by Protein Intake." *Journal of Nutrition 102*: 1297–1302, 1972.

Warmer, Rebecca, et al. *Off Diabetes Pills, A Diabetic's Guide to Longer Life.* Washington: Public Citizens' Health Group, 1978.

Yoon, J. W. "Isolation of a Viris from the Pancreas of a Child with Ketocidosis." *New England Journal of Medicine 300:* 1173–1179, 1979.

INDEX

About the author

Julian M. Whitaker, M.D. is the founder of the Whitaker Wellness Institute and the author of *Reversing Heart Disease* and *Reversing Health Risks*. A staff member of Nathan Pritikin's Longevity Center, he graduated from Emory University in 1970 with a degree in medicine and continued his education with graduate studies in surgery at the University of California at San Francisco. At the Whitaker Wellness Institute in Newport Beach, California, he has successfully treated over four thousand patients with the programs described in this book and, in almost all of his diabetic patients, has been able to reduce or eliminate dependency on insulin or drugs.